"WHAT IS THE BABY'S NAME?"

"When it comes to naming your baby, you want to get it right. You want to strike a fine balance between uniqueness and familiarity, honor a family member, reflect your ethnic heritage, avoid horrible nicknames, ensure that your child's name will never be misspelled. You'd like to name him for Granddad, but Granddad's name was Elmer. You thought Sally sounded nice until your best friend asked you if you're naming her for Gidget. The baby's due in six weeks and your spouse has vetoed every single suggestion. So you do what you always swore you wouldn't, and buy . . ."

20,001 NAMES FOR BABY

"There are many baby name books on the market. They give varying numbers of names, and varying amounts of information about the names. I believe that when it comes to picking a name, more is more. More choices can help you make *your* choice."

Carol McD. Wallace

Avon Books by
Carol McD. Wallace

THE GREATEST BABY NAME BOOK EVER
20,001 NAMES FOR BABY

20,001
NAMES
FOR BABY

REVISED AND UPDATED

Carol McD. Wallace

AVON BOOKS
An Imprint of HarperCollinsPublishers

AVON BOOKS
An Imprint of HarperCollins*Publishers*
10 East 53rd Street
New York, New York 10022-5299

Copyright © 1992 by Carol McD. Wallace
ISBN: 0-380-76227-7
www.avonbooks.com

First Avon Books paperback printing: March 1992

Avon Trademark Reg. U.S. Pat. Off. and in Other Countries, Marca
Registrada, Hecho en U.S.A.
HarperCollins ® is a trademark of HarperCollins Publishers Inc.

Printed in the U.S.A.

56 55 54 53 52

My heartfelt thanks go to my agent, Lynn Seligman, who long ago urged me to write this book; to Rick, for his eternal patience; and to Sarah Durand at Avon Books, who sets new standards for cheerful efficiency.

I am also grateful to the researchers in this field whose work I leaned on, notably Leslie Dunkling and William Gosling, authors of *The Facts on File Dictionary of First Names,* and Connie Lockhart Ellefson, author of *The Melting Pot Book of Baby Names*. Finally, the Social Security Administration keeps fascinating records of recent fashions in American baby names, which I consulted frequently in compiling this book.

CONTENTS

ABBREVIATIONS

Arab	Arabic	*ME*	Middle English
Celt	Celtic		
Dan	Danish	*Nor*	Norwegian
Eng	English	*OE*	Old English
Fr	French	*OF*	Old French
Gael	Gaelic	*OG*	Old German
Gk	Greek	*ONorse*	Old Norse
Haw	Hawaiian	*Per*	Persian
Heb	Hebrew	*Pol*	Polish
Hung	Hungarian	*Port*	Portuguese
Ir. Gael	Irish Gaelic	*Scan*	Scandinavian
It	Italian	*Scot*	Scottish
Jap	Japanese	*Scot. Gael*	Scottish Gaelic
Lat	Latin		
Lith	Lithuanian	*Teut*	Teutonic

INTRODUCTION

One of the first questions anyone asks about a newborn is, "What is the baby's name?" Faced with this tiny pink scrap of humanity, we want to put a name to it as if, by doing so, we welcome it to the realm of individuals. We always name the things we love. A small child will give names to even his tiniest toys or his well-chewed blanket, and the difference between "Blankie" and "the blanket" is an entire personality.

So when it comes to naming your baby, you want to get it right. You want to strike a fine balance between uniqueness and familiarity, honor a family member, reflect your ethnic heritage, avoid horrible nicknames, ensure that your child's name will never be misspelled. You'd like to name him for Granddad, but Granddad's name was Elmer. You thought Rosie sounded nice until your best friend asked if you're naming her for Rosie O'Donnell. The baby's due in six weeks and your spouse has vetoed every single suggestion. So you do what you always swore you wouldn't, and buy a baby name book.

There are many baby name books on the market. They give varying numbers of names, and varying amounts of information about the names. I believe that when it comes to picking a name, more is more. More choices can help you make *your* choice. I also think a simple alphabetical listing is easiest to use. I suspect most people simply browse through these books in the hope that the perfect selection will leap off the page at them. And who knows? Maybe sometimes it does.

More often, though, parents arrive at their final selection by a process of elimination. They rule out the bizarre names, the unfashionable names, the names that remind them of a second-grade bully. The process is highly emotional, because every name is wreathed with a cluster of associations that we may not even be aware of. Some of these associations are with public figures, which is why books like this one include examples of famous people under most listings. If you connect the name Molly with a kind of freckled cuteness, that is probably because you saw Molly Ringwald in *Pretty in Pink*, even if you don't remember this momentous event.

We are also swayed, whether or not we'd like to think so, by fashion and class. Certain kinds of names are the ones used by any group at a certain time. In the 1980s, for instance, WASPy unisex names were enormously popular. The parents who named their babies Ashley or Whitney may not have been aware that they were following a trend, but these names would not even have occurred to most parents twenty years earlier.

America takes its basic naming traditions, along with its language, from the British Isles. Before the Norman invasion in the eleventh century, England was inhabited by a mix of Germanic and Scandinavian groups, with Celts at the outer edges. Many Old English names (like Albert or Randolph) are rooted in German languages. They tend to be attribute names, often characterizing prowess in battle. (The girls' names surviving from this era are usually later feminizations of the old forms, like Alberta.)

The Norman conquest brought French names to England, and the gradual conversion of Britain to Christianity ushered in the use of saints' and Latin names, like Agnes or Vincent. But the great change in the Middle Ages was the formation of last names. The population increased, and a first name was no longer sufficient identification. John could mean one of three or four people in a community: but John Baker was the John who made the bread. Many of our last names and a good percentage of masculine first names come from this period. By and large, they are place names (John Woods) or occupational names (John Weaver), descriptive names (John White) or son-of names (Joe Johnson). The place names especially give a vivid glimpse of what life must have been like for the average Englishman at the time. The points of reference are humble, a stump or a willow tree or a stream that would nevertheless have been major landmarks in rural life.

The next great upheaval in naming practices came with the Reformation. Puritans felt it was popish to use saints' names so they ransacked the Old Testament, bringing names like Ezra and Rebecca into fashion. Of course, there are many fewer female than male names in the Bible, so the Puritans also named their daughters for admired qualities or virtues like Constance or Hope. Since New England was settled by ardent Protestants, these names also took root in the northeastern colonies, and many of them survived well into the nineteenth century.

Through much of the eighteenth century America was still identified with Britain and followed its naming practices, which included the addition of a few Germanic names like Adelaide that were brought in the wake of the Hanoverian kings. But by the middle of the nineteenth century the habits of the two countries diverged. In England the middle class turned to the past and revived many of the Old English names that had been unused for centuries. At the same time many last names were adopted for use as first names, resulting in a generation of little boys named Carpenter or Wakefield. Meanwhile girls were often given flower names like Rose or Violet or Daisy, perfectly appropriate for the Victorian concept of girlhood.

In the United States, however, immigration began to make a mark. Irish, German, and Italian-born parents gave their children names that were redolent of the homeland, though the well-assimilated second generation often chose anglicized names. This tendency was particularly marked among Jewish immigrants several decades later who picked out Anglo-Saxon names like Sheldon and Alvin for their sons.

The elaborate three-syllable names of the turn of the century gave way to increasingly streamlined models as the twentieth century progressed. Made-up names like Darlene flourished, and children's names were increasingly drawn from popular culture. For instance, some parents consciously named a son Rick for the hero of *Casablanca*, while others, having seen the movie three nights before the baby's birth, no doubt decided to name the baby for Uncle Richard, and thought Rick would make a handy nickname. The popularity of certain names (like Samantha) closely followed the careers of a movie star or TV show. If nothing else, a star's fame guarantees that her name has been widely heard, so it doesn't sound completely outlandish when it's suggested for a baby.

Outlandish names, though, did become popular in the 1960s and 1970s. Cher Bono named her daughter Chastity. Frank Zappa's children are Moon Unit and Dweezil. Individuality was critical to counterculture parents, and traditional names began to drift out of favor.

This urge to uniqueness is still with us. Gone are the days of Tommy and Margaret and Susan and Peter. The names on kindergarten cubbies today are a dizzying cocktail of obscure Old Testament prophets, proud ethnic selections, creatively spelled favorites, and sheer inventions. Parents of the twenty-first century want to be sure their children's names stand out.

There is already a countertrend afoot, though. Hospital nurseries are still full of babies names Chiarra or Zane, but the occasional truly old-fashioned choice is sneaking in. Abigail is back. So is William. I know little girls named Violet and Maisie. They're still unusual, but they come with a distinguished provenance. I think these are the names we'll be seeing more of in the next few years, though a parent who really wanted his baby to have an unusual name would choose, believe it or not, John or Mary.

Pick a Name, Any Name

There are any number of ways to choose a name for a baby. One of the most common is to use an old family name. If the family tie is strong enough, parents are often willing to overlook an unfashionable aura or an unpleasant meaning. If all the menfolk for five generations have been named Brendan, who are you to complain that the name means "stinking hair?"

But inspiration need not be limited to a family tree. Pick an attribute (brilliant mind: Hubert). Pick a birthstone (Ruby) or an astrological connection (Pisces, the water sign: Undine). Pick an ethnic favorite or the name of the Italian city where the baby was conceived. Name the baby for your favorite poet or an interesting saint.

Or simply leaf through this book and make a list, then pare the list down. Cut out the choices that won't work well with the baby's last name, or that may have unacceptable nicknames. For instance, you might insist on calling your son Hugh, but sooner or later someone is going to call him Huey, and it may stick. If you're using a middle name, make sure the three initials together don't spell something odious. And when you're down to a handful of finalists, try the playground test. Can you imagine yourself bellowing the name across a crowded playground? If you feel self-conscious, it will never do.

As the pregnancy moves into its later months, you'll hear two questions over and over: "Do you know what you're having?" and "Have you thought about names?" You'll answer these questions as you like, of course. But bear in mind that people will feel perfectly free to tell you what they think about your choice of names—*before* you have the baby. If you wait until after the infant's already been named Osbert, nobody will be rude enough to criticize. If you're set on an unusual name, this might be the best strategy.

There's no use starting on the process too early. Maybe you can settle on the perfect name by the thirty-fourth gestational week, but there are plenty of parents who start doing their Lamaze breathing without a final selection. There's nothing wrong with making your choice after you've met the little one. And even if you think you've decided, it wouldn't hurt to tuck this book into your hospital bag just in case you have second thoughts.

Finding the perfect name for your baby can be difficult, but the beauty of the process is this: By the time the baby is a few months old, his personality erases all other associations the name may hold. The second-grade bully or the much-loved poet fade away, and the name becomes, quite simply, the name of your child. And you will have made the right choice.

If it's a
GIRL

Abarrane (Basque. Fem. **Abraham**) Heb. "Father of many."

Abame

Abebi Nig. "She came after asking."

Abelia (Fem. **Abel**) Fr. from Heb. "Sigh."

Abella, Abelle

Abellona (Fem. **Apollo**) Dan. In Greek myth, Apollo is the sun god. See **Apolline**.

Aberdeen Place name: city in northeast Scotland.

Abia Arab. "Great."

Abida Arab. "She who worships" or Heb. "My father knows."

Abiela Heb. "My father is the Lord."

Abigail Heb. "My father is joyful." Biblical name adopted by the Puritans and popular through the 18th century. After a hundred years of obscurity, it was revived with the trend toward old-fashioned names beginning in the 1970s. Abigail Adams, wife of President John Adams; advice columnist Abigail Van Buren.

Abagael, Abagail, Abagale, Abagil, Abaigeal, Abbe, Abbey, Abbi, Abbie, Abbigael, Abbigail, Abbigale, Abby, Abbye, Abbygael, Abbygail, Abbygaie, Abegale, Abigael, Abigal, Abigale, Abigall, Abigil, Abigayle, Gael, Gail, Gaila, Gal, Gale, Gayel, Gayle

Abijah Heb. "God is my father."

Abeedja, Abeeja, Abeesha, Abisha, Abishah

Abilene Place name: town in Texas, and also, in early Christian times, an area in Lebanon near Damascus.

Abalene, Abalina, Abilena, Abiline

Abina Ghanaian. "Born on Thursday."

Abir Arab. "Scent."

Abeer

Abital Heb. "My father is dew." Currently popular in Israel.

Abeetal, Avital

Abra (Fem. **Abraham**) Heb. "Father of many" or Arab. "Example, lesson." King Solomon's favorite concubine was named Abra.

Abame, Abarrane, Abrahana

Acacia Gk. Name of a blossoming tree that symbolized resurrection. Uncommon even in Greece, though the derivatives like **Casey** occur often in the U.S.

Cacia, Cacie, Casey, Casha, Casia, Cassie, Cassy, Caysha, Kacey, Kacie, Kasey, Kasi, Kassja, Kassy

Acadia Place name: The French settlers of Nova Scotia called it Acadia after the name of a river there. When the French inhabitants were driven out by the English in the 18th century, many of them settled in Louisiana and became known as "Cajuns."

Accalia Lat. In myth, the name of the human foster mother of Romulus and Remus, the twins who founded Rome. Legend has it that after their abandonment as infants, they were initially suckled by a she-wolf, whose name is not known. Accalia was her replacement.

Aceline (Fem. **Acelin**) Fr. "Highborn."

Asceline

Achsah Heb. "Ankle bracelet."

Achsah

Acima (Fem. **Acim**) Heb. "The Lord will judge."

Acimah, Achima, Achimah

Acquanetta Invented name related to the particle *aqua*, which is Latin for "water." Possibly derived from the name of the hairspray "AquaNet."

Acquanette, Aquanette, Aquannette

Ada Ger. "Noble, nobility." Originated as a short form of names like **Adelaide,** and popular in the last quarter of the 19th century, though infrequently used now.

Adan, Adda, Addi, Addie, Addiah, Addy, Adey, Adi, Adia, Adiah, Adie, Aida, Aidah

Adah Heb. "Ornament, adornment." Biblical name. Unusual, but brought to prominence in the 19th century by American actress Adah Isaacs Mencken.

Adalia Heb. "God is my refuge"; OG. "Noble one." See also **Adelaide**.

Adal, Adala, Adalee, Adali, Adalie, Adalley, Addal, Addala

Adamina (Fem. **Adam**) Heb. "Child of the red earth." In the Bible God created Adam out of the "red earth" and breathed life into him. This unusual feminine version of the name is Scottish in origin.

Ada, Adameena, Adamine, Adaminna, Addie, Ademina, Ademeena, Mina, Minna

Adara Gk. "Beauty" or Arab. "Virgin."

Adra

Addie Dim. **Adelaide, Adeline,** or **Addison.** A nostalgic-sounding nickname.

Addy

Addison OE. "Son of Adam."

Addeson, Adison, Adisson

Addula Teut. "Noble cheer."

Adelaide OG. "Noble, nobility." First popular in England after the reign (1830-37) of William IV and Queen Adelaide. The city of Adelaide, Australia, founded in 1836, was named for her.

Adalaide, Adalayde, Addala, Addalla, Addey, Addi, Addie, Addy, Adel, Adela, Adelaida, Adelais, Adele, Adelheid, Adelina, Adeline, Adelice, Adelicia, Adelis, Adelle, Adey, Adi, Ado, Ady, Aline, Aliosha, Alline, Alyosha, Del, Della, Delle, Delli, Delly, Edeline, Eline, Heidi, Lady, Laidey

Adele OG. "Noble, nobility." See **Adelaide.** Nutritionist Adelle Davis; writer Adela Rogers St. John.

Adelia, Adell, Adella, Adellah, Adelle, Edelle

Adelinda Teut. "Noble, sweet." Com. form **Adele** and **Linda.**

Adele, Adeline, Adelinde, Linda

Adeline OG. "Noble, nobility." See **Adelaide.** Adelina enjoyed a burst of popularity during the career of operatic soprano Adelina Patti, in the late 19th century.

Adalina, Adaline, Adallina, Adelina, Adelind, Adella, Adellah, Ahdella, Aline, Dahlina, Dalina, Daline, Dallina, Delina, Deline, Dellina, Delly, Delyne, Edelie, Lina

Adelpha Gr. "Beloved sister."

Adena Heb. "Decoration."
 Adene, Adina, Adinah, Deena, Denah, Dina, Dinah

Adeola Nig. "Crown."
 Adola, Dola

Adesina Nig. "She paves the way."

Adiba Arab. "Cultured, refined."
 Adeeba, Adibah

Adiella Heb. "The Lord's adornment."

Adima Teut. "Noble, renowned."

Adin Heb. Meaning unclear: possibly "delicate and slender." Appears in the Old Testament as a male name.
 Adina, Adeana

Adira Heb. "Noble, powerful."
 Adeera, Edira

Aditi Hindi. "Boundless." In Hindu cosmology, Aditi is the mother of the gods.

Adiva Arab. "Agreeable, gentle."

Adlai Arab./Heb. "Just." More familiar to us as a man's name made famous by U.S. Senator Adlai Stevenson.

Adolpha (Fem. **Adolph**) Ger. "Noble wolf."
 Adolfa, Adollfa

Adoncia Sp. "Sweet."
 Doncia

Adonia (Fem. **Adonis**) Gk. In Greek myth Adonis was a young man so beautiful that Aphrodite, goddess of love, became enamored of him. The name Adonis has come to epitomize male beauty.

Adora Lat. "Adored."
 Adorabelle, Adorae, Adoray, Adoré, Adorée, Adoria, Adorlee, Dora, Dorae, Dori, Dorie, Dorri, Dorrie, Dorry, Dory

Adra Arab. "Virgin."
 Adara

Adrian Lat. Place name: Adria was a North Italian city. First popular in the 1950s in Britain, and more common as a man's name. Hollywood costume designer Adrian (*Queen Christina, The Philadelphia Story*) and 12th-century Pope Adrian IV (the only English pope) both predate its use as a girl's name. Fashion designer Adrienne Vittadini.

Adrea, Adreea, Adria, Adriah, Adriana, Adrianah, Adriane, Adrianna, Adriannah, Adrianne, Adrie, Adrien, Adriena, Adrienah, Adrienne, Aydrian, Aydrienne, Hadria, Hadrienne

Afra Arab. "Color of earth" or Heb. "Young deer" or "Dust."
Affera, Affery, Affra, Aphra

Afraima Arab./Heb. "Fertile."

Africa Place name; the continent.
Affrica, Affricah, Affrika, Affrikah, Africah, Afrika, Afrikah, Aifric, Aifrica, Aphria, Aphfrica, Apirka, Apirkah

Afton OE. Place name: There is a town called Afton in southern Scotland. Like so many place names that have become first names, this one was first a name for boys.
Affton

Agapi Gk. "Love, affection."
Agape, Agappe

Agate OF. A semiprecious stone. Can be considered either one of the jewel names so popular in the 19th century, or a variant of **Agatha**. The agate, though not a particularly beautiful stone, was once believed to have numerous magical and curative powers.

Agatha Gk. "Good." Saint Agatha was a 3rd-century Christian who refused to marry a Roman consul. She was tortured and ultimately martyred. Her name was popular in the early years of the Christian Church, but not again until the late 19th century. It now has an unfashionable ring, but some of the international variants are pretty. Writer Agatha Christie.
Ag, Agace, Agacia, Agafia, Agafon, Agapet, Agapit, Agata, Agathe, Agathi, Agatta, Aggi, Aggie, Aggy, Aggye, Agi, Agie, Agota, Agotha, Agueda, Agy, Agye

Agave Gk. "Illustrious, noble."

Aglaia Gk. In Greek myth, one of the three Graces, epitomizing brilliance. **Thalia** (blossoming) is still sometimes used; Euphrosyne (joy) is obsolete.

Agnes Gk. "Pure, virginal." Another early Christian saint's name. She was a virgin martyr, and her emblem in art is a lamb (the Latin for "lamb" is *agnus*). Very popular in England between the 12th and 16th centuries, Agnes is uncommon now, perhaps because of its connotations of homeliness. A French variant, **Anaïs**, is currently very popular in France. Choreographer Agnes De Mille; actress Agnes Moorhead; writer Anaïs Nin; film director Agnieska Holland.

Ag, Agafi, Agafia, Agafon, Aggi, Aggie, Aggye, Aghna, Agi, Agie, Agna, Agnah, Agnella, Agnellah, Agnelle, Agnese, Agnesse, Agneta, Agnetta, Agnettah, Agnola, Agnolah, Agot, Agota, Agote, Agoti, Agy, Agye, Aigneis, Aina, Ainah, Anas, Annais, Anneyce, Annis, Annisa, Annisah, Annise, Ina, Inah, Ines, Inessa, Inez, Nessa, Nessah, Nesi, Nessie, Nessy, Nesta, Nestah, Nevsa, Nevesah, Neysa, Oona, Oonagh, Oonah, Senga, Una, Unah, Ynes, Ynez

Agnola It. "Angel." Also a variant of **Agnes**.
Agnolla, Agnolle

Agrafina Rus. "Born feet first." See **Agrippa**.

Agrippa Lat. "Born feet first." The name of a 1st-century Roman Emperor, the son of Herod. A man's name possibly transferred to female use because of the "-a" ending.
Agrafina, Agrippina, Agrippine

Agrippina Lat. Sister of the corrupt Roman Emperor Caligula and mother of the equally unsavory Roman Emperor Nero, who had her murdered. Not a common name, for obvious reasons.

Ahava Heb. "Loved one."
Ahouva, Ahuva, Ahuda

Aibhlin Ir. Gael. form of **Evelyn** or **Helen**.

Aida Arab. "Reward, present." Name of an immensely popular opera by Giuseppe Verdi.
Aeeda, Ayeeda, Ieeda, Iyeeda

Aidan Ir. Gael. "Fire." Saint Aidan was a 7th-century Irish monk. The name used to be more common for men than for women, but in the last ten years, has become as well used for girls as more familiar names like **Molly** and **Catherine**.

Adan, Aden, Aiden, Aydan, Ayden, Aydenn

Aiko Jap. "Little loved one."

Ailbhe Ir. "Noble, bright."

Alva, Alvy, Elva, Elvy

Aileen Ir. Var. **Helen** (Gk. "Light"). This form has been most popular in Scotland.

Aila, Ailee, Ailene, Ailey, Ailli, Ailie, Aleen, Alene, Aline, Alleen, Allene, Alline, Eileen, Eleen, Elleen, Ellene, Ileana, Ileane, Ileanna, Ilone, Iliana, Iliane, Ilianna, Illeanne, Illene, Leana, Leanah, Leanna, Leannah, Lena, Lenah, Liana, Lianna, Liannah, Lina, Linah

Ailith OE. "Seasoned warrior."

Aldith, Eilith

Ailsa Scot. The name has two possible sources. As a homonym for **Elsa,** a diminutive of **Elizabeth,** it means "Pledge from God." An alternate source is the tiny Scottish island Ailsa Craig.

Ailis, Ailse, Elsa, Elsha, Elshe

Aimée Fr. "Beloved." See **Amy.** Evangelist Aimée Semple McPherson.

Aimie, Aimey, Amey, Amie

Aina Scand. "Forever."

Aine Celt. "Happiness."

Ainsley Scot. Gael. Place name: "One's own meadow." A last name converted to a first name, used by both sexes.

Ainslee, Ainsleigh, Ainslie, Ansley, Aynslee, Aynsley, Aynslie

Airlea Gk. "Ethereal."

Airlia

Aisha Arab. "Woman" or Swahili. "Life." Aisha was the favored wife of Mohammed, hence the name's current popularity among Muslim families.

Aeesha, Aeeshah, Aesha, Aeshah, Aiesha, Aieshah, Aishah, Aisia, Aisiah, Asha, Ashah, Ashia, Ashiah, Asia, Asiah, Ayeesa, Ayeesah, Ayeesha, Ayeeshah, Ayeisa, Ayeisah, Ayeisha, Ayeishah, Ayisa, Ayisah, Ayisha, Ayishah, Ieasha, Ieashah, Ieashia, Ieashiah, Iesha, Ieshah, Ieesha, Ieeshah, Ieeshia, Ieeshiah, Yiesha, Yieshah

Aislinn Ir. Gael. "Dream."
  Aisling, Ashling, Isleen
Aithne (Fem. **Aidan**) Ir. Gael. "Fire." Not to be confused, despite its sound, with the name of the Sicilian volcano.
  Aine, Aithnea, Eithne, Ena, Ethnah, Ethnea, Ethnee
Aiyana Native American. "Forever flowering."
Akela Haw. "Noble." A form of **Adele**.
Akilina Gk./Rus. "Eagle."
  Acquilina, Acuqileena, Aquilina
Akiva Heb. "Protect, shelter."
  Akeeva, Keeva, Keevah, Kiba, Kibah, Kiva, Kivah, Kivi
Alaia Arab. "Sublime."
Alaine (Fem. **Alan**) Fr. from Gael. Possibly "Rock" or "Comely." Not actually used in France, where it would be very easily confused with **Hélène**.
  Alaina, Alayna, Alayne, Aleine, Alenne, Allaine, Allayne, Alleine, Allene, Alenne, Aleyne
Alala Gk. In Greek mythology, the sister of Ares, the god of war.
Alamea Haw. "Ripe, precious."
Alanna (Fem. **Alan**) Gael. "Rock" or "Comely." Also a possible derivative of **Elaine** (OF. "Bright, shining") or **Helen** (Gk. "Light"). Singer Alanis Morrissette; actress Lana Turner.
  Alaina, Alaine, Alana, Alane, Alanis, Alannah, Alayne, Alène, Aleyna, Aleyne, Alleen, Allena, Allene, Allyna, Alleynah, Alleyne, Allina, Allinah, Allyn, Lana, Lanah, Lanna, Lannah, Aleyna, Aleynah
Alaqua Native American. "Sweet gum tree."
Alarice (Fem. **Alaric**) OG. "Noble king." Alaric was a king of the Visigoths who sacked Rome.
  Alarica, Alaricka, Alarieka
Alastair Scot. Var. **Alexander** (Gk. "Man's defender"). More generally used as a man's name.
  Alasdair, Alastrina, Alastriona
Alaula Haw. "Light of daybreak."
Alba Lat. "White." See **Albinia**.
  Albane, Albina, Albine, Albinia, Albinka, Alva

Alberga Lat. "White" or OG. "Noble." Also closely related to the French and Italian words for "inn."
Alberge, Elberga, Elberge

Alberta OE. "Noble-shining." Rare and old-fashioned now, it was most widely used during the lifetime of Queen Victoria's Prince Consort, Albert. Also the name of a western Canadian province, and a very popular strain of peach.
Alberthine, Albertina, Albertine, Ali, Alli, Allie, Ally, Auberta, Auberte, Aubertha, Auberthe, Aubine, Berrie, Berry, Bert, Berta, Berte, Berti, Bertie, Berty, Elberta, Elbertha, Elberthina, Elberthine, Elbertina, Elbertine

Albinia (Fem. **Alban, Albin**) Lat. "White, fair."
Alba, Albina, Alva, Alvina, Aubine

Albreda (Fem. **Aubrey**) OG. "Counsel from the elves."

Alcestis Gk. In Euripides' play of the same name, Alcestis descends to Hades in place of her husband, and is then rescued by Hercules.

Alcina Gk. In Greek myth, a sorceress who rules over a magical island. When she tired of her lovers, Alcina turned them into animals, trees, or stones. Despite this startling role model the name occurs from time to time.
Alcine, Alcinia, Allcine, Allcinia, Alseena, Alsina, Alsinia, Alsyna, Alzina

Alda (Fem. **Aldo, Otto**) OG. "Old, prosperous."
Aldabella, Aldea, Aldina, Aldine, Aleda, Alida

Aldara Gk. "Winged gift."

Aldis OE. "Battle-seasoned."
Aldith, Ailith

Aldonza Sp. "Sweet."

Aleeza Heb. "Joy."
Aleezah, Alieza, Aliezah, Aliza, Alizah, Alitza

Alegria Sp. "Happiness, joy." For related names, see **Hilary, Felicity, Bliss**. A charming choice for a much-wanted child.
Alagria, Alegrya, Allegria

Alena Rus. Var. **Helen** (Gk. "Light").

Alesia Gk. "Help, aid."
Alessia

Aleta Gk. "Footloose."

Aletta, Alette, Alletta, Allette, Eletta, Elletta, Ellette, Lettee, Lettie, Letty

Alethea Gk. "Truth." Unusual name that first appeared in Britain in the 17th century.

Alathia, Aleethia, Aleta, Aletea, Aletha, Alethia, Aletta, Alette, Alithea, Alithia, Elethea, Elithia

Alexandra (Fem. Alexander) Gk. "Man's defender." Became very popular in Britain after the Prince of Wales (later Edward VII) married the Danish Princess Alexandra in 1863. Still used in the English royal family and its many branches. Ballet dancer Alexandra Danilova; fashion designer Zandra Rhodes.

Alastrina, Alastriona, Alejanda, Alejandra, Alejandrina, Aleka, Aleki, Alesandare, Alesandere, Alessanda, Alessandra, Alessandre, Alessandrina, Alessandrine, Alessia, Alex, Alexa, Alexanda, Alexandere, Alexanderia, Alexanderina, Alexanderine, Alexandre, Alexandrea, Alexandreana, Alexandrena, Alexandrene, Alexandretta, Alexandria, Alexandrina, Alexandrine, Alexea, Alexena, Alexene, Alexia, Alexina, Alexine, Alexis, Ali, Aliki, Alissandre, Alissandrine, Alista, Alix, Alla, Allejandra, Allejandrina, Allessa, Allessandra, Alle, Allexa, Allexandra, Allexandrina, Allexina, Allexine, Alli, Allie, Allix, Ally, Anda, Cesya, Elena, Ellena, Lesy, Lesya, Lexi, Lexie, Lexine, Lissandre, Lissandrine, Sanda, Sande, Sandi, Sandie, Sandra, Sandrina, Sandrine, Sandy, Sandye, Sanndra, Sasha, Sashenka, Shura, Shurochka, Sohndra, Sondra, Xandra, Zahndra, Zanda, Zanndra, Zohndra, Zondra

Alexis Gk. "Helper." Usually thought of as a short form of **Alexandra**, though it has a different etymological root. Actress Alexis Smith.

Alessa, Alessi, Alexa, Alexi, Alexia, Lexi, Lexie, Lexy

Alfonsine (Fem. Alfonso) OG. "Noble and ready for battle."

Alfonsia, Alonza, Alphonsine

Alfreda (Fem. **Alfred**) OE. "Elf power." Actress Alfre
Woodard.
**Alfi, Alfie, Alfre, Alfredah, Alfredda, Alfreeda, Alfri,
Alfried, Alfrieda, Alfryda, Alfy, Allfie, Allfreda,
Allfredah, Allfredda, Allfrie, Allfrieda, Allfry, Allfryda,
Allfy, Elfie, Elfre, Elfrea, Elfredah, Elfredda, Elfreeda,
Elfrida, Elfrieda, Elfryda, Elfrydah, Ellfreda, Ellfredah,
Ellfredda, Ellfreeda, Ellfrida, Ellfrieda, Ellfryda,
Ellfrydah, Elva, Elvah, Freda, Freddi, Freddie, Freddy,
Fredi, Fredy, Freeda, Freedah, Frieda, Friedah, Fryda,
Frydah**

Alice OG. "Noble, nobility." See **Adelaide**. An old standby
name since the Middle Ages that became enormously
popular after the 1865 publication of Lewis Carroll's
Alice's Adventures in Wonderland. Its popularity waned in
the 1930s, and it now has a pleasantly old-fashioned air.
Ballerina Alicia Markova; writers Alice Walker, Alice Se-
bold; actresses Ali McGraw, Ally Sheedy, Alicia Silver-
stone; singer Alicia Keys.
**Adelice, Ailis, Ala, Aleceea, Alecia, Aleetheea,
Aleethia, Ali, Alica, Alicah, Alicea, Alicen, Alicia, Alid,
Alie, Alika, Alikah, Aliki, Alis, Alisa, Alisah, Alisann,
Alisanne, Alisha, Alison, Alissa, Alisz, Alitheea, Alitia,
Aliz, Alla, Allecia, Alleece, Alleeceea, Alles, Alless,
Alli, Allice, Allicea, Allie, Allis, Allison, Allissa,
Allisun, Allisunne, Allsun, Ally, Allyce, Allyceea, Allys,
Allyse, Allysia, Allysiah, Allyson, Allyssa, Allysson,
Alyce, Alyceea, Alys, Alyse, Alysia, Alyson, Alyss,
Alyssa, Elissa, Elli, Ellie, Ellissa, Ellsa, Elsa, Illyssa,
Ilysa, Ilysah, Ilyssa, Ilysse, Leece, Leese, Licha,
Lichah, Lissa, Lyssa**

Alida Lat. "Small winged one."
**Adela, Adelina, Adelita, Adellyna, Adellyta, Adelyna,
Adelyta, Alaida, Alda, Aldina, Aldine, Aldona,
Aldonna, Aldyne, Aleda, Aleta, Aletta, Alette, Alidah,
Alidia, Alita, Allda, Alldina, Alldine, Alldona,
Alldonna, Alldyne, Alleda, Allida, Allidah, Allidia,
Allidiah, Allyda, Allydah, Alyda, Alydah, Dela, Della,**

Dila, Dilla, Elida, Elita, Leda, Ledah, Lida, Lidah, Lita,
Lyda, Lydah, Oleda, Oleta, Oletta, Olette

Alima Arab. "Cultured."

Alina Slavic. Var. **Helen** (Gk. "Light").
Aleen, Aleena, Alena, Alenah, Alene, Aline, Alleen,
Allena, Allene, Alline, Allyna, Allynah, Allyne, Alyna,
Alynah, Alyne, Leena, Leenah, Lena, Lenah, Lina,
Linah, Lyna, Lynah

Alisa Heb. "Great happiness."
Alisah, Alissa, Alissah, Aliza, Allisa, Allisah, Allissa,
Allissah, Allysa, Allysah, Alyssa, Alyssah

Alison Dim. **Alice** (OG. "Noble, nobility"). Actress Allison
Janney.
Aili, Alisann, Alisanne, Alisoun, Alisun, Allcen,
Allcenne, Allicen, Allicenne, Allie, Allisann, Allisanne,
Allison, Allisoun, Allsun, Ally, Allysann, Allysanne,
Allyson, Allysoun, Alysan, Alysann, Alysanne, Alyson,
Alysoun

Alix OG. "Noble." See **Alexandra**.
Alex, Alexa, Alexis, Aliki, Alissandre, Alissandrine,
Lissandre

Aliya Arab. "Highborn." Pop musician Aaliyah.
Aaliya, Aaliyah, Alia, Aliah, Aliyah, Aliye, Allia, Alliah

Allegra It. "Joyous." The musical term *allegro* means
"quickly, with a happy air." Ballerina Allegra Kent.
Alegra, Allegretta, Alegria, Legra, Leggra

Allena (Fem. **Allen**, **Alan**) Ir. Possible meaning "Rock" or
"Comely." See **Alanna**.
Alana, Alanice, Alanis, Alanna, Alena, Alene, Allene,
Alleyne, Allynn, Allynne, Allyn, Alynne

Allyriane Fr. from Gk. "Lyre." The lyre was a stringed instrument, a predecessor of today's harp or guitar.

Alma Lat. "Giving nurture"; It. "Soul"; Arab. "Learned."
Also the name of a river in the Crimea where a famous
19th-century battle was fought, bringing it into prominence as a first name. The more common usage, of course,
is "alma mater" for a college or university. Composer's
wife Alma Mahler.

Almah, Allma

Almarine OG. "Work ruler."

Almeria, Almerine

Almeda Lat. "Goal-directed, ambitious."

**Allmeda, Allmedah, Allmeta, Allmetah, Allmida,
Allmidah, Allmita, Allmitah, Almedah, Almeta,
Almetah, Almida, Almidah, Almita, Almitah, Maelle**

Almera (Fem. **Elmer**) Arab. "Aristocratic lady."

**Allmeera, Allmeria, Almeera, Almeeria, Almeria,
Almire, Almirah, Almyra, Ellmera, Ellmeria, Elmeera,
Elmeeria, Elmera, Elmeria, Elmira, Elmyra, Elmyrah,
Mera, Meera, Mira, Mirah, Myra, Myrah**

Almodine Lat. "Precious stone."

Aloha Haw. "Love, kindness, affection." The familiar
Hawaiian greeting.

Aloisia (Fem. **Aloysius**) OG. "Famous fighter."

Aloysia, Eloisia, Eloysia

Alona Heb. "Oak tree." The many different spellings of this
name attest to its use all over Europe.

Allona, Allonia, Alonia, Elona, Ilona, Ilonka

Alonsa (Fem. **Alonso**) Sp./OG. "Ready for battle."

Alonza

Alpha Gk. First letter of Greek alphabet, corresponding to
A. Appropriate for a first daughter.

Alfa

Alphonsine (Fem. **Alphonse**) Fr. from OG. "Ready for
battle."

Alta Lat. "Elevated."

Alita

Altair Arab. "Bird." Also the name of the brightest star in
the constellation Aquila. It is about ten times as bright as
the sun.

Althea Gk. "With healing power." Tennis star Althea Gibson.

**Altha, Althaia, Altheda, Althelia, Althia, Eltha, Elthea,
Thea**

Altheda Gk. "Like a blossom."

Alura OE. "Godlike adviser." Same sound as **Allura,** but
completely different source.

Alurea, Allura, Ellura

Alva Sp. "Blond, fair-skinned." See **Alba, Albina.** Also Heb. "Foliage." Better-known as a man's name, as in Thomas Alva Edison.

Alba, Albina, Albine, Albinia, Alvah, Alvit

Alvar OE. "Army of elves." Also used as a man's name, but very unusual.

Alverdine OE. "Counsel from the elves." A rare feminine variant of **Alfred. Alfreda** is more common.

Alvina (Fem. **Alvin**) OE. "Noble friend" or "Elf-friend."

Alveena, Alveene, Alveenia, Alvine, Alvineea, Alvinia, Alwinna, Alwyna, Alwyne, Elveena, Elvena, Elvene, Elvenia, Elvina, Elvine, Elvinia, Vina, Vinni, Vinnie, Vinny

Alvita Lat. "Lively."

Alysia Gk. "Entrancing."

Alyssa Gk. "Rational." Also the name of a bright yellow flower, alyssum, and its use may have been influenced by the 19th-century vogue for flower names. Also see the variants of **Alice.**

Alissa, Allissa, Alysa, Ilyssa, Lyssa

Alzena Arab. "Woman."

Alzeena, Alzeina, Alzina, Elzeena, Elzina

Ama Ghanaian. "Born on Saturday."

Amabel Lat. "Lovable, amiable." Somewhat popular in the 19th century.

Ama, Amabelle, Belle, Mab, Mabel

Amada Lat. "Loved one."

Amata

Amadea (Fem. **Amadeus**) Lat. "God's beloved." Amadeus was Mozart's middle name, given great prominence by Peter Shaffer's play and the subsequent film.

Amadée, Amedée

Amadore It. "Gift of love."

Amadora

Amal Arab. "Hope."

Amahl, Amahla, Amala

Amalida OG. "Hardworking woman." See **Amelia.**

Amaleeda, Amelida

Amana Heb. "Loyal, true."

Amanda Lat. "Much-loved." Regularly used since the 17th century, and extremely fashionable in the U.S. during the 1980s and 1990s. Use is dwindling now, however. Actresses Amanda Plummer, Amanda Peet; pop musician Mandy Moore.

Amandi, Amandie, Amandine, Amandy, Amata, Manda, Mandaline, Mandee, Mandi, Mandie, Mandy

Amara Gk. "Lovely forever."

Amargo, Amargoe, Amargot, Amarinda, Amarra, Amarrinda, Mara, Marra

Amarantha Gk. "Deathless." Also the name of both a mythical and a real plant. The mythical one was supposed to be immortal.

Amarande, Amaranta, Amarante, Amaranthe

Amaris Heb. "Pledged by God."

Amariah, Amarit

Amaryllis Gk. "Fresh." Also the name of a flower. Used in 18th-century poetry to refer to an unspoiled rural beauty like an idealized shepherdess.

Amarilis

Amber OF. Name of the gold-brown semiprecious stone. Jewel names were popular in the 19th century, but Amber came to prominence again in the 1960s, prompted by the Kathleen Winsor novel and film, *Forever Amber*. Perhaps because it is a good descriptive name for a golden-skinned baby, Amber is quite well used today. Model Amber Valletta.

Ambar, Amberetta, Amberly, Ambur

Ambika Hindi. "Mother." Also one of many names for the goddess Devi, wife of Shiva. She has both positive and negative forms, with names for each.

Ambeeka, Ambeika

Ambrosine (Fem. **Ambrose**) Gk. "Ever-living." Like other names with an "-ine" ending, this one has a French air.

Ambrosia, Ambrosina, Ambrosinetta, Ambrosinette, Ambrosiya, Ambrozetta, Ambrozia, Ambrozine

Amelia OG. "Industrious." See **Emily**. 18th-century Princess Amelia brought the name to Britain, where it was

popular in the 19th century. Dress reformer Amelia
Bloomer; aviatrix Amelia Earhart.

**Aimiliona, Amalea, Amalee, Amaleta, Amalia, Amalie,
Amalija, Amalina, Amaline, Amalita, Amaliya, Amalya,
Amalyna, Amalyne, Amalyta, Amelie, Amelina,
Ameline, Amelita, Ameliya, Amelyna, Amelyne,
Amelyta, Amilia, Amy, Em, Emelie, Emelina, Emeline,
Emelita, Emma, Emmeline, Emmie, Emmy, Mali,
Malia, Malika, Melia, Meline, Millie, Milly**

Amelinda Lat./Sp. Com. form "Beloved" and "Pretty."
Amalinda, Amalynda, Amelindah, Amellinda

Amethyst Gk. "Precious wine-colored jewel." An unusual
jewel name, though appropriate for a February baby, since
amethyst is that month's birthstone.
Amathyst, Amatista, Amethist, Amethiste

Amica Lat. "Friend." Very unusual. Closely related to Spanish *amiga* or Italian *amica,* the everyday words for
"friend" in those languages.
Amicah, Amice, Amika

Amilia Lat. "Amiable." Also possible variant spelling for
Amelia or **Emilia.**
Amiliya, Amillia, Amilya

Amina Arab. "Honest, trustworthy." Mother of the prophet
Muhammad.
Ameena, Aminah, Amyna

Aminta Lat. "Protector." Aminta was the heroine of a well-
known pastoral play of the Renaissance, but her name was
not much used in real life.
Amintah, Amynta, Eminta, Minta, Minty

Amira Arab. "Highborn girl." Currently popular in the
Arabic-speaking countries.
**Ameera, Ameerah, Amera, Amerah, Amirah, Amyra,
Amyrah, Meera, Meerah, Mera, Merah, Mira, Mirah**

Amisa Heb. "Companion, friend."
Amissa

Amita Heb. "Truth" or It. "Friendship." See **Amica, Amy**.

Amitola Native American. "Rainbow."

Amity Lat. "Friendship, harmony."
Amitie

Amor Sp. "Love."
   Amora, Amore, Amorra
Amorette Fr. "Little love."
   Amoretta
Amy Lat. "Loved." In spite of the prominence given the name by Louisa May Alcott's *Little Women,* and the 1995 film version, it didn't become a favorite until the 1950s. Hugely popular (along with Jennifer) in the 1970s. Amy is a top-ten name in both Scotland and Ireland. Poet Amy Lowell; evangelist Aimée Semple McPherson; singer Amy Grant; actress Amy Sedaris.
   Aimée, Aimie, Amada, Amata, Amé, Amecia, Ami, Amia, Amiah, Amice, Amie, Amii, Amye, Esma, Esmé
Anastasia Gk. "Resurrection." Indelibly associated with the daughter of Czar Nicholas II who was rumored to have escaped death when her family was assassinated during the Russian Revolution. The 1956 film starring Ingrid Bergman popularized her story, but the name is still something of a mouthful. Short forms like **Stacey** are much more common. Actress Nastassja Kinski.
   Ana, Anastaise, Anastase, Anastasie, Anastasija, Anastasiya, Anastassia, Anastay, Anasztaizia, Anasztasia, Anestassia, Anstass, Anstice, Asia, Nastassia, Nastassiya, Nastassja, Nastassya, Nastya, Stace, Stacey, Stacia, Stacie, Stacy, Stasiya, Stasja, Stasya, Taisie, Tasenka, Tasia, Tasiya, Tasja, Tasya
Anatola Gk. "From the east." Anatolia is a region of Turkey.
   Anatolia, Anatolya
Ancelote Fr. Feminine form of **Lancelot,** the famous knight of the Round Table.
Andrea (Fem. **Andrew**) Gk. "A man's woman." Used very steadily without ever becoming truly fashionable. Actresses Andie MacDowell, Andrea McArdle.
   Aindrea, Andee, Andere, Anderea, Andi, Andie, Andra, Andre, Andreana, Andreas, Andrée, Andrel, Andresa, Andrewena, Andrewina, Andri, Andria, Andriana, Andy, Aundrea, Ohndrea, Ohndreea, Ohndria, Ondrea, Ondreea, Ondria, Onndrea, Onndreea, Onndria

Andromeda Gk. In Greek myth, the beautiful daughter of Cassiopeia (now famous as a constellation), she was chained to a rock as a sacrifice to a sea monster until Perseus rescued her. She, too, became a star. Also the name of a spring-blooming shrub.

Anemone Gk. "Breath." In Greek myth, Anemone was the name of a nymph who was turned into a flower, which is also called a windflower.

Anemona, Ann-Aymone, Anne-Aymone

Angela Gk. "Messenger from God, angel." **Angel** was originally used as a name for men, and in Latin countries **Angelo** is still popular. Angela came into frequent use in the early 20th century. Actresses Angela Lansbury, Angie Dickinson, Angela Bassett, Angelina Jolie, Angie Harmon.

Aingeal, Ange, Angel, Angele, Angeleta, Angelica, Angelika, Angeliki, Angelina, Angeline, Angelique, Angelita, Angelle, Angellina, Angie, Angil, Angiola, Angy, Angyola, Anjel, Anjela, Anjelica, Anjelika, Anngela, Anngil, Anngilla, Anngiola, Annjela, Annijilla, Gelya

Angelica Lat. "Angelic." See **Angela**. Actress Anjelica Huston.

Angelika, Angelique, Angyalka, Anjelica, Anjelika

Anisah Arab. "Friendly, congenial."

Anisa, Annissa

Anita Sp. form of **Ann**. Most common in 1950s, possibly because of the popularity of Swedish actress Anita Ekberg. Actress Anita Pallenberg; writers Anita Loos, Anita Brookner.

Anitra, Annita, Annitra, Annitta

Ann Anglicization of **Hannah** (Heb. "Grace"). One of the most frequently used names for girls until the mid-19th century, when it became less popular. When Elizabeth II of England named her daughter Anne in 1950, it became more prominent, but is still more common as a middle name (Betty Ann, etc.). Though the name Ann may seem plain to many, its numerous derivatives offer plenty of variety. The European form **Anna** is now much more fashionable than plain old Ann in the United States, and is a top-ten name in Germany, while **Anya** is popular in Russia. Saint Anne (mother of the Virgin Mary); Anne Boleyn, Queen of England; ballerina Anna Pavlova; Wild West sharpshooter Annie Oakley; actresses Anouk Aimée, Anne Bancroft, Anne Heche, Anna Paquin; writer Ayn Rand; diarist Anne Frank; tennis player Anna Kournikova; golfer Annika Sorenstam.

Aine, Ana, Anci, Anechka, Anet, Anett, Anette, Ania, Anica, Anika, Aniko, Anissa, Anita, Anitra, Anka, Anke, Anki, Anna, Annabel, Annabella, Annabelle, Annaelle, Annelle, Annelore, Annetta, Annette, Anni, Annice, Annick, Annie, Annimae, Annina, Annis, Annise, Annora, Annus, Annuska, Anny, Anona, Anouche, Anouk, Anoushka, Anouska, Anushka, Anuska, Anya, Anyoushka, Anyshka, Anyu, Asya, Ayn, Hajna, Hana, Hanja, Hanka, Hanna, Hannah, Hanneke, Hannelore, Hanni, Hannie, Hanny, Nan, Nana, Nance, Nancee, Nancey, Nanci, Nancie, Nancy, Nanete, Nanette, Nanice, Nanine, Nanni, Nannie, Nanny, Nanon, Nanor, Neti, Nettia, Nettie, Netty, Nina, Ninette, Ninon, Ninor, Nita, Nona, Nonie

Annabel Possibly com. form **Anna** and **Belle** : "Graceful" and "Beautiful." Also mutation of **Amabel**. Most famous bearer was Edgar Allan Poe's Annabel Lee, in the poem of the same name.

Anabel, Anabella, Anabelle, Annabal, Annabelinda, Annabell, Annabella, Annabelle

Annamaria Com. form **Ann** and **Mary**. **Annemarie** is the most popular variation, especially since the 1950s. The reverse form, **Marianne**, is also frequently used. The popularity of the pairing may originate in Roman Catholic veneration of Saint Anne and Saint Mary, mother and daughter.

Annamarie, Annemarie, Annmaria

Annelise Com. form **Ann** and **Lise**.

Analeisa, Analiesa, Analiese, Analise, Anelisa, Anelise, Annaleisa, Annalie, Annaliesa, Annaliese,

Annalise, Annelie, Anneliese, Annelisa, Annelise, Annissa

Annemae Com. form. **Ann** and **May**.

Annamae, Annamay, Annemie

Annette Dim. **Ann**. Elaborated forms like **Annetta** may also be considered variations of **Agnes**. Actress Annette Bening.

Anet, Anett, Anetta, Annetta

Annis Gk. "Finished, completed." See also variants of **Ann**. Also easily confused by the ear with **Agnes**, a point prospective parents might keep in mind.

Anissa, Annes, Annice, Annys

Annora Lat. "Honor." A phonetic version of **Honora**.

Anora, Anorah, Honor, Honora, Onora, Nora, Norah

Annot Heb./Scot. "Light."

Anonna Lat. Name of the Roman goddess of the annual harvest. An appropriate name for an October or November baby.

Anona, Nona

Annunciata Lat. Allusion to the Annunciation, when the Virgin Mary learned she would be Jesus' mother. Sometimes given to a girl born in March, the logical month for such an announcement.

Anonciada, Annunziate, Anunciacion, Anunciata, Anunziata

Anselma (Fem. **Anselm** OG. "Godly helmet"). The short forms are much more common.

Selma, Zelma

Ansonia (Fem. **Anson**). Unclear origin and meaning. Possibly "Son of Ann," though "Son of the divine" seems more likely

Annesonia, Annsonia, Annsonya, Ansonya

Anthea Gk. "Flowerlike." Used by English 17th-century poets to symbolize spring, but occurring infrequently in real life.

Annthea, Anthe, Antheia, Antheya, Antia, Thia

Anthemia Gk. "In bloom." From the same Greek root as **Anthea**.

Antheemia, Anthemya, Anthymia

Antje Ger. Var. **Ann** (Heb. "Grace").

Antigone Gk. In myth, the daughter of Oedipus.

Antoinette (Fem. **Anthony**) Lat. "Beyond price, invaluable." Also a diminutive of **Ann**. Irresistibly associated with the ill-fated French Queen Marie Antoinette. Ballerina Antoinette Sibley.
Antonetta, Antonia, Antonie, Antonietta, Antonina, Antonine, Antwahnette, Antwanetta, Antwinett, Netta, Netti, Nettie, Netty, Toinette, Toni, Tonia, Tonie, Tony, Tonye

Antonia Lat. "Beyond price, invaluable." Also a diminutive of **Ann**. Willa Cather novel *My Antonía*; English writer Antonia Fraser.
Antoinette, Antonetta, Antonie, Antonietta, Antonija, Antoniya, Antonina, Antonya, Netta, Nettie, Netty, Toinette, Tonechka, Tonette, Toni, Tonia, Tonie, Tony, Tonya

Anwen Welsh. "Very fair."
Anwyn

Anwar Arab. "Rays of light." Most familiar as a man's name borne by Egyptian President Anwar Sadat.

Aphra Heb. "Dust." The English Puritans actually used both Dust and Ashes as first names in the 17th century. Playwright Aphra Behn.
Affera, Affery, Afra

Apolline (Fem. **Apollo**) Gk. The god of the sun in Greek mythology. Saint Apollonia was an early Christian martyr. Her teeth were knocked out as part of her martyrdom. In art she is often portrayed with a pair of tongs and an outsized molar.
Abbeline, Abbelina, Appoline, Appolinia, Apollinia, Apollonia, Apollyne, Appolonia

Aponi Native American. "Butterfly."
Aponee

April Lat. "Opening up." First used as a name in the 20th century, and occurs most often for a girl born in that month. Curiously, only the months April, **May,** and **June** are used regularly for names, with June the most popular. Pop musician Avril Lavigne.

Aipril, Aprilete, Aprill, Aprille, Averel, Averell, Averil, Averill, Averyl, Averyll, Averylle, Avril, Avrill

Aquilina (Fem. **Aquilino**) Sp. "Like an eagle."

Ara Arab. "Brings rain."

Ari, Aria, Arria

Arabella Lat. "Answered prayer." Unusual name that occurs most frequently in England.

Ara, Arabel, Arabela, Arabele, Arabelle, Arbela, Arbell, Arbella, Arbelle, Bel, Bella, Belle, Orabel, Orabella, Orabelle, Orbel, Orbella, Orbelle

Arachne Gk. In myth, a young maiden who challenged the goddess Athena to a weaving contest and was turned into a spider for her presumption.

Arakne, Archna

Araminta Com. form **Arabella** and **Aminta**. Invented by an 18th-century English playwright, and very unusual.

Arcadia Gk. Originally the place name of a region in Greece which eventually came to stand for the home of simple pastoral happiness.

Arcadie

Arcelia Sp. "Treasure chest."

Aricelia, Aricelly

Arda Heb. "Bronze."

Ardah, Ardath

Ardelle Lat. "Burning with enthusiasm." See **Arden**.

Arda, Ardeen, Ardelia, Ardelis, Ardella, Ardene, Ardia, Ardine, Ardis, Ardra

Arden Lat. "Burning with enthusiasm." The Forest of Arden in Shakespeare's *As You Like It* was a magically beautiful place. Most famous in modern times as the surnames of cosmetics queen Elizabeth Arden and actress Eve Arden.

Ardeen, Ardena, Ardenia, Ardin, Ardis

Arella Heb. "Messenger from God, angel."

Arela, Arelle

Arete Gk. "Woman of virtue." Singer Aretha Franklin has put an indelible stamp on her version of this name.

Areta, Aretha, Arethusa, Aretina, Aretta, Arette, Oreta, Oretha, Oretta, Orette, Retha

Argenta Lat. "Silvery." The country of Argentina is named for the silver its early Spanish settlers hoped to find there—but did not.

Argentia, Argentina

Aria It. "A melody." In the classical operatic form, arias are solos performed by the leading characters.

Ariadne Gk. The mythological daughter of Cretan King Minos, who gave Theseus a thread to guide him out of the mazelike prison known as the Labyrinth. Theseus married, then abandoned, her. Also the subject and title of a Richard Strauss opera.

Arene, Ariadna, Ariana, Ariane, Arianie, Arianna, Arianne, Aryana, Aryane, Aryanie, Aryanna, Aryanne

Ariana Welsh. "Like silver." This is also the Italian version of **Ariadne**. Political commentator Arianna Stassinopolous Huffington.

Ariane, Arianna

Ariel Heb. "Lioness of God." In Shakespeare's *The Tempest,* Ariel is a sprite who can disappear at will. The name has the connotation of something otherworldly, and though Shakespeare's Ariel is male, the name is used mostly for girls.

Aeriel, Aeriela, Aeriell, Ariela, Ariella, Arielle, Ariellel

Arista Gk. "The best."

Aristella, Aristelle

Arlene Derivation unclear. Possibly Dim.**Charles** (OE. "Man") or Fem. **Arlen** (related to Gael. "Pledge"). The name first appeared in the mid-19th century, and was popular by the 1930s. Actresses Arlene Francis, Arlene Dahl.

Arla, Arlana, Arlee, Arleen, Arlen, Arlena, Arleta, Arlette, Arleyne, Arlie, Arliene, Arlina, Arlinda, Arline, Arluene, Arly, Arlyn, Arlyne, Arlynn, Lena, Lene, Lina

Arlette Fr. From **Charles** (OE. "Man").

Arlot, Arletta

Arlise (Fem. **Arliss**) Heb. "Pledge."

Arlyse, Arlyss

Armida Lat. "Little armed one."

Armina (Fem. **Armand**) It. from OG. "Army man." **Her-**

man is another masculine form of the name that both **Armande** and **Armina** are based on.

Armantine, Armeena, Armine, Arminie, Armyne, Erminia, Erminie, Ermyne

Arnalda (Fem. **Arnold**) OG. "Eagle-strength."

Arnolda

Arnina (Fem. **Aaron**) Heb. "On high."

Arna, Arona, Arnice, Arnit

Artemisia Gk./Sp. "Perfect." Also a version of Artemas, a man's name that occurs in the Bible.

Artemesia

Arthuretta (Fem. **Arthur**) Celt. Possibly "Bear" or "Rock." A 19th-century version of the man's name that was very popular until about 1920. The women's forms never really caught on.

Artheia, Arthelia, Arthene, Arthurene, Arthurette, Arthurina, Arthurine, Artia, Artice, Artina, Artis, Artlette, Artrice

Asención Sp. Literally "ascension," marking Christ's ascension into heaven, which is commemorated 40 days after Easter.

Asunción

Ashanti Af. Area in West Africa where many American slaves came from. Used in modern American black families.

Ashanta, Ashantae, Ashantay, Ashante, Ashantee, Ashaunta, Ashaunte, Ashauntee, Ashaunti, Ashuntae, Shantee, Shanti, Shauntae, Shauntee

Ashira Heb. "Rich" or "I will sing."

Asheera, Ashirah

Ashley OE. Place name: "Ash-tree meadow." Originally a surname that migrated to first-name status, possibly helped along by Ashley Wilkes in Margaret Mitchell's *Gone With the Wind*. Though originally used for boys, it is now tremendously popular for girls, having been in the top ten female names for the last dozen years. Actresses Ashley Judd, Ashley Olsen.

Ashely, Ashla, Ashlay, Ashlan, Ashlee, Ashleigh, Ashlen, Ashli, Ashlie, Ashly

Asia Name of the continent. The feminine "-ia" ending lends itself to adaptation as a girl's name.
Aja, Asiah, Azha

Asima Arab. "Guardian."

Aspasia Gk. "Welcoming." The famous Athenian statesman Pericles had a mistress named Aspasia, who was noted for her beauty and wit. Surprisingly the name enjoyed mild popularity in the straitlaced 19th century. Almost unknown now.

Asphodel Gk. "Lily." Flower name, albeit an unusual one. The asphodel is a member of the lily family.
Asfodel, Asfodelle, Asphodelle

Asta Gk. "Like a star." Also short form of **Anastasia, Astrid, Augusta,** etc. The most famous Asta is probably the terrier owned by Nick and Nora Charles in the famous Thin Man movies of the 1930s.
Astera, Asteria, Asti, Astra, Estella, Esther, Estrella, Etoile, Hadassah, Hester, Stella

Astra Lat. "Starlike, of the stars." First appeared in the 1940s, though other "star names," like Estella, have been around longer.
Asta, Astera, Asteria, Asterina, Astraea, Astrea, Astri, Astria

Astraea Gk. The goddess of justice in classical mythology. When she retired from the earth, according to legend, she became the constellation Virgo. A clever name for a girl born under that sign.
Astraeia

Astrid ONorse. "Beautiful like a god." Unusual in English-speaking countries, but occurs in the royal families of Norway and Belgium. Brazilian singer Astrud Gilberto.
Assi, Astra, Astri, Astride, Astrud, Astryr, Atti

Asunción Sp. Marking the Virgin Mary's ascent into Heaven, which is commemorated on August 15.
Asención

Atalanta (Fem. **Atlas**) Gk. "Immovable." In Greek myth, Atalanta was an extremely athletic young maiden who refused to marry any man who couldn't beat her in a foot race. In the end, she was defeated by a ruse involving three golden apples.

Atlanta, Atlante

Atara Heb. "Diadem."

Atera, Ateret

Athalia Heb. "The Lord is exalted." In the Old Testament, Athalia was wife of the King of Judah. She murdered 42 princes to win the throne for herself, and after a reign of six years, was ultimately killed by a mob.

Atalee, Atalia, Atalie, Athalee, Athalie, Attalie

Athanasia (Fem. **Athanasius**) Gk. "Immortal."

Atanasia, Atanasya, Athenasia

Athena Gk. The goddess of wisdom in Greek myth. She was a virgin goddess who sprang fully armed from Zeus's head, and Homer, in the *Odyssey,* frequently refers to her as "gray-eyed Athena." A daunting name to live up to.

Athenais, Athene, Athie, Athina, Attie

Atifa Arab. "Empathy, affection."

Ateefa, Ateefah, Atifah

Aubrey OF. "Elf ruler." Originally a man's name that arrived in England with the Norman Conquest. For a girl, the ear will readily confuse it with **Audrey.**

Aubary, Aubery, Aubree, Aubreigh, Aubrette, Aubrie, Aubry, Aubury

Auda OF. "Prosperous."

Aud, Aude

Audrey OE. "Noble strength." Also the root, via Saint Audrey, for the word "tawdry." (In England, cheap and gaudy necklaces used to be sold at Saint Audrey's Fair.) Most popular in the 1920s and 1930s, now out of fashion. Actress Audrey Hepburn.

Audi, Audie, Audra, Audre, Audree, Audreen, Audria, Audrie, Audry, Audrye

Audris OG. "Lucky."

Audriss

Augusta (Fem. **Augustus**) Lat. "Worthy of respect." Imported to England by the German mother of George III. Though common enough in the 18th and 19th centuries, it is little used now. P.G. Wodehouse's foppish hero Bertie

Wooster had a terrifying Aunt Augusta, and she may be responsible for the slightly intimidating connotations of the name.

Auguste, Augustia, Augustina, Augustine, Augustyna, Augustyne, Austina, Austine, Austyna, Austyne, Gus, Gussie, Gusta, Tina

Aura Gk. "Soft breeze"; Lat. "Gold." Most familiar now, perhaps, in its psychic sense, meaning the atmosphere surrounding an individual.

Aure, Aurea, Auria, Oria

Aurelia Lat. "Gold." Originally a name used by Roman clans, it resurfaced as a first name in the 19th century, but is seldom seen now.

Aranka, Aural, Auralia, Aurea, Aurel, Aureliana, Aurélie, Aurelina, Aurita, Ora, Oralia, Orel, Orelee, Orelia

Auriel Lat. Dim. "Golden." Not to be confused with **Ariel**. A name used for slaves in the Roman Empire, possibly as a descriptive term. The 19th-century penchant for unusual names brought it back to occasional use, but it is rare now.

Aureola, Aureole, Auriol, Oriel, Oriole

Aurora Lat. "Dawn." Aurora was the Roman goddess of sunrise. Used by 19th-century poets such as Byron and Browning, but never common.

Aurore, Ora, Rora, Rory, Zora, Zorica

Austine (Fem. **Austin** or **Augustine**) Lat. "Worthy of respect."

Autumn Season name, only recently used as a first name.

Ava Lat. "Like a bird." May have originated as a form of **Eva**. Actress Ava Gardner.

Avis

Avalon Celt. "Island of apples." In Celtic myth, Avalon is an island paradise. In Arthurian legend, it is the island where King Arthur took refuge after his final defeat, and whence he will reappear.

Ave Lat. "Hail."

Avena Lat. "Field of oats."

Avichayil Heb. "Strong father." The Anglicized version is **Abigail**.

Abichail, Avigail, Avigayil

Aviva Heb. "Springlike, fresh, dewy."

Avivah, Avivi, Avivit, Viva, Auvit

Avril A French version of **April,** the month name. Also possibly a version of the name of a 7th-century saint, Everild. Pop musician Avril Lavigne.

Averel, Averell, Averil, Averill, Averyl

Axelle (Fem. **Axel**) OG. "Father of peace."

Axella

Aya Heb. "Bird."

Ayla

Ayanna Recently invented name that may be considered an elaboration of **Anna,** or of the typically feminine "-ana" ending. Probably popular because it sounds pretty.

Aiyana, Aiyanna, Ayana, Ayania, Ayannia, Iana, Ianna

Ayesha Per. "Small one."

Aza Arab. "Comfort."

Azalea Lat. "Dry earth." More familiar to us as the name of the shrub that produces brilliant blooms in the spring.

Azalia, Azaleia

Azelia Heb. "Aided by God."

Aziza Heb. "Mighty" or Arab. "Precious."

Azuba Meaning unknown. Biblical name, used occasionally from the 17th through 19th centuries.

Azubah, Zuba, Zubah

Azura OF. "Azure, sky blue." A good attribute name for a blue-eyed baby.

Azor, Azora, Azure, Azzura, Azzurra

B **Babe** Dim. **Barbara** (Gk. "Foreign"). Also short for "baby," as in "See ya, babe." Socialite Babe Paley.

Babette Fr. Dim. **Barbara** (Gk. "Foreign").

Baila Sp. "Dance."
Beyla, Byla

Bailey OE. "Law enforcer, bailiff." A surname that metamorphosed into a first name in the 19th century, though uncommon. Used more often for boys than for girls.
Bailee, Baily

Balbina Lat. "Little stutterer."
Balbine

Bambi It. "Child." Short for bambina. Of course, the most famous Bambi is Walt Disney's cartoon deer, who happens to be male.
Bambalina, Bambie, Bambina, Bamby

Baptista Lat. "One who baptizes."
Baptiste, Batista, Battista, Bautista

Bara Heb. "To select."
Barah, Bari, Barra, Barrie

Barbara Gk. "Foreign." The adjective was originally applied to anyone who did not speak Greek; it has the same root as "barbarian." The early Christian martyr Saint Barbara was imprisoned in a tower by her father; she is patroness of engineers and architects. The name had its greatest popularity in the 19th-20th centuries, peaking around 1925, when in the U.S. it was second only to **Mary**. Use since then has dropped off dramatically, and in one 1989 poll it didn't even make the top 100. Many people may associate this name with the popular doll Barbie. Actress Barbara Stanwyck; singer Barbra Streisand; writer Barbara Tuchman; First Lady Barbara Bush.
Bab, Baba, Babara, Babb, Babbett, Babbette, Babbie,

**Babe, Babett, Babette, Babita, Babs, Baibin, Bairbre,
Barb, Barbary, Barbe, Barbee, Barbette, Barbey,
Barbi, Barbie, Barbra, Barbro, Barby, Barra, Basha,
Basia, Baubie, Bauby, Beba, Berbera, Berberia,
Berberya, Berbya, Bobbe, Bobbee, Bobbi, Bobbie,
Bobby, Bonni, Bonnie, Bonny, Varvara, Varina**

Barrie A place name (Barry Islands, Wales) turned into a
surname turned into a first name used by both sexes. Possibly influenced by the fame of Sir James Barrie, author
of Peter Pan, since it first appeared as a given name during the height of his renown. It can also be considered a
more feminine version of **Barry**.

Bari, Barri

Bartha OG. "Shining, brilliant." Var. **Bertha**.

Barta

Basha Pol. "Stranger." From the same root as **Barbara**.

Basia, Basja

Basilia (Fem. **Basil**) Gk. "Royal, regal." Common in the
Middle Ages, but very unusual now.

**Baseele, Baseelia, Baseelle, Bazeele, Bazeelia,
Bazeelle, Basile, Basilie, Basille, Bazile, Bazille,
Bazilia**

Bathilda OG. "Woman warrior." Saint Bathild was a young
English girl who became queen of the Franks in the 7th
century. She was apparently canonized for opposing the
then-flourishing slave trade, and also for founding a con-
vent.

**Bathild, Bathilde, Batilda, Batilde, Berthilda,
Berthilde, Bertilda, Bertilde**

Bathsheba Heb. "Daughter of the oath." Biblical name:
Bathsheba was the mistress and later the wife of King
David. Surprisingly (given her history), the name was
used often by the Puritans. Now rare.

**Bathseva, Bathshua, Batsheba, Batsheva, Batshua,
Batya, Bethsabee, Sheba, Sheva**

Bathshira Arab. "Seventh girl-child." Unlikely to be appropriate in this age of small families.

Batya Heb. "God's daughter."

Bitya, Basha

Beata Lat. "Blessed." First word of the Latin version of the famous "beatitudes" section of the biblical Sermon on the Mount: "Blessed are the poor in spirit . . ." A popular name in Northern Europe.

Bea, Beate

Beatrice Lat. "Bringer of gladness." The original form, **Beatrix,** was often found in the Middle Ages in England, then forgotten until its Victorian revival as Beatrice. Its popularity was no doubt boosted by Queen Victoria's naming one of her daughters Beatrice. It fell out of fashion after the 1920s and is very rare today. Heroine of Dante's *Divine Comedy* and of Shakespeare's *Much Ado About Nothing*; entertainer Beatrice Lillie; writer Beatrix Potter; actress Bea Arthur; Queen Beatrix of the Netherlands.

Bea, Beah, Beatrisa, Beatrix, Bebe, Bee, Beea, Beeatrice, Beeatris, Beeatrisa, Beeatriss, Beeatrissa, Beeatrix, Beitris, Beitriss, Trix, Trixi, Trixie, Trixy

Bebba Heb. "God's pledge."

Becky Dim. **Rebecca** (Heb. "Noose"). Often used as an independent first name. Becky Sharp, heroine of William Thackeray's novel *Vanity Fair.*

Beda OE. "Battle maid."

Bedelia Ir. var. **Bridget** (Ir. Gael. "Strength, power") by way of **Biddy**. Actress Bonnie Bedelia.

Bedeelia, Bidelia, Delia

Bee Dim. **Beatrice** (Lat. "Bringer of gladness"). Also the name of an obscure 7th-century English saint. There is an English village called Saint Bees.

Behira Heb. "Shining, bright."

Belinda Unclear origin; possibly com. form **Belle** and **Linda**. Since the name first occurs in 18th-century English poet Alexander Pope's *The Rape of the Lock,* that derivation seems unlikely. It may be related to the Old German for "dragon." Has upper-class English connotations. Pop singer Belinda Carlisle.

Bel, Belle, Bellinda, Bellynda, Belynda, Linda, Lindie, Lindy

Belita Sp. "Little beauty."

Bellita

Bell Dim. **Isabel** (Heb. "Pledged to God"). Also, surname used as a first name.

Bella Lat. "Beautiful." Or Dim. **Isabella** (Heb. "Pledged to God"). Used as early as the Middle Ages, but not popular until the 18th century. Politician Bella Abzug.

Bell, Belle, Bellette

Bellanca It. "Blond."

Bianca, Blanca

Belle Fr. "Beautiful." Enjoyed a brief fad in the 1870s, but almost unheard-of since then. Author Belva Plain.

Belinda, Belisse, Bell, Bella, Bellina, Belva, Belvia, Billie, Billy

Bellona Lat. "Goddess of battle.

Ballona, Belona

Bena (Fem. **Ben**) Heb. "Wise."

Benedicta (Fem. **Benedict**) Lat. "Blessed." Extremely rare. **Benita** is the more common form.

Benedetta, Bénédicte, Benedictine, Benedikta, Benetta, Benita, Benoite, Bennie, Dixie

Benigna Lat. "Kindly, benevolent."

Benita Sp. Var. **Benedicta**. More common than Benedicta, but very unusual in English-speaking countries. Soprano Benita Valente; writer Benita Eisler.

Bendite, Benedetta, Benedicta, Benedikta, Benetta, Benni, Bennie, Benny, Benoite, Binnie, Binny

Bentley OE. "Meadow of ben (grass)." Place name become surname become first name, more common for boys. Irresistibly linked in most minds with the luxurious English cars.

Bentlea, Bentlee, Bentleigh, Bently

Bera Teut. "Bear."

Berdine OG. "Bright or glowing maiden."

Berengaria OE. "Maiden of the bear-spear." The wife of English King Richard the Lion-Heart.

Berit Scan. "Gorgeous, splendid, magnificent." Currently popular in Sweden.

Beret

Bernadette (Fem. **Bernard**) Fr. "Bear/courageous." Made famous by Saint Bernadette of Lourdes, a miller's daughter who in 1858 repeatedly saw visions of the Virgin Mary. By the time she was canonized in 1933, Lourdes had become a world-famous destination for pilgrims. The name was popular among Catholic families especially after the 1943 movie *Song of Bernadette,* but is now unusual in English-speaking countries. Actress Bernadette Peters.

Benadette, Bennie, Benny, Berna, Bernadeena, Bernadene, Bernadett, Bernadetta, Bernadina, Bernadine, Bernadyna, Bernardina, Bernardine, Bernee, Berneta, Bernetta, Bernette, Bernie, Bernina, Bernita, Berny

Bernice Gk. "She who brings victory." From the same root as **Veronica**. The name appears in the New Testament and first occurred in Britain in the 16th century, but its only real popularity came at the end of the 19th century. Little used today.

Barri, Barrie, Barry, Beranice, Beraniece, Beranyce, Bereniece, Berenice, Berenyce, Berneece, Bernelle, Bernetta, Bernette, Bernee, Berni, Bernie, Berniece, Berny, Bernyce, Berri, Berrie, Berry, Bunni, Bunnie, Bunny, Nixie, Veronica, Veronika, Veronike, Veronique

Berry Nature name. Also diminutive of **Bernice, Bernadette,** etc. Flower names enjoyed a vogue, especially in Britain, in the 1880s. Berry is also used for men, in that case more often as a transferred surname or a diminutive for **Bernard**. Photographer Berry Berenson.

Berree, Berrie

Bertha OG. "Bright." Also related to the name of a Teutonic goddess. Very popular in the late 19th century, but almost unheard of since 1920. This disuse may be explained by the fact that a German cannon used in World War I was nicknamed "Big Bertha" after Bertha Krupp, daughter of the family that manufactured the weapon. In Spain, **Berta** is currently fashionable.

Berrta, Berrte, Berrti, Berrtina, Berrty, Berta, Berte, Berthe, Berti, Bertie, Bertina, Bertine, Bertuska, Berty, Bird, Birdie, Birdy, Birta, Birtha

Bertilde Bertilde OG. "Bright warrior maiden."

Bertina Ger. "Bright, shining." Dim. **Bertha**.

Bertrade OE. "Bright adviser."

Berura Heb. "Pure."

Beruria Heb. "God-selected."

Beryl Gk. "Pale green gemstone." The beryl was considered a token of good luck. The name first appeared with the fashion for jewel names in the late 19th century. Its popularity peaked in the 1920s, and it is now rare. Author Beryl Markham.

Berri, Berrie, Berry, Beryle, Berylla, Beryn

Beta Gk. Second letter of the Greek alphabet. Also a middle-European variant of **Beth**.

Beth Heb. "House." Dim. **Elizabeth** (Heb. "pledged to God"), **Bethany**. In Louisa May Alcott's *Little Women*, Beth is the sweet, gentle sister who dies young.

Bethany Biblical: the name of the village near Jerusalem where Lazarus lived with his sisters Mary and Martha. In some cases a variant on the combined form **Beth-Ann**.

Bethanee, Bethaney, Bethanie, Bethanne, Bethannie, Bethanny, Betheney, Betheny

Bethell Heb. "House of God." Another biblical place name: the spot where Abraham built an altar. Unusual as a first name.

Bethel, Bethell, Bethelle, Bethuel, Bethuna, Bethune

Bethesda Heb. "House of mercy." Bethesda pool in Jerusalem was supposed to have healing powers after being stirred by an angel.

Bethia Heb. "Daughter of Jehovah." Popular in the eras, such as the 17th century, when Old Testament names have been intensively used.

Betia, Bithia

Bettina Dim. **Elizabeth** (Heb. "Pledged to God"). Spanish or Italian in origin, and briefly popular in the sixties. One of photographer William Wegman's canine models was named Battina.

Battina, Betiana, Betina, Bettine

Betty Dim. **Elizabeth** (Heb. "Pledged to God"). A nickname with great popularity in its own right. It first became common in the 18th century, and after a spell of disuse, by the 1920s was one of the top names in every English-speaking country. Now it appears most often in combination with other names: Betty Lou, Betty Ann, etc. Actresses Betty Grable, Betty Buckley, Bette Davis; singer Bette Midler; First Lady Betty Ford.

Bett, Betta, Bette, Betti, Bettie, Bettina, Bettine

Beulah Heb. "Married." Also used to refer to Israel, and in John Bunyan's *The Pilgrim's Progress,* Beulah is the promised land. It first became a girl's name in the late 16th century. References to "Beulah land" appear in American spirituals.

Beula, Bewlah, Byulah

Beverly OE. Place name: "Beaver-stream." Originally an English place name and a surname, then used for both sexes as a first name. Probably still most famous as a place name, referring to Beverly Hills. The English spelling is usually **Beverley.** Singer Beverly Sills.

Bev, Beverle, Beverlee, Beverley, Beverlie, Beverlye, Bevlyn, Bevverlie, Bevverly, Bevvy, Buffy, Verlee, Verlie, Verly, Verlye

Bevinn Ir. Gael. "Singer." More commonly a man's name, although Ireland's famous 11th-century king Brian Boru had a daughter with the name.

Bevan

Bianca It. "White." The meek younger daughter in Shakespeare's *The Taming of the Shrew,* and subject of a song in the spin-off musical *Kiss Me, Kate.* The most famous Bianca in recent times is former Rolling Stone wife Bianca Jagger.

Biancha, Bianka, Blanca, Blancha

Bibi Arab. "Lady." Actress Bebe Neuwirth.

Bebe, Beebee

Bibiana Sp. Var. **Vivian** (Lat. "Alive").

Bibiane, Bibianna

Bienvenida Sp. "Welcome."

Billie OE. Dim. **Wilhelmina** (OG. "Will-helmet"). Feminine use of what is generally considered a man's name; more popular in the South, though uncommon now.

Singer Billie Holliday; actress Billie Burke; tennis player Billie Jean King.

Billa, Billee, Billi, Billina, Billy, Willa

Bina Heb. "Knowledge, perception." Also dim. **Albina, Sabina,** etc.

Binah, Buna

Bird Eng. Unusual nature name.

Birdey, Birdie, Byrd, Byrdie

Birgit Nor. "Splendid." Var. **Bridget.**

Birget, Birgetta, Birgitt, Birgitta, Birgitte, Byrget, Byrgitt

Bithron Heb. "Daughter of song."

Blaine Ir. Gael. "Slender." Surname now used as a first name, more usually for boys. Cropped up as a first name in the 1930s. Socialite Blaine Trump.

Blane, Blayne

Blair Scot. Gael. Place name referring to a plain or flat area. Surname now used as a first name, again more common for boys. Like many similarly transferred names, Blair was used for girls in greater numbers in the 1980s and '90s. Actress Blair Brown.

Blaire, Blayre

Blaise Lat. "One who stutters." Used for both sexes, though more common for men. The alternate spelling of **Blaze** probably refers to fire instead.

Blaize, Blase, Blasia, Blaze

Blake OE. Paradoxically, could mean either "pale-skinned" or "dark." Surname used as a first name for either sex, but more common for boys.

Blakelee, Blakeley, Blakely, Blakenee, Blakeney, Blakeny

Blanche Fr. "White, pale." Very popular in America at the end of the 19th century, but unusual now.

Bellanca, Bianca, Blanca, Blanch, Blanka, Blinny, Branca

Blanchefleur Fr. "White flower."

Blanda Lat. "Smooth, seductive." Saint Blandina was a 2nd-century martyr, a slave girl who was gored to death by a bull.

Blandina, Blandine
Blasia Var. **Blaise** (Lat. "One who stutters").
Blaise, Blaisia, Blasya, Blaysia
Blessing OE. "Consecration."
Blimah Heb. "Blossom."
Blimah, Blime
Bliss OE. "Intense happiness."
Blisse, Blyss
Blodwen Welsh. "White flower." Literal translation into Welsh of **Blanchefleur**. Little used outside Wales.
Blodwyn, Blodwynne
Blondelle Fr. "Little pale one."
Blondell, Blondie, Blondy
Blossom OE. "Flowerlike." Generic flower name, used mostly at the turn of the 20th century.
Bluebell Flower name popular in the 19th century, though when it became the typical name for a cow (like Rover for a dog), it dropped out of human use.
Blythe OE. "Happy, carefree." Made famous by the opening lines of Shelley's poem "To a Skylark" ("Hail to thee, blithe spirit!") and Noel Coward's play *Blithe Spirit*. Actress Blythe Danner.
Blithe
Bo Chinese. "Precious." More often used as a masculine diminutive for names like **Robert**. Actress Bo Derek.
Beau
Boadicea Name of a heroic queen of early Britain, who led a massive army against Roman invaders. Has rather intimidating connotations.
Bobbie Dim. **Roberta** (OE. "Bright renown"). Like **Billie,** a feminine version of a man's nickname, often used in combination with a monosyllabic second name, and more common in the South. Also derives from **Barbara** (Gk. "Stranger"). Author Bobbie Ann Mason.
Bogdana Pol. "Gift from God."
Bogna, Bohdana
Bolade Nig. "The coming of honor."
Bolanile Nig. "This house's riches."
Bonfilia It. "Good daughter."

Bonita Sp. "Pretty." Popular in the early 1940s, but unusual now.

Bo, Bonie, Bonnie, Bonny, Nita

Bonnie Scot. "Good, fair of face." The Scots adopted the French word *bonne,* meaning "good." Its most common use as an adjective is the fond nickname "Bonnie Prince Charlie." The old nursery rhyme claims that "the child who is born on the Sabbath Day/Is bonny and blithe and good and gay," which makes this an appropriate name for a Sunday's child. Actress Bonnie Hunt; Olympic speed-skater Bonnie Blair.

Bonne, Bonnebell, Bonnee, Bonni, Bonnibel,
Bonnibell, Bonnibelle, Bonny, Bunni, Bunnie, Bunny

Borbala Hung. "Foreigner." Var. **Barbara** (Gk. "Stranger").

Bora, Boriska, Borka, Borsala, Borsca

Bradley OE. Place name: "Broad field." Surname now used as a first name for either sex, though more common for boys. Little seen outside America.

Bradlea, Bradlee, Bradleigh, Bradly

Brandy Name of a liquor. In the early 1980s, one of the most popular names for American girls, reaching the top ten in some surveys. Like most trendy names, it has lost favor rather rapidly. Pop singer Brandy.

Brandais, Brande, Brandea, Brandee, Brandi,
Brandice, Brandie, Brandye, Branndais, Brannde,
Branndea, Branndi, Branndie

Brenda (Fem. **Brendan**) OE. "Burning." One source translates the Irish as "stinking hair," though the origin may also be a Norse word for "sword." Brenda was originally a Scottish name and was particularly fashionable in the 1940s. Actress Brenda Vaccaro; comic strip heroine Brenda Starr.

Bren, Brenn, Brennda, Brenndah

Brenna Ir. Gael. "Raven; black-haired." Also dim. **Brendan.**

Bren, Brenn, Brenne, Brennah, Brinna, Brynna,
Brynne

Brett Lat. "From Britain." Surname transferred to first name. Still more common for boys.

Brette, Britt

Brianna (Fem. **Brian**) Ir. Gael. Meaning obscure, possibly "Strong" or "Hill."

Brana, Breana, Breanne, Breeann, Breeanna, Breeanne, Breena, Bria, Briana, Brianne, Brina, Briney, Brinn, Brinna, Briny, Bryana, Bryann, Bryanna, Bryanne, Bryn, Bryna, Brynne

Brice Obscure origin, possibly OE. "Noble" or Celt. "Swift." Originally a surname.

Bryce

Bridget Ir. Gael. "Strength, power." May also derive from the name of a goddess of ancient Ireland. Very popular name in Ireland from the 18th century to the 1950s, so much so that in the late 19th century in the U.S. the stock figure of the Irish housemaid (in plays, cartoons, etc.) was frequently called Bridget. In France, **Brigitte** is currently popular. Saint Brigid of Kildare, patroness of Ireland; opera star Birgit Nilsson; actresses Brigitte Bardot, Brigitte Nielsen, Bridget Fonda; model Bridget Hall.

Beret, Berett, Berget, Bergett, Bergette, Biddie, Biddy, Birget, Birgett, Birgit, Birgitt, Birgitta, Birgitte, Birkita, Birkitta, Birkitte, Birte, Bitta, Breeda, Bride, Bridee, Bridey, Bridgett, Bridgette, Bridgit, Bridgitt, Bridgitta, Bridgitte, Bridie, Bridy, Brietta, Briget, Brigett, Brighid, Brigid, Brigida, Brigidine, Brigit, Brigitt, Brigitta, Brigitte, Brijet, Brijit, Brijitte, Brita, Britt, Britta, Britte, Brydie, Brydget, Brydgit, Brydgitta, Brydgitte, Brydjette, Brydjitt, Bryget, Brygette, Brygid, Brygit, Brygitte, Bryjet, Bryjit

Brie Fr. Place name for a region in France most famous for the production of its cheese.

Bree, Briette

Brier Fr. "Heather." Unusual botanical name. Though the personal name derives from the French term for heather, the word in English usually describes a wild rose with small, prickly thorns. In some versions of *Sleeping Beauty,* Prince Charming has to cut through a hedge of briers to reach the princess.

Briar

Brina (Fem. **Brian**) Slavic. "Defender."
Brinn, Bryn, Bryna, Brynn, Brynna, Brynne
Brit Celt. "Spotted, freckled." Also a diminutive of **Brittany.**
Britt
Britannia Lat. "Britain." Personification of Britain or the British Empire. She first appeared on a coin in the 2nd century A.D. For zealous Anglophiles.
Brites Port. "Power."
Brittany Lat. "From England." According to records kept by the U.S. government, this was the sixth most popular girl's name in America in the 1990s, though it has been sliding down the lists since 1990. Singer Britney Spears; actress Brittany Murphy.
Brett, Brit, Briteny, Britiney, Britney, Britni, Britny, Britt, Britta, Brittan, Brittaney, Brittani, Britteny, Brittin, Brittiny, Brittnee, Brittney, Brittni, Brittny, Britton
Bronwyn Welsh. "Fair breast." Use of Welsh-language names such as Bronwyn, **Blodwyn,** and the like may be related to periodic surges of separatist or nationalistic feeling in Wales.
Bronnie, Bronny, Bronwen, Bronya
Brooke OE. Place name: "Small stream." Also a surname, and originally more common for boys. Now clearly a feminine name. Actress Brooke Adams; philanthropist Brooke Astor.
Brook, Brookie, Brooks, Brooky
Brucie (Fem. **Bruce**) OF. "Thicket of brushwood." The man's name was first common in Scotland, after a 14th-century king. The feminine variant is little used.
Brucina, Brucine
Bruna (Fem. **Bruno**) It. "Brown-skinned, brown-haired."
Brunella OF. "Little one with brown hair."
Brunelle, Brunetta, Brunette
Brunhilda OG. "Armor-wearing fighting maid." Heroine of the Siegfried legend popularized in the Ring cycle of operas by Richard Wagner. Brunhilda is one of the Valkyrie, maidens who ride into battle.

**Brinhild, Brinhilda, Brinhilde, Brunhild, Brunhilde,
Brunnhilda, Brunnhilde, Brynhild, Brynhilda,
Brynhilde, Brynnhild, Brynnhilda, Brynnhilde, Hilda,
Hilde, Hildi, Hildie, Hildy**

Bryony Botanical name. Bryony is a vine native to Europe
that has large leaves and small flowers.
Bryonie, Briony

Bryn Welsh. "Mount." Another place name converted to a
Christian name in the 20th century.
Brinna, Brynn, Brynna, Brynne

Buena Sp. "Good, excellent."

Bunny Nickname deriving from a number of "B" names
such as **Barbara** or **Bernice**. Has come to be a child's
name for a rabbit, of course. Likely to be associated with
the famous Playboy Bunnies, the now defunct mid-20th-
century emblem of a slightly licentious good time.
Bunnee, Bunni, Bunnie

C

Cadence Lat. "With rhythm."
**Cadena, Cadenza, Kadena, Kadence,
Kadenza**

Cady OE. Last name of uncertain meaning. It
may have been successfully adopted as a girl's first name
because of its resemblance to other popular girls' names
like **Katie**. Women's rights pioneer Elizabeth Cady Stanton.
**Cade, Cadee, Cadey, Cadi, Cadie, Cadye, Caidie,
Kade, Kadee, Kadi, Kadie, Kady, Kadye**

Cai Viet. "Feminine."

Caitlin Ir. See **Catherine**. Along with **Megan,** Caitlin has
been very popular recently among families with no Irish
ties whatsoever, though it is a top-ten name in Ireland.

Caitilin, Caitlan, Caitlann, Caitlinn, Caitlyn, Caitlynn, Catelan, Catelinn, Catelynn, Catlin, Catlinn, Cayelin, Caylin, Kaitlan, Kaitlann, Kaitlin, Kaitlinn, Kaitlyn, Kaitlynn, Katelan, Katelin, Katelynn, Kayelin, Kayelyn

Cala "Castle, fortress."

Calandra Gk. "Lark."
Cal, Calandre, Calandria, Calendre, Callee, Calley, Calli, Callie, Cally, Kalandra

Calantha Gk. "Lovely flower."
Cal, Calanthe, Callee, Calley, Calli, Callie, Cally, Kalantha

Caledonia Lat. "From Scotland." Place name adapted to first name, probably because of its typically feminine "-ia" ending. The Caledonian Canal runs through Northern Scotland, while New Caledonia consists of a group of tiny islands in the South Pacific.

Calida Sp. "Heated, with warmth."
Calla, Calli, Callida

Calla Gk. "Beautiful." Also the name of a flower, though the calla lily, with its smooth, sculptured lines, was not fashionable at the same time as the general vogue for flower names.

Callidora Gk. "Gift of beauty."

Calligenia Gk. "Daughter of beauty." A subtle compliment to the baby's mother.

Calliope Gk. Muse of epic poetry. See **Clio**. Also the name of a musical instrument typically seen at circuses and carnivals.
Callia, Callyope, Kalliope

Callista Gk. "Most beautiful." Actress Callista Flockhart.
Cala, Calesta, Calista, Calla, Callesta, Calli, Callie, Cally, Callysta, Calysta, Kala, Kalesta, Kalista, Kalla, Kallesta, Kalli, Kallie, Kallista, Kally, Kallysta

Callula Lat. "Small beauty."

Caltha Lat. "Golden flower."

Calvina (Fem. **Calvin**) Lat. "Hairless." Very unusual.
Calvine

Calypso Gk. "She who hides." In Greek myth the nymph

Calypso held Odysseus captive on an island for seven years. The name is also applied to the lilting music of the West Indies.
Calipso, Callypso, Kallypso

Camellia Flower name first used in the 1930s, when the rather exotic blooms were quite fashionable. Its root is actually distinct from the more common **Camille**.
Camellia, Cammelia, Kamelia

Cameo It. from Middle French. "Skin." A stone or shell (frequently pinkish), carved with a picture, often a tiny portrait. Cameos have been very popular as jewelry at various periods, most recently the Victorian era.
Cammeo

Cameron Scot. Gael. "Crooked nose." Clan name derived from the facial feature. Little used as a first name, even for boys, until the middle of this century. Actresses Cameron Diaz, Camryn Manheim.
Camaran, Camren, Camron, Camryn, Kameren, Kameron, Kamryn, Kamrynn, Kamrynne

Camille Lat. Meaning unclear, though some sources trace it to the young girls who assisted at pagan religious ceremonies. The heroine of Alexandre Dumas's famous play *Camille* was actually named Marguerite (see **Camellia**, above). The name has been used consistently since the 19th century, usually in the form **Camilla**. Camille has been more common in the U.S., is a top-ten name in France. Friend of royalty Camilla Parker-Bowles.
Cam, Cama, Camala, Cami, Camila, Camile, Camilla, Cammi, Cammie, Cammilla, Cammille, Cammy, Cammylle, Camyla, Camylla, Camylle, Kamila, Kamilka, Kamilla, Kamille, Kamyla, Milla, Mille, Millee, Milli, Millie, Milly

Candace Possibly Lat. "Brilliantly white." Historically the name was the ancient title of the queens of Ethiopia before the 4th century. Not much used until the mid-20th century. Actress Candice Bergen; author Candace Bushnell.
Candaice, Candase, Candayce, Candee, Candi, Candie, Candis, Candiss, Candy, Candyce, Dace,

Dacee, Dacey, Dacie, Dacy, Kandace, Kandice, Kandiss, Kandy

Candida Lat. "White." Popular in the early Christian era, then very rare until this century, when it has been used occasionally. Journalist Candida Crewe.

Candi, Candide, Candie, Candy

Candra Lat. "Glowing."

Cantara Arab. "Little bridge."

Caprice It. "Ruled by whim."

Capreece, Capricia, Caprise

Capucine Fr. "Cowl." French form of an Italian word for a cloak with a deep collar, characteristic of a certain order of Franciscan monks. A French actress who worked in Hollywood in the 1960s gave the name some exposure in the U.S., but it is rare.

Cara Lat. "Darling." Began to be fashionable from the 1970s onward.

Caralie, Caretta, Carina, Carine, Carrie, Carry, Kara, Karina, Karine, Karrie, Karry

Carey Welsh. Place name: "Near the castle." A name used for both men and women. In this form it is a transferred surname, but, especially for women, it may be considered a diminutive of **Caroline**. Actress Carey Lowell.

Carrey, Cary

Carina It. "Dear little one." Dim. **Cara**. Often used in Italy in the exclamation *"Che carina!"* meaning, "How darling!" or even "How cute!"

Careena, Caren, Carena, Carin, Carine, Kareena, Karena, Karina, Karine

Carinthia Place name: an idyllic region of southern Austria.

Carissa Gk. "Grace." See Charis. Also possibly another variation of Cara.

Caresa, Caressa, Carisa, Charissa, Karisa, Karissa, Kharissa

Carita Lat. "Beloved." Also possibly derived from the Latin word for charity, *caritas*. Occasionally used in the last hundred years.

Caritta, Karita

Carla (Fem. **Carl**) Dim. **Caroline** (OG. "Man"). A European-sounding version of the many names that derive from **Charles**.

Carlah, Carlana, Carlette, Carlia, Carlla, Karla, Karlla

Carlie (Fem. **Charles**) Dim. **Caroline, Charlotte** (OG. "Man"). The form **Carleen** (or **Carlene**) was primarily a product of the 1960s; this shorter version is now more popular. Singer Carly Simon.

Carlee, Carleen, Carleigh, Carlene, Carley, Carli, Carline, Carlita, Carly, Carlye, Carlyne, Carlyta, Karlee, Karlene, Karli, Karlie, Karline, Karlita, Karly, Karlyta

Carlin Gael. "Little champion."

Carling

Carmel Heb. "Garden." Biblical place name: Mount Carmel is in Israel, and is often referred to as a kind of paradise. The name has been used by Catholic families for some hundred years, though the form **Carmen** is much more common. Editor Carmel Snow.

Carma, Carman, Carmania, Carmanya, Carmela, Carmeli, Carmelina, Carmelit, Carmelita, Carmia, Carmie, Carmiela, Carmina, Carmine, Carmit, Carmiya, Carmy, Karmel, Karmela, Karmelit, Karmen, Lina, Lita, Melina, Melita, Mina

Carmen Lat. "Song." A derivation of **Carmel**. One of the titles of the Virgin Mary is Santa Maria del Carmen (meaning Saint Mary of Mount Carmel), and this form of the name honors her. The most famous Carmen, of course, is the ill-fated heroine of Bizet's opera. Dancer Carmen Miranda; model Carmen Kass.

Carma, Carmelia, Carmelina, Carmelita, Carmencita, Carmia, Carmie, Carmina, Carmine, Carmita, Carmyna, Carmyta, Charmaine, Karmen, Karmia, Karmina, Karmita, Lita, Mina

Carna Lat. "Horn." See **Cornelia**.

Carniela, Carniella, Carnyella, Karniela, Karniella, Karnyella

Carnation Lat. "Becoming flesh." Unusual flower name.

Carol (Fem. **Carl, Charles**) OG. "Man." Originally a short

form of **Caroline,** not an adoption of "Christmas carol." It
first appeared about a hundred years ago, and by mid-20th
century was enormously popular, possibly influenced by
the career of actress Carole Lombard. It is sometimes
paired with a monosyllabic second name, most commonly
Ann, as in Carol-Ann. The popularity of the name peaked
in the mid-sixties, and it is now out of style. Actresses
Carol Burnett, Carol Channing; skater Carol Heiss; playwright Caryl Churchill.

**Carel, Carey, Cari, Carla, Carleen, Carlene, Carley,
Carlin, Carlina, Carline, Carlita, Carlota, Carlotta,
Carly, Carlyn, Carlynn, Carlynne, Caro, Carola,
Carole, Carolena, Carolin, Carolina, Carolinda,
Caroline, Caroll, Caroly, Carolyn, Carolynn,
Carolynne, Carri, Carrie, Carroll, Carrolyn, Carry,
Cary, Caryl, Caryll, Charla, Charleen, Charlena,
Charlene, Charlotta, Charmain, Charmaine,
Charmian, Charmion, Charyl, Cheryl, Cherlyn, Ina,
Karel, Kari, Karla, Karleen, Karli, Karlie, Karlina,
Karlinka, Karlote, Karlotta, Karole, Karolina, Karyl,
Karyll, Karryl, Karryll, Kerril, Kerryl, Keryl, Lola,
Loleta, olita, Lotta, Lotte, Lotti, Lottie, Sharleen,
Sharlene, Sharline, Sharmain, Sharmian**

Caroline (Fem. dim. **Carl, Charles**) OG. "Man." A rather
stately diminutive with royal connotations. The name was
brought to England by George II's queen and was popular
until the end of the 19th century. It is now enjoying a revival. Princess Caroline of Monaco; fashion designers
Carolina Herrera, Carolyne Roehm; First Daughter Caroline Kennedy Schlossberg; comedian Caroline Rhea.

**Caraleen, Caraleena, Caraline, Caralyn, Caralyne,
Caralynn, Carla, Carleen, Carleena, Carlen, Carlene,
Carley, Carlin, Carlina, Carlita, Carlota, Carlotta,
Carly, Carlyn, Carlyna, Carlyne, Carlynn, Carlynne,
Carol, Carola, Carole, Carolin, Carolina, Carolyne,
Carolynn, Carolynne, Carri, Carrie, Caroll, Carollyn,
Cary, Charla, Charleen, Charleena, Charlena,
Charlene, Charline, Charlyne, Ina, Karaleen,
Karaleena, Karalina, Karaline, Karalyn, Karalynna,**

Karalynne, Karla, Karleen, Karlen, Karlena, Karlene,
Karli, Karlie, Karlina, Karlinka, Karolina, Karoline,
Karolinka, Karolyn, Karolyna, Karolyne, Karolynn,
Karolynne, Leena, Lina, Sharla, Sharleen, Sharlena,
Sharlene, Sharline, Sharlyne

Carys Welsh. "Love." A Welsh name dating from the 1960s.

Casey Ir. Gael. "Watchful." Made famous by the song about
the engineer of the Cannon Ball Express, Casey Jones.
Used for both boys and girls. Can be considered a diminutive of **Acacia**.

Cacey, Cacie, Caisee, Caisey, Caisi, Caisie, Casee,
Casi, Casie, Caycee, Caycey, Cayci, Caycie, Caysee,
Caysey, Caysi, Caysie, Kacey, Kacie, Kacy, Kacyee,
Kasey, Kaycee, Kaycey, Kayci, Kaycie, Kaysee,
Kaysey, Kaysi, Kaysie, Kaysy, Kaysyee

Casilda Lat. "Dwelling place." Also Spanish from German,
"Warlike, a fighter."

Cassilda

Cassandra Gk. Perhaps a version of **Alexander**. In Greek
myth, she was the daughter of King Priam of Troy. Apollo
gave her the gift of foresight but, because she spurned his
advances, decreed that her prophecies would never be believed. In vain she warned the besieged Trojans against
accepting the gift of a gigantic wooden horse presented by
their Greek enemy; it was full of Greek soldiers, who took
the city captive. The name now indicates someone who is
always prophesying doom and gloom.

Casandera, Casandra, Cass, Cassandre, Cassandry,
Cassaundra, Cassi, Cassie, Cassondra, Cassy,
Kasandera, Kassandra, Kassi, Kassie, Kassy, Sande,
Sandee, Sandera, Sandi, Sandie, Sandy, Saundra,
Sohndra, Sondra, Zandra

Cassia Gk. "Cinnamon."

Cassidy Ir. "Clever." Surname transferred to male first
name transferred to girl's name.

Cassady, Cassidey, Kassadey, Kassidy, Kassodey

Catherine Gk. "Pure." One of the oldest recorded names,
with roots in Greek antiquity. Almost every Western country has its own form of the name, and phonetic variations

are endless. It has been borne by such illustrious women as Saint Catherine of Alexandria, the early martyr who was tortured on a spiked wheel; Empress Catherine the Great of Russia; and three of Henry VIII's six wives. It is currently very popular in England and France, and was one of the top ten American girls' names in the 1980s. It is still a favorite; Social Security records indicate that if you grouped together the most popular spellings of the name (Katherine, Kathryn, and Catherine) as one name, it would have ranked as the eighth most popular girl's name of the 1990s. Actresses Catherine Oxenberg, Catherine Deneuve, Katharine Hepburn, Catherine Zeta-Jones, Cate Blanchett; Australian track star Cathy Freeman.

Cait, Caitey, Caitie, Caitlin, Caitlinn, Caitrin, Caitrine, Caitrinn, Caitriona, Caitrionagh, Caity, Caren, Cari, Carin, Caron, Caronne, Carren, Carri, Carrin, Carron, Caryn, Carynn, Cass, Cassey, Cassi, Cassie, Cassy, Cat, Cataleen, Cataleena, Catalin, Catalina, Cataline, Catarina, Catarine, Cate, Cateline, Caterina, Catey, Catha, Cathaleen, Cathaline, Catharin, Catharina, Catharine, Catharyna, Catharyne, Cathe, Cathee, Cathelin, Cathelina, Cathelle, Catherin, Catherina, Catherinn, Catheryn, Cathi, Cathie, Cathirin, Cathiryn, Cathleen, Cathlene, Cathline, Cathlyne, Cathrine, Cathrinn, Cathryn, Cathrynn, Cathy, Cathye, Cathyleen, Cati, Catia, Catie, Catina, Catlaina, Catreena, Catrin, Catrina, Catrine, Catriona, Catrionagh, Catryna, Caty, Cay, Caye, Cazzy, Ekaterina, Kait, Kaitey, Kaitie, Kaitlin, Kaitlinne, Kaitrin, Kaitrine, Kaitrinna, Kaitriona, Kaitrionagh, Kaity, Karen, Karena, Kari, Karin, Karon, Karri, Karrin, Karyn, Karynn, Kasia, Kasienka, Kasja, Kaska, Kass, Kassey, Kassia, Kassy, Kasya, Kat, Kata, Kataleen, Katalin, Katalina, Katarina, Katchen, Kate, Katee, Katell, Katelle, Katenka, Katerina, Katerinka, Katey, Katinka, Katha, Katharine, Katharyn, Katharyne, Kathee, Kathelina, Katheline, Katherin, Katherina, Katherine, Katheryn, Katherynn, Kathi, Kathie, Kathileen, Kathiryn, Kathleen,

Kathlene, Kathleyn, Kathline, Kathyleen, Kathrine, Kathrinna, Kathryn, Kathryne, Kathy, Kathyrine, Kati, Katica, Katie, Katina, Katka, Katla, Katlaina, Katleen, Katoushka, Katrena, Katrine, Katrina, Katriona, Katrionagh, Katryna, Katushka, Katy, Katya, Kay, Kaye, Kit, Kittee, Kittie, Kitty, Trina, Trine, Trinette, Yekaterin, Yekaterina

Cathleen Ir. Var. **Catherine** (Gk. "Pure").

Cecilia (Fem. **Cecil**) Lat. "Blind one." From a Roman clan name. Saint Cecilia is the patroness of music. The name was used in Roman times, then resurfaced in the Victorian era, possibly given a boost by the fame of industrialist (and founder of Rhodesia) Cecil Rhodes. The form **Cecily** was briefly popular in the 1920s, but neither name has been used much since. Actress Cicely Tyson; soprano Cecilia Bartoli.

Ceceley, Cecely, Cecil, Cecile, Ceciley, Ceciliane, Cecilija, Cecilla, Cecily, Cecilyann, Cecyl, Cecyle, Cecylia, Ceil, Cela, Cele, Celia, Celie, Celli, Cellie, Cesia, Cesya, Cicely, Cicily, Cile, Cilka, Cilia, Cilla, Cilly, Cissie, Kikelia, Kikylia, Sacilia, Sasilia, Sasilie, Seelia, Seelie, Seely, Sesilia, Sessaley, Sesseelya, Sessile, Sessilly, Sessily, Sheila, Sile, Sileas, Sisely, Siselya, Siseel, Sisile, Sisiliya, Sissela, Sissie, Sissy

Celandine Gk. Botanical name: a yellow-blossomed wild-flower.

Celadonia, Celida, Cellandine, Selodonia, Zeledonia

Celena Gk. Goddess of the moon, later identified with Artemis. A version of the more common **Selina,** although neither name is frequently used.

Cela, Celeena, Celina, Celinka, Cesia, Cesya, Saleena, Salena, Salina, Selena, Selina

Celeste Lat. "Heavenly." Unusual in any of its forms, and probably most familiar through the fame of actress Celeste Holm. Parents may associate the name with Queen Celeste, wife of Jean and Laurent de Brunhoff's children's book character Babar, the Elephant. Casting agent Celestia Fox.

Cela, Celesta, Celestena, Celestene, Celestia, Celestijna, Celestina, Celestine, Celestyne, Celia,

Celie, Celina, Celinda, Celine, Celinka, Celka,
Celleste, Celyna, Saleste, Salestia, Seleste, Selestia,
Selestina, Selestine, Selestyna, Selestyne, Silesta,
Silestena, Silestia, Silestijna, Silestina, Silestyna,
Silestyne, Tina, Tinka

Celine Fr. Var. **Celeste**. Singer Celine Dion.

Celinda, Celinde, Salinda, Salinde, Selinda, Selinde,
Seline

Celosia Gk. "Aflame."

Cenobia "Power of Zeus." A Spanish form of the slightly
more common **Zenobia**.

Cerelia Lat. "Relating to springtime." A nice name for a
spring baby.

Cerella, Sarelia, Sarilia

Cerise Fr. "Cherry." See **Cherry**.

Cerisse, Charisse, Cherise, Sarese, Sherise

Cesarina (Fem. **Caesar**) Lat. Probably "Hairy, hirsute."

Cesarea, Cesarie, Cesarine, Kesare

Chanah Heb. "Grace." See **Hannah**.

Chaanach, Chaanah, Chana, Chanach

Chandra Sanskrit "Like the moon." The greatest Hindu
goddess Devi is also known as Chandra.

Candra, Chandi, Shandra

Chanel Fr. Surname of the legendary fashion designer
Coco Chanel, and by extension, the name of a number of
famous perfumes. Began to be used as a first name in the
1980s.

Chanelle, Channelle, Shanel, Shanell, Shanelle,
Shannel, Shannelle, Shenelle, Shynelle

Chantal Fr. Originally a place name meaning "stony spot,"
but possibly also derived from the verb *chanter,* "to sing."
A top-ten name in France, but unusual in the U.S.

Chantalle, Chantel, Chantelle, Chantele, Shantal,
Shantalle, Shantel, Shantell, Shantelle, Shontel,
Shontelle

Charis Gk. "Grace." One of the mythological Three
Graces.

Chareesse, Charisse, Charysse, Karas, Karis, Karisse

Charity Lat. "Brotherly love." One of the three cardinal

virtues, along with Faith and Hope. They have survived
better than many of the other virtue names (Temperance,
Fortitude, Humility, Chastity, Mercy, Obedience) popular
among the Puritans in the 17th century.

**Carissa, Carita, Chareese, Charis, Charissa, Charisse,
Charita, Charitee, Charitey, Charitye, Chariza, Charty,
Cherri, Cherry, Sharitee, Sharitey, Sharity, Sharitye**

Charlotte Fr. "Little and womanly." One of the most popular feminine forms of **Charles.** Like **Caroline,** Charlotte
was popularized in England by a queen (George III's
wife) and was much used from the 18th century to the beginning of the 20th. In the U.S. its use peaked in the
1870s, but with the recent return to "old-fashioned"
names, it has been dusted off for a reappearance. Currently very popular in England. In E. B. White's *Charlotte's Web,* the heroine of the title is a spider. Novelist
Charlotte Brontë; actress Charlotte Rampling; singer
Charlotte Church.

**Carla, Carleen, Carlie, Carline, Carlota, Carlotta,
Carly, Carlyne, Char, Chara, Charill, Charla,
Charlaine, Charleen, Charlene, Charlet, Charlette,
Charline, Charlot, Charlotta, Charly, Charlyne,
Charmain, Charmaine, Charmian, Charmion, Charo,
Charty, Charyl, Cherlyn, Cheryl, Cheryll, Karla,
Karleen, Karlene, Karli, Karlicka, Karlie, Karlika,
Karline, Karlota, Karlotta, Karlotte, Karly, Karlyne,
Lola, Loleta, Loletta, Lolita, Lolotte, Lotta, Lottchen,
Lotte, Lottey, Lotti, Lottie, Lotty, Sharel, Sharil,
Sharla, Sharlaine, Sharleen, Sharlene, Sharlet,
Sharlette, Sharline, Sharlot, Sharmain, Sharmayne,
Sharmian, Sharmion, Sharyl, Sheri, Sherie, Sherrie,
Sherry, Sherye, Sheryl**

Charmaine From a Latin clan name; also possibly related
to **Carmen** and **Caroline.** Enjoyed bursts of popularity in
the 1920s and 1950s.

**Charmain, Charmane, Charmayne, Charmian,
Charmion, Charmyan, Charmyn, Sharmain, Sharman,
Sharmane, Sharmayne, Sharmian, Sharmion,
Sharmyn**

Charmian Gk. "Joy." A distinctly separate name from Charmaine, though they are often confused. Because of its Greek origin, Charmian should be pronounced with a hard *C*, but it rarely is. Actress Charmian Carr.

Charmin, Charmiane, Charmyan, Charmin, Sharmian, Sharmiane, Sharmyan, Sharmyane

Chasidah Heb. "Devout woman."

Chastity Lat. "Purity." A virtue name that has, for obvious reasons, fallen out of favor, though Cher used it for her daughter.

Chasaty, Chasity, Chassity, Chastitee, Chastitey

Chava Heb. "Life."

Chabah, Chaya, Chayka, Eva, Hava, Haya, Kaija

Chaviva Heb. "Beloved."

Eva

Chelsea OE. "Port or landing place." Place name; possibly owes some of its appeal to British pop culture of the late 1960s. First Daughter Chelsea Clinton.

Chelcie, Chelsee, Chelseigh, Chelsey, Chelsie, Chelsy

Chepzibah Heb. "My delight is in her." See **Hepzibah**.

Cher Fr. "Beloved." For most people, inseparable from the singer and actress who uses this name alone, without a surname. Somewhat popular in the late 1960s and early 1970s.

Chere, Cherée, Cherey, Cheri, Cherice, Cherie, Cherise, Cherish, Cherrie, Cherry, Chery, Cherye, Cherylee, Cherylie, Sher, Sherelle, Sherey, Sheri, Sherice, Sherie, Sherry, Sheryll

Cherry OF. "Cherry." The 19th-century vogue for botanical names did not usually extend to fruit, so when Cherry occurs, it is most likely a variant of **Charity** or **Cheryl**.

Chere, Cheree, Cherey, Cherida, Cherise, Cherita, Cherrey, Cherri, Cherrie

Cheryl Familiar form of **Charlotte** or **Cherry**. A 20th-century development that first became popular in the 1940s, and increased in use into the 1960s. Like most 30-year-old fashions, it is now quite dated. Pop musician Sheryl Crow.

Charil, Charyl, Cheriann, Cherianne, Cherryl, Cheryll,

Cherylle, Cherilynn, Chryil, Chyrill, Sharil, Sharyl, Sharyll, Sheral, Sherianne, Sheril, Sherill, Sheryl, Shyril, Shyrill

Cherilyn Form of **Cheryl**. Names that are modern developments seem more susceptible to widely variable spellings, as this one is.

Charalin, Charalyn, Charalynne, Charelin, Charelyn, Charelynn, Charilyn, Charilynn, Cheralin, Cheralyn, Cherilin, Cherilynn, Cherilynne, Cherralyn, Cherrilin, Cherrilyn, Cherrylene, Cherrylin, Cherryline, Cherrylyn, Cherylin, Cheryline, Cheryllyn, Cherylyn, Sharalin, Sharalyn, Sharelyn, Sharelynne, Sharilynn, Sheralin, Sheralynne, Sherilin, Sherralin, Sherrilyn, Sherrylene, Sherryline, Sherrylyn, Sherylin, Sherylyn

Chesna Slavic. "Peaceful."

Chessa, Chessy

Chiara It. "Light." See **Claire**.

Chiarra, Kiara, Kiarra

Chiquita Sp. "Little one." Most parents will probably associate this name with the heavily advertised Chiquita banana.

Chickie, Chicky, Chiqueeta, Chiquin

Chloe Gk. "Young green shoot." Appears in the Bible, and as a name in literature, especially in the tale of Daphnis and Chloe, set to music by Ravel. Enormously popular throughout Great Britain and in France, but only occasionally used in the US. Actresses Chloe Webb, Chloe Sevigny.

Chloe, Clo, Cloe, Cloey, Khloe, Khloey, Kloe

Chloris Gk. "Pale." Another name from Greek mythology, though an obscure one. Actress Cloris Leachman.

Chloress, Cloris, Khloris, Kloris

Cholena Delaware Indian. "Bird."

Christabel Lat./Fr. "Fair Christian." Use has been primarily literary, as in Samuel Taylor Coleridge's poem of the same name, in which the heroine is an example of innocent purity. Used occasionally in Britain.

Christabella, Christabelle, Christobel, Chrystabel, Chrystabelle, Chrystobel, Cristabel, Cristabella, Cristabelle, Crystabel, Crystabella

Christina (Fem. **Christian**) Gk. "Anointed, Christian."
Christian was used for women in medieval times, but by
the 18th century Christina was the more common form. It
was superseded in the 1930s by the French form **Christine,** which was very popular in the fifties and sixties, but
the cycle of fashion has now brought Christina back to
solid but not trendy popularity. **Christiane** is currently
very popular in Germany. Queen Cristina of Sweden; poet
Christina Rossetti; tennis star Chris Evert; model Christie
Brinkley; pop singer Cristina Aguilera; actress Christina
Ricci.

**Chris, Chrissie, Chrissy, Chrissta, Chrisstan,
Chrissten, Chrissti, Chrisstie, Chrissty, Christa,
Christan, Christeen, Christel, Christen, Christi,
Christian, Christiana, Christiane, Christianna,
Christie, Christin, Christine, Christini, Christinn,
Christmar, Christy, Christyna, Chrystal, Chrystalle,
Chrystee, Chrystel, Chrystelle, Chrystle, Cris, Crissey,
Crissie, Crissy, Crista, Cristal, Cristel, Cristelle,
Cristen, Cristena, Cristi, Cristie, Cristin, Cristina,
Cristine, Cristiona, Cristy, Crysta, Crystena,
Crystene, Crystie, Crystina, Crystine, Crystyna,
Khristeen, Khristena, Khristina, Khristine, Khristya,
Kirsten, Kirstin, Kit, Kris, Krissy, Krista, Kristeen,
Kristel, Kristen, Kristi, Kristijna, Kristin, Kristina,
Kristy, Krysta, Krystka, Krystle, Stina, Teena, Teyna,
Tina, Tiny**

Christmas OE. Name of the holiday, used occasionally
through the 19th century for Dec. 25 babies, but now more
usually replaced by the French, and somewhat subtler
form, **Noel.**

Chryseis Lat. "Golden daughter." A very beautiful young
girl named Chryseis appears in Homer's *Iliad.*
Chrysilla

Chumani Sioux. "Drops of dew."

Cinderella Fr. "Little ash-girl." The name from the fairy
tale. Very rare.
Cendrillon, Cenerentola, Cindie, Cindy, Ella

Cindy Originally a nickname for **Cynthia** (Gk. "Goddess

from Mt. Cynthos") or **Lucinda** (Lat. "Light"). Popular
for children born in the fifties and sixties, but rarely used
since. Singer Cyndi Lauper; model Cindy Crawford.
**Cindee, Cindi, Cindie, Cyndee, Cyndi, Cyndie, Cyndy,
Sindee, Sindi, Sindie, Sindy, Syndi, Syndie, Syndy**

Cipriana It. "From Cyprus."
**Chipriana, Chiprianna, Cipriane, Ciprianna, Cypriana,
Cyprienne, Sipriana, Sipriane, Siprianne, Sypriana,
Syprianne**

Claire Lat. "Bright." The original form was **Clare,** as in
Saint Clare, 13th-century founder of a Franciscan order of
nuns. In the 19th century **Clara** became fashionable,
but since the 1960s, the French form Claire has
dominated. Writer Clare Booth Luce; actresses Clara
Bow, Claire Bloom, Claire Danes.
**Ceara, Cearra, Cheeara, Chiara, Ciara, Ciarra, Clair,
Claire, Claireen, Clairene, Claireta, Clairette, Clairey,
Clairice, Clairinda, Clairissa, Clairita, Clairy,
Clarabel, Clarabelle, Clare, Clarene, Claresta,
Clareta, Claretta, Clarey, Clari, Claribel, Claribella,
Claribelle, Clarice, Clarie, Clarinda, Clarine, Clarissa,
Clarisse, Clarita, Claritza, Clarrie, Clarry, Clary,
Claryce, Clayre, Clayrette, Clayrice, Clayrinda,
Clayrissa, Clerissa, Cliara, Clorinda, Klaire, Klara,
Klaretta, Klarissa, Klaryce, Klayre, Kliara, Klyara,
Seara, Searra**

Clara Lat. "Bright." Another version of **Claire,** but one that
has been very rare for some time. It was at its most popular in the 19th century, but is popular in Spain at the moment.
**Clarabelle, Claretha, Claribel, Clarice, Clarie,
Clarinda, Clarine, Clarita, Claritza, Clarry, Klara,
Klarra**

Claramae Eng. A compound form of **Clara,** probably dating from the late 19th century, when **May** was also a popular name.
Claramay

Clarice Variant of **Claire** which enjoyed a flurry of popularity around the turn of the 20th century. **Clarissa** is a La-

tinized version made famous by Samuel Richardson's 18th-century novel *Clarissa.*
Claris, Clarise, Clarisse, Claryce, Clerissa, Clerisse, Cleryce, Clerysse, Klarice, Klarissa, Klaryce

Clarimond Lat./Ger. "Shining defender."
Claramond, Claramonda Claramonde, Clarimunde

Claudia (Fem. **Claude, Claudius**) Lat. Clan name probably meaning "lame." The name has never been very popular in English-speaking countries in any of its forms, in spite of the exposure given it by Colette's novels (*Claudine at School,* etc.) and the career of actress Claudette Colbert. It is currently used quite a bit in Germany. Actress Claudia Cardinale; model Claudia Schiffer.
Claude, Claudella, Claudelle, Claudetta, Claudette, Claudie, Claudina, Claudine, Claudey, Claudy, Clodia, Klaudia, Klodia

Clea Unknown derivation, but possibly invented by author Lawrence Durrell, for a character in his famous *Alexandria Quartet.* See also **Cleopatra, Clio.**
Claea, Klea

Clelia Lat. "Glorious." A maiden who figures in the legendary history of Rome. Her story was retold (in 10 volumes!) by the 17th-century French novelist Mlle. de Scudéry.

Clematis Gk. "Vine or brushwood." Flower name, from the blossoming vine with white or purple blooms.
Clematia, Clematice, Clematiss

Clementine Lat. "Mild, giving mercy." **Clemence** and **Clemency** were both Puritan virtue names, but are now unheard-of. **Clementia** was used until the 19th century, when it was replaced by **Clementina**. The well-known song "My Darling Clementine" would make it hard to use that version of the name with a straight face.
Clem, Clemence, Clemency, Clementia, Clementina, Clementya, Clementyna, Clementyn, Clemmie, Clemmy, Klementijna, Klementina

Cleopatra Gk. "Her father's renown." There were actually generations of Egyptian princesses of this name, but the most famous is the intriguer who enthralled both Caesar and Antony. Very rare.

Clea, Cleo, Cleona, Cleone, Cleonie, Cleta

Cleva (Fem. **Cleve, Clive**) ME. "Hill-dweller." Place name transferred to a surname and thence to a first name used for men. This feminine form is unusual.

Cliantha Gk. "Glory-flower."

Cleantha, Cleanthe, Clianthe, Kliantha, Klianthe

Clio Gk. Mythological name of the muse of history. There are nine muses, the daughters of Zeus and Mnemosyne, and each represents an art or science. **Calliope** (epic poetry), **Terpsichore** (choral song and dance), and **Thalia** (comedy) have survived as first names.

Klio

Clorinda Lat. Literary name coined by 16th-century Italian poet Tasso. Possibly derived from **Claire** or **Chloe**.

Chlorinda

Clotilda Ger. "Renowned battle." Saint Clothilde was the wife of Frankish King Clovis I in the 6th century, and supposedly went into battle by his side. One of Paris's most fashionable churches is named for her.

Clothilda, Clothilde, Clotilde, Klothilda, Klothilde

Clover OE. Flower name. Perhaps because of the modest nature of the flower, the name occurred in the 19th century more commonly as a nickname.

Clymene Gk. "Renowned one." In Greek myth, most notably the daughter of Oceanus and mother of Atlas and Prometheus, though several other legendary figures also bear this name.

Clytie Gk. "Lovely one." Another mythological figure whose unrequited love for the sun god resulted in her being changed into a heliotrope, or sunflower, which turns to follow the sun's path.

Cochava Heb. "Star."

Cody OE. "Pillow." This is an example of the kind of unisex name that was popular in the '90s. Cody remains more usually masculine.

Codee, Codey, Codi, Codie, Kodee, Kodey, Kodie, Kody

Colette Dim. **Nicole** (Gk./Fr. "People of victory"). Used mostly since the 1940s, though never widespread. Probably made familiar by the French writer Colette, whose last name it was.

Coletta, Collet, Collete, Collette, Nicolette

Coline (Fem. **Colin,** derived from **Nicholas**) Gk. "People of victory."

Colena, Colene, Coletta, Colina, Collina, Colline, Nicoleen, Nicolene, Nicoline, Nicolyne

Colleen Ir. Gael. "Girl." In use since the 1940s in English-speaking countries *except* Ireland. A vogue in the early 1960s faded rapidly. Actress Colleen Dewhurst; writer Colleen McCullough.

Coleen, Collie, Colline, Colly, Kolleen, Kolline

Columba Lat. "Dove." Saint Columba, 6th-century Irish saint, founded an influential monastery on the Scottish island of Iona, and is supposed to have exorcised the River Ness of a monster. Though the Irish Columba was a man, two other saints of that name were both women.

Collie, Colly, Colombe, Columbia, Columbine

Columbine Lat. "Dove." Columbine is also a literary character who appears in traditional Italian comedy and English pantomime as Harlequin's beloved. Also a flower name for a delicate two-colored blossom.

Comfort Fr. "To strengthen and comfort." In the Bible the Holy Ghost is referred to as the "Comforter." It was a surname in the Middle Ages, then popular among the Puritans. Almost unused since the 18th century.

Concepción Lat. "Conception." Used mostly in Latin American countries to honor the Immaculate Conception and, by extension, the Virgin Mary.

Cetta, Chiquin, Chita, Concetta, Concha, Concheta, Conchissa, Conchita

Conchita Dim. **Concepción.**

Conchata, Conchissa

Concordia Lat. "Peace, harmony." In classical myth, Concordia was the goddess of peace succeeding a battle.

Concord, Concorde

Conradine (Fem. **Conrad**) OG. "Brave counsel."

Connee, Connie, Conny, Conrada, Conradeen, Conradina

Constance Lat. "Steadfastness." Used often in the early Christian and medieval eras, then by the Puritans (usually as **Constant** or **Constancy**). After a brief revival at the beginning of this century, it lapsed back into obscurity. Singer Connie Francis.
Con, Conetta, Connee, Conney, Conni, Connie, Conny, Constancia, Constancy, Constanta, Constantia, Constantija, Constantina, Constantine, Constantya, Constanz, Costanza, Konstance, Konstantija, Konstantina, Konstanze, Kosta, Kostatina, Tina

Consuelo Sp. "Consolation, comfort." Honors Santa Maria del Consuelo. In 1842 George Sand, a popular French author, published an historical novel called *Consuelo*. The heroine, a gypsy, became a successful opera singer.
Chela, Chelo, Consolata, Consuela

Cora Gk. "Maiden." Though some sources trace the name to classical myth, its modern form was probably coined by American writer James Fenimore Cooper in *The Last of the Mohicans* (1826). It grew in popularity through the 19th century, but now its variant forms are more often used. Civil rights activist Coretta Scott King.
Corabel, Corabella, Corabelle, Corabellita, Coree, Corella, Corena, Corene, Coretta, Corey, Cori, Corie, Corilla, Corine, Corinna, Corinne, Corita, Correen, Corrella, Correlle, Correna, Correnda, Correne, Correy, Corri, Corrie, Corrina, Corrine, Corrissa, Corry, Corynna, Corynne, Coryssa, Kora, Korabell, Kore, Koreen, Korella, Koretta, Korey, Korilla, Korina, Korinne, Korry, Koryne, Korynna, Koryssa

Coral Lat. Nature name: first appeared during the Victorian vogue for jewel names, usually in England. Actress Coral Browne.
Coralee, Coralena, Coralie, Coraline, Corallina, Coralline, Coraly, Coralyn, Coralyne, Koral, Korall, Koralie, Koralline

Corazón Sp. "Heart." Corazón Aquino, former president of the Philippines.

Cordelia Derivation unclear, but probably related to Latin *cor* or "heart." In Shakespeare's *King Lear,* Cordelia is the youngest and only lovable daughter of the tragic king.
Cordelie, Cordella, Cordelle, Cordey, Cordi, Cordie, Cordy, Delia, Delie, Della, Kordelia, Kordella, Kordelle

Corey Ir. Gael. Place name: "the hollow." Place name transferred to surname. Author Corrie ten Boom.
Cory, Cori, Corrie, Corry, Cory, Korie, Korrey, Korri, Korry

Corinne French form of **Cora,** used since the 1860s.
Carinna, Carinne, Carine, Carynna, Carynne, Corenne, Corin, Corina, Corinda, Corine, Corinn, Corinna, Correna, Corrianne, Corrienne, Corrinda, Corrine, Corrinn, Corrinna, Karinne, Karynna, Koreen, Korina, Korinne, Korrina

Corliss OE. "Benevolent, cheery."
Corlee, Corless, Corley, Corlie, Corly

Cornelia (Fem. **Cornelius**) Lat. "Like a horn." Comes from a famous Latin clan name, and was often used in the Roman Empire. Modern use is sparing, dating from mid-19th century.
Cornalia, Corneelija, Cornela, Cornelija, Cornelya, Corelie, Cornella, Cornelle, Cornie, Korneelia, Korneelya, Kornelia, Kornelija, Kornelya, Neel, Neely, Nela, Nelia, Nell, Nella, Nellie, Nelly

Corona Sp. "Crown." A spate of English use occurred around the coronation of King Edward VII in 1902, but this sentimental homage to royalty was not repeated at subsequent coronations. Also the name of a very popular Mexican beer, which would seem to limit its further use as a given name.
Coronetta, Coronette, Coronna

Corvina Lat. "Like a raven."
Corva, Corveena, Corvetta

Cosette Fr. Probably a feminine diminutive of **Nicholas** (Gk. "People of victory").
Cosetta

Cosima (Fem. **Cosmo**) Gk. "Order." Very unusual in

English-speaking countries. The composer Richard Wagner married (as his second wife) Cosima Liszt, daughter of the composer Franz Liszt. Two of their children were named Siegfried and Isolde, after characters in two of his operas.

Cosma, Cosmé, Kosma

Courtney OE. "Court-dweller." Surname transferred to first name; usually feminine in U.S. Immensely popular in the 1990s, probably owing to upper-class connotations. Actresses Courteney Cox, Courtney Love.

Cordney, Cordni, Cortenay, Corteney, Cortland, Cortnee, Cortneigh, Cortney, Cortnie, Cortny, Courtenay, Courteneigh, Courteney, Courtland, Courtnay, Courtnee, Courtnie, Courtny, Kordney, Kortney, Kortni, Kourtenay, Kourtneigh, Kourtney, Kourtnee, Kourtnie

Crescent OF. "Increasing, growing." Also, by extension, the shape of the crescent moon.

Crescence, Crescenta, Crescentia, Cressant, Cressent, Cressentia, Cressentya

Cressida Gk. Heroine of a tale (*Troilus and Cressida*) that has been told by Boccaccio, Chaucer, and Shakespeare.

Crispina (Fem. **Crispin**) Lat. "Curly-haired."

Cristina Lat. "Anointed, Christian." See **Christina**.

Crystal Gk. "Ice." Transferred use of the word, mostly modern, and increasing since the 1950s. Curiously enough, Crystal was considered a man's name in Scotland hundreds of years ago, where it was a diminutive of **Christopher**. See **Christina**.

Christal, Christalle, Chrystal, Chrystalle, Chrystel, Chrystle, Cristal, Cristel, Cristle, Crysta, Crystel, Khristalle, Khrystle, Kristle, Krystal, Krystalle, Krystle

Csilla Hung. "Defenses."

Cyanea Gk. "Sky blue."

Cybele Gk. Asian goddess, also known in Greek myth as Rhea, and in Rome as "Great Mother of the Gods." In legend she was originally bisexual, but made female by the Olympian gods.

Cynara Gk. "Thistly plant." Made famous by the late-19th-century English poet Ernest Dowson, who is in turn largely remembered by the line "I have been faithful to thee, Cynara! in my fashion."
Zinara

Cynthia Gk. "Goddess from Mount Cynthos," i.e., Artemis, the moon goddess, who was supposed to have been born there. Used as a literary name in the 17th century, and by American slave owners in the early 19th century. Enjoyed a period of popularity from the 1920s to 1950s, then was replaced by its nickname, **Cindy,** which is now rare. Many of the diminutives are also variants of **Lucinda.** Ballerina Cynthia Gregory; actress Cynthia Nixon.
Cinda, Cindee, Cindi, Cindie, Cindy, Cinnie, Cinny, Cinthia, Cintia, Cinzia, Cyn, Cynda, Cyndee, Cyndia, Cyndie, Cyndra, Cyndy, Cynnie, Cynthea, Cynthie, Cynthya, Cytia, Kynthia, Kynthija, Sindee, Sindi, Sindy, Sindya, Sinnie, Sinny, Synda, Syndee, Syndi, Syndy, Syntha, Synthee, Syntheea, Synthia, Synthie, Synthya

Cypris Gk. "From the island of Cyprus."
Cipriana, Cypriane, Ciprienne, Cyprianne, Cyprien, Cyprienne, Sipriana, Siprianne

Cyra (Fem. **Cyrus**) Per. "Sun" or "Throne." Author Cyra McFadden.

Cyrilla (Fem. **Cyril**) Lat. "Lordly."
Ciri, Cirilla, Siri, Sirilla, Syrilla

Cytherea Gk. "From the island of Cythera," i.e., Aphrodite or Venus, who is supposed to have come ashore there after being born of seafoam.

D

Dacey Ir. Gael. "From the south."
   Dacee, Dacia, Dacie, Dacy, Daicee, Daicy, Daisey
   Dacia Lat. Place name: Dacia was a Roman province which existed where Romania is now.

Dada Nig. "Curly-haired."

Daffodil OF. Flower name for the familiar yellow blossom; an inventive name for a spring baby.

Dagmar OG. Meaning unclear, though possibly "Day's glory." In Denmark Dagmar is a royal name, but it appears only rarely in English-speaking countries.

Dahlia Scan. Flower name of fairly recent vintage, first used in numbers since the 1920s. The flower itself was named in honor of the 18th-century Swedish botanist Anders Dahl.
   Dahiana, Dayha, Daleia, Dalia, Dalla

Dai Jap. "Great."

Daisy OE. "Eye of the day." One of the most popular of the 19th-century flower names. It was often used as a nickname for **Margaret,** since in France the flower is called a *marguerite.* It was such a popular name that, when Henry James was writing the story of the typical American girl in Europe, he named her *Daisy Miller.* Little used in the modern era, but this is the kind of name that nostalgia may resurrect. Actress Daisy Fuentes.
   Daisee, Daiscy, Daisie, Dasle

Dale OE. Place name: "Valley." Originally a surname meaning "One who lives in the valley." The term "dale" is still used in parts of England. Most popular as a first name in the 1930s. Actress Dale Evans.
   Dael, Dail, Daile, Dalla, Dayle

Dalila Swahili. "Delicate."
   Lila

Dallas Scot. Gael. Place name of a village in northeastern Scotland, used as a first name since the 19th century. Apparently unrelated to Dallas, Texas, which was named for a U.S. Vice President.

Dalles

Dalmace Lat./Fr. Place name: Dalmatia is a region of northeastern Italy, extending down into coastal Croatia, and the supposed origin of dalmatian dogs, white-haired with black spots.

Dalma, Dalmassa, Dalmatia

Damaris Gk. "Calf" is the most commonly proposed meaning though another source suggests "to tame." A Damaris in the New Testament was converted by Saint Paul, and the Puritans adopted the name with enthusiasm, if not uniformity in spelling. Many variants exist, though the name is very unusual.

Damalas, Damalis, Damalit, Damalla, Damara, Damaress, Dameris, Damerys, Dameryss, Damiris, Damris, Demaras, Demaris, Demarys, Mara, Mari, Maris

Damia Gk. Meaning not clear; possibly "To tame," although the Greek root is also close to the word for "Spirit." The masculine form, **Damian,** is more often seen.

Damian, Damiana, Damiane, Damienne, Damya, Damyan, Damyana, Damyen, Damyenne

Damita Sp. "Little noblewoman."

Dama

Dana OE. "From Denmark." Also a surname, used as a boy's first name in the 19th century, but now almost exclusively a girl's name, and a specifically American one. Actress Dana Delany.

Danaca, Danay, Dane, Danet, Dania, Danica, Danna, Danya, Dayna, Donnica

Danaë Gk. A character in Greek myth, whom Zeus visited in the form of a shower of gold (a popular subject for Old Master painters). The child of this union was the heroic Perseus.

Dee, Denae, Dene, Dinae, Dinay, Donnay

Danielle (Fem. **Daniel**) Heb. "God is my judge." Uncommon until the middle of the 20th century, when, following a revival of Daniel, it became more fashionable. Novelist Danielle Steele.

Daanelle, Danee, Danele, Danella, Danelle, Danelly, Danette, Daney, Dani, Dania, Danica, Danice, Danie, Daniela, Daniella, Danijela, Danila, Danit, Danita, Danitza, Danna, Dannette, Danney, Danni, Danniella, Dannielle, Danny, Dannyce, Dany, Danya, Danyell, Danyella, Danyelle

Daphne Gk. "Laurel tree." In Greek myth Daphne was a nymph who, attempting to flee an amorous Apollo, was turned into a laurel tree. Though used under the Roman Empire, the name disappeared until the 18th century. It came to the U.S. as a slave name, and enjoyed a brief English vogue between 1900 and 1930. Author Daphne Du Maurier.

Daffi, Daffie, Daffy, Dafna, Dafne, Dafnee, Dafneigh, Dafnie, Danfy, Daphna, Daphney, Daphnie

Dara Heb. "Nugget of wisdom." In the New Testament, a man's name, but its occasional modern use is for girls. Its resemblance to the familiar **Sarah** and **Farrah** probably works in its favor. Olympic swimmer Dara Torres.

Darda, Daria, Darian, Darragh, Darrah, Darya

Daralis OE. "Beloved."

Daralice, Darelis

Darby OE. Place name: "Park with deer." Derived from **Derby,** a surname used as a first name, almost exclusively for boys. Darby is also usually masculine.

Darb, Darbee, Darbey, Darbie, Darrbey, Darrbie, Darrby

Darcie Ir. Gael. "Dark." Also Norman place name, "From Arcy." In Britain, usually a boy's name, but in the U.S., more likely to be feminine. Ballerina Darci Kistler.

D'Arcy, Darcee, Darceigh, Darcey, Darcy, Darice, Darsee, Darseigh, Darsey, Darsie, Darsi

Daria (Fem. **Darius**) Gk. "Rich."

Dari, Darian, Darice, Darien, Darya, Dhariana, Dorian, Doriane

Darlene Modern adaptation of "Darling" used for a given name. First used in the late 1930s and extremely fashionable by the 1950s in the U.S. Now out of style, and unlikely to be revived soon.
Dareen, Darelle, Darla, Darleen, Darlenny, Darline, Darlinn, Darlyn, Darlyne, Darrelle, Darryleen, Darrylene, Darryline

Daron (Fem. **Darren**) Modern use. Darren may be a transferred Irish surname, first used widely in the 1950s as a given name. Daron can be considered a feminine form because of its similarity to **Sharon** (also popular in that era).

Daryl Transferred surname, possibly originated as a French place name, like **Darcy**. Actress Daryl Hannah; fashion designer Darryl Kerrigan.
Darel, Darille, Darrel, Darrell, Darrelle, Darrill, Darrille, Darrylene, Darryline, Darryl, Darrylin, Darryline, Darrylyn, Darylin, Daryline, Darylyne, Derrill

Davina (Fem. **David**) Heb. "Loved one." The most commonly used feminine variant of the hugely popular masculine name.
Daveen, Daviana, Daviane, Davida, Davidina, Davine, Davinia, Davita, Devina, Divina, Divinia

Dawn OE. "Dawn." Modern use of the word for a name. **Aurora,** the Latin term, dates back some fifteen hundred years, but Dawn first appeared in the late 1920s. Opera singer Dawn Upshaw; comedian Dawn French; basketball player Dawn Staley.
Dawna, Dawnita, Dawnyelle, Dawnysia, Dowan, Duwan, Dwan

Day OE. "Day." Possibly use of the word as a name, like **Dawn,** but more likely to be a transferred surname.

Daya Heb. "Bird of prey." Specifically, a kind of hawk known as a kite.
Dayah

Dea Lat. "Goddess."

Deanna OE. Place name "Valley" or occupational name "Church leader." Feminine of **Dean,** which only came into use as a first name in the 1950s. Could also be considered a version of **Diana**. Actress Deanna Durbin.

Deana, Deann, Deanne, Deeann, Deeanna

Deborah Heb. "Bee." One of the few significant women's names to figure in the Old Testament; in the Book of Judges, she was an important prophetess and judge. Predictably, the Puritans latched on to the name, but it was not widely used until the 1950s, possibly influenced by the career of actress Deborah Kerr. Actresses Debbie Reynolds, Debra Winger, Debra Messing; Olympic figure skater Debi Thomas; TV journalist Deborah Norville.

Deb, Debb, Debbee, Debbera, Debbey, Debbi, Debbie, Debbra, Debby, Debee, Debera, Deberah, Debi, Debor, Debora, Debra, Debrah, Debs, Devora, Devorah, Dobra

Decima Lat. "Tenth girl." Unlikely to be used in these days of small families.

Decia

Dee Welsh. "Swarthy." Dim. **Deirdre, Diana, Delia**, etc.

Dede, Dedie, DeeDee, DeeAnn, Didi

Deifilia Lat. "God's daughter."

Deirdre Ir. Possible meanings are "Fear" or "Raging woman." In Irish myth, Deirdre was the most beautiful woman in Ireland, whose tragically complex love life caused several deaths, including her own. The name has only been in use since the 1920s. Actress Deidre Hall.

Dede, Dedra, Dee, DeeDee, Deedre, Deidra, Deidre, Deidrie, Derdre, Didi, Dierdrey

Delaney Ir. Gael. "Offspring of the challenger."

DeLaina, Delaine, Delainey, Delainy, Delane, Delanie, Delany, DeLayna

Delia Gk. "From Delos." In Greek myth, the goddess Artemis was born in Delos, so Delia could be an allusion to her. It may also be a diminutive of **Cordelia** or **Adelaide**. Though it has never had a period of great popularity, it has never faded from sight either. Author Delia Ephron.

Deelia, Delya

Delicia Lat. "Delight." Used in the Roman Empire, and occasionally since then, but never common.

Dalicia, Dalise, Dalisha, Dalisse, Dee, DeeDee, Dela, Delice, Delis, Delise, Delisha, Delissa, Deliz, Della, Dellis, Dellise, Delyse, Delysia, Didi

Delight OF. The emotion as a name. Scarce.

Delilah Heb. "Lovelorn, seductive." In the Old Testament, mistress of Samson. The familiar story of how she cuts off his hair to sap his strength probably limits use of her name.

Dalila, Delila, Lila, Lilah

Della Short for **Adelle, Adeline, Adelaide**. Used as an independent name since the 1870s. Singer Della Reese.

Delle, Dellene, Delline

Delores Sp. "Sorrows." Var. **Dolores**.

Delphine Gk. "Dolphin." This is a French form of a name with a complex origin. It alludes to the Greek town of Delphi, home of a famous oracle. The Greeks believed that Delphi was the earth's womb; the dolphin's shape resembles that of a pregnant woman. The larkspur flower, whose center resembles a dolphin, is also known as delphinium, so in some respects this is a flower name. French actress Delphine Seyrig.

Delfa, Delfin, Delfine, Delfyne, Delpha, Delphina, Delphinea, Delphinia

Delta Fourth letter of the Greek alphabet, thus a name for a fourth child. May also be a place name, as in the Mississippi Delta. Actress Delta Burke.

Dellta

Demetria Gk. In Greek myth, Demeter was goddess of corn, and mother of Persephone, whose abduction to Hades led to the cycle of seasons.

Demeter, Demetra, Demetria, Demetris, Dimitra, Dimitria

Demelza Cornish. "Fort on the hill." First used as a given name in the 1950s, probably because of its pretty sound.

Dena OE. Place name. "Valley." Use of Dena followed the popularity of **Dean** in the 1950s.

Deana, Deane, Deanna, Deena, Dene, Denna, Denni, Dina

Denise (Fem. **Dennis**) Fr. "Follower of Dionysius."
Though there is an ancient Latin form of the name
(**Dionysia**) this variation dates back only to the 1920s. It
was very popular in the 1950s, but since the mid 1960s,
has been eclipsed. Actress Denise Richards.
> **Deneigh, Denese, Dennet, Dennette, Deney, Deni,
> Denice, Daniece, Denisse, Denize, Denni, Dennie,
> Dennise, Denny, Denyce, Denys, Denyse, Dinnie,
> Dinny**

Deolinda Port. "Beautiful God."

Derinda Modern name, probably formed from **Derek** and
Linda.
> **Darinda, Dorinda**

*Derora Heb. "A bird, a swallow."
> **Derorit, Drora, Drorah, Drorit, Droriya**

Deryn Welsh. "Bird." Dates from the 1950s, and its popularity mirrors names like **Karen** and **Sharon**. Unusual
after the 1970s.
> **Derran, Deren, Derhyn, Deron, Derrin, Derrine,
> Derron, Derrynne**

Desdemona Gk. "Wretchedness." In Shakespeare's *Othello,* Desdemona is the beautiful, innocent heroine,
wrongly accused of adultery by her husband, who then
murders her, and commits suicide in a fit of remorse. Little used, for obvious reasons.
> **Desmona**

Desirée Fr. "Much desired." The Puritans used **Desire** as a
given name, though its connotations in the 17th century
were religious rather than erotic. The French form is more
usual today.
> **Desarae, Deseray, Desideria, Desir, Desirae, Desirat,
> Desiray, Desirea, Desiri, Disirae, Dezirae, Deziray**

Desma Gk. "Binding oath."
> **Desmé**

Detta Dim. **Benedetta** (Lat. "Blessed").

Deva Hindi. "Godlike." In Hindu myth, Deva is another
name for the moon goddess.
> **Devi**

Devin Ir. Gael. "Poet."

Deva, Devinne, Devvin, Devyn

Devon OE. Place name: a county in Southern England. More common for girls than for boys. **Devin** may also be considered a variant.

Devan, Deven, Devenne, Devona, Devondra, Devonne, Devvon

Dextra (Fem. **Dexter**) OE. "Dyer." Lat. "Right-handed." Dexter, like most occupational names, was originally a surname. Dextra could also mean "skillful, dextrous."

Dextera

Diamond Unusual jewel name, first used in the 1890s but not as common then as **Ruby, Emerald,** etc. The gem is the birthstone for April.

Diamanta, Diamante

Diana "Divine." The Roman goddess of the moon, corresponding to the Greek Artemis. Used steadily since the 16th century, though the French version **Diane** eclipsed it in the mid-20th century. The vogue for Diane faded after the 1960s, and the apotheosis of Lady Diana Spencer as Princess of Wales in 1980 gave Diana new charm for prospective parents, especially in Britain. French courtesan Diana de Poitiers; actresses Diahann Carroll, Dyan Cannon, Diane Keaton, Diane Lane, Dianne Wiest.

Danne, Dayann, Dayanna, Dayanne, Deana, Deane, Deandra, Deanna, Dede, Dee, DeeDee, Deeana, Deeane, Deann, Dena, Di, Diahann, Diahanne, Dian, Diandra, Diane, Diann, Dianna, Dianne, Didi, Dyan, Dyana, Dyane, Dyann, Dyanna, Dyanne

Dianthe Gk. "Flower of the gods."

Diandra, Diandre, Diantha

Didi Var. **Diana, Deirdre.** Actress Didi Conn.

DeeDee

Didiane Fr. Feminine form of **Didier,** which is in turn a form of **Desirée,** through the Latin **Desideratus.**

Didiana, Didianna, Didiere

Dido Gk. In Virgil's *Aeneid,* the queen of Carthage who falls in love with the wandering Aeneas, and commits suicide when he leaves her. The name's origins are obscure: Virgil may have coined it. Pop musician Dido.

Didrika (Fem. **Dietrich**) OG. "People's ruler."
Diedericka, Diedricka, Diedrika

Dielle Fr. "God." Probably a female version of the French *dieu*. Unusual.
Diella

Digna Lat. "Worthy."
Deenya, Dinya

Dilys Welsh. "Reliable." Somewhat older than many names now popular in Wales, since it dates from the mid-19th century.
Dillys, Dylis, Dyllis, Dylys

Dinah Heb. "Justified." Old Testament name. In the U.S., has been popular in the South. Dina may also be considered a diminutive of names like **Claudina**. Actress Dina Merrill; singer Dinah Shore.
Dina, Dyna, Dynah

Dionne Two possible sources: Dione, in Greek myth, is the mother of Aphrodite. The name can also be a feminine version of **Dion** (Gk. "Follower of Dionysus"). It is also a homonym for the French pronunciation of **Diane**. Singer Dionne Warwick.
Deiondra, Deonne, Dion, Diona, Diondra, Dione, Dionetta, Dionis, Dionna

Dionysia Lat. Form of **Denise** (Gk. "Follower of Dionysus").
Deonisia, Deonysia, Dinicia, Dinisha, Dinitia, Dionisia

Dita Var. **Edith** (OE. "Prosperity/battle").

Divina It. "Divine, heavenly." Also var. **Davina** (Heb. "Loved one").
Divine, Divinia

Dixie Fr. "Tenth." The term "Dixie" for the Southern states, made popular by the song, is mysterious. It might come from the Mason-Dixon line, or from Louisiana dollars printed in French with the word *dix* on them (hence, "the land of 'dixies' "). Actress Dixie Carter.
Dix, Dixee

Docila Lat. "Biddable."

Dodie Heb. "Well loved." Familiar form of **Dora, Dorothy** (Gk. "Gift of God"). Author Dodie Smith.

Doda, Dodee, Dodey, Dodi, Dody

Dolly Familiar form of **Dorothy**. As an independent name, it was most popular at the turn of the century, but never a favorite. First Lady Dolley Madison; country singer Dolly Parton.

Dollee, Dolley, Dollie

Dolores Sp. "Sorrows." An allusion to the Virgin Mary, Santa Maria de los Dolores. Actress Dolores Del Rio.

Dalores, Delora, Delores, Deloria, Deloris, Dolorcita, Dolorcitas, Dolorita, Doloritas, Lola, Lolita

Domina Lat. "Lady."

Dominique (Fem. **Dominic**) Lat. "Lord." French form of a Latin name, rather fashionable in the last 25 years. Could be used for a child born on Sunday, "the Lord's day." Olympic gymnasts Dominique Dawes, Dominique Moceanu.

Domaneke, Domanique, Domenica, Domeniga, Domenique, Dominga, Domineek, Domineke, Domini, Dominica, Dominie, Dominika, Dominizia, Domino, Domitia, Meeka, Mika, Domorique

Donalda Scot. Gael. "World mighty." One of many attempts to form a feminine of **Donald,** a Scottish name particularly popular in the first half of the 20th century.

Dona, Donaldette, Donaldina, Donaline, Donelda, Donetta, Donia, Donita

Donata Lat. "Given."

Donatila, Donatilia

Donna It. "Lady." The original meaning is closer to "lady of the home." Strictly modern use as a given name, dating from the 1920s. Very popular in the 1950s, but little used now. Actress Donna Reed; swimming champion Donna Devarona; fashion designer Donna Karan; singer Donna Summer.

Dona, Donalie, Donella, Donelle, Donetta, Donia, Donica, Donielle, Donita, Donnell, Donnella, Donnelle, Donni, Donnica, Donnie, Donnisse, Donny, Ladonna

Dora Gk. "Gift." Probably originated as a diminutive of names like **Theodora,** and introduced as an independent name by a character in Charles Dickens's *David Copper-field*. Its heyday in the U.S. came at the turn of the century, but it is currently popular in Greece.

Dodee, Dodi, Dodie, Dody, Doralee, Doraleene, Doralia, Doralice, Doralicia, Doralina, Doralisha, Doralyn, Doralynn, Dore, Dorea, Doree, Doreen, Dorelia, Dorelle, Dorena, Dorene, Doretta, Dorette, Doreyda, Dori, Dorie, Dorita, Dorrie, Dory

Dorcas Gk. "Gazelle." New Testament name, Greek version of **Tabitha**. Saint Peter raised her from the dead. Predictably, well used by the Puritans, but uncommon since.

Dorcass, Dorcia, Dorkas

Dorée Fr. "Gilded."

Dorae, Doraie, D'Oray, Dore, Doree, Dorey, Dory

Doreen Several possible origins, including Ir. Gael. "Brooding," Fr. "Gilded," and an elaboration of **Dora**. In the top ten in Britain in the 1920s, now unusual.

Dorene, Doreyn, Dorine, Dorreen, Doryne

Doretta Gk. "Gift from God." Variant of **Dora** or **Theodora**.

Doria Gk. Place name: "from Doris," an area in Greece. Also feminine of **Dorian**; var. **Dorothy, Theodora** (Gk. "Gift from God").

Dori, Dorian, Doriane, Dorianne, Dorria, Dory

Dorinda Gk./Sp. Var. **Dora**. English poets in the 18th century coined a number of names with the "-inda" suffix. This one has enjoyed a small revival in this century.

Derinda, Dorrinda, Dyrinda

Doris (Fem. **Dorian**) Gk. Place name: "From Doris," an area in Greece. This form is more common than **Doria**, having been hugely popular between 1900 and the 1930s, when it subsided. Actress Doris Day; writer Doris Lessing.

Dori, Doria, Dorice, Dorisa, Dorita, Dorrie, Dorry, Dorrys, Dory, Dorys, Doryse

Dorothy Gk. "Gift of God." **Theodora,** never as popular, simply reverses the order of the Greek words. Has had two periods of popularity, around 1500 to 1700, and 1900 to the mid-1920s. The latter vogue may have been inspired by the heroine of Frank Baum's *The Wonderful Wizard of Oz,* published in 1900. Writers Dorothy Parker, Dorothy Sayers; actresses Dorothy Gish, Dorothy Lamour.

Dasha, Dasya, Dodie, Dody, Doe, Doll, Dolley, Dolli, Dollie, Dolly, Doortje, Dora, Doretta, Dori, Dorika, Dorinda, Dorit, Dorita, Doritha, Dorlisa, Doro, Doronit, Dorota, Dorotea, Doroteya, Dorothea, Dorothée, Dorrit, Dorthea, Dorthy, Dory, Dosha, Dosya, Dot, Dottey, Dottie, Dotty, Tea, Thea

Dorrit Dim. **Dorothy.** Another example of the influence of popular culture on names, as it probably stems from Charles Dickens's novel *Little Dorrit.*

Dorita, Doritt

Dory Fr. "Gilded." Also dim. **Dorothy, Isadora.**

Douce Fr. "Sweet."

Drew Dim. **Andrew** (Gk. "Masculine"). More commonly used for boys. When used as a girl's name, it is probably a transferred surname. Actress Drew Barrymore.

Drusilla Lat. Feminine version of a Roman clan name which appears in the New Testament. Very unusual nowadays. Philanthropist Drue Heinz.

Drewsila, Dru, Drucella, Drucie, Drucilla, Drucy, Drue, Druesilla, Druscilla, Drusella, Drusy

Duane Ir. Gael. "Swarthy." Dates from the 1940s. More common for boys. Socialite Duane Hampton.

Duana, Duna, Dwana, Dwayna, Dwayne

Duena Sp. "Chaperone."

Dulcie Lat. "Sweet." Roman name revived for some years at the turn of the 20th century, but extremely unusual now. Cervantes used a slightly different form when he named the heroine of *Don Quixote* **Dulcinea.**

Delcina, Delcine, Delsine, Dulce, Dulcea, Dulci, Dulcia, Dulciana, Dulcibella, Dulcibelle, Dulcine, Dulcinea, Dulcy, Dulsea, Dulsia, Dulsiana, Dulsibell, Dulsine

Dusty (Fem. **Dustin**) An English place name transferred to first name. Probably popularized in this century by English singer Dusty Springfield.

Dustan, Dustee, Dustie, Dustin

Dylana (Fem. **Dylan**) Welsh. "Born from waves." Use of Dylan tends to be a tribute to the poet Dylan Thomas. Most parents today would not hesitate to use the original, masculine name for a girl. Entrepreneur Dylan Lauren.
Dillan, Dillon, Dylane, Dyllan

Dympna Ir. Gael. Saint's name of obscure origin. Many cures of epilepsy and other mental disturbances were attributed to her, and she became known as patroness of the insane. A medieval mental hospital in Belgium, in the town where her bones were discovered, is still going strong.
Dymphna

Earla (Fem. **Earl**) OE. "Nobleman, leader." Several English aristocratic titles such as Duke, Earl, and Baron have been turned into proper names, a sterling example of wishful thinking. Feminine variants are more uncommon.
Earldena, Earldene, Earldina, Earleen, Earlene, Earletta, Erlette, Earley, Earlie, Earline, Erlene, Erletta, Erlette, Erlina, Erline, Erlinia, Ireleen, Irelene, Irelina, Irelene

Eartha OE. "Earth." Used by the Puritans in the 17th century, but obsolete since then. Singer Eartha Kitt.
Erda, Ertha, Herta, Hertha

Easter Name of the holiday, transferred to use as a Christian name predominantly in the 19th century. (Some sources trace it to a variation of **Esther**.) A more common Eastertide name is the French **Pascale**.

Eberta Teut. "Bright."

Ebony Name of the wood, which is prized for its black color. In use since the 1970s with African-American families.

Ebboney, Ebbony, Ebonee, Eboney, Ebonney, Ebonni, Ebonny, Eboni, Ebonie, Ebonyi

Echo Gk. Name of a mythological nymph who was a disembodied voice. One version of her story holds that she pined away of love for Narcissus until only her voice was left.

Eda OE. "Wealthy, happy." Also possibly a variation of Edith.
Ede

Edana (Fem. **Aidan**) Gael. "Fire." Saint Aidan was a 7th-century Irish monk. Although Aidan is still primarily a boy's name (and chugging up the popularity charts at a rapid rate), it is increasingly used for girls as well.
Aidana, Aydana

Edeline OG. "Noble, nobility." Var. **Adeline**.
Edelina

Eden Heb. "Pleasure, delight." It is a short step from the Hebrew meaning of the word to its general association with Paradise. The name is used, infrequently, for boys as well as girls.
Eaden, Eadin, Edenia, Edin

Edina OE. Possibly a form of **Edwina**, or a literary term meaning "From Edinburgh," the capital city of Scotland. Fashion designer Edina Ronay.
Adena, Adina, Edeena, Edyna

Edith OE. "Prosperity/battle." Anglo-Saxon name that continued to be used after the Norman Conquest, and was revived along with other ancient names in the 19th century. By the 1870s it was one of the ten most popular girls' names in Britain, but has been steadily displaced since the 1930s. Writer Edith Wharton; singers Eydie Gorme and Edith Piaf; actresses Dame Edith Evans, Edie Falco.
Dita, Eadie, Eadith, Eda, Ede, Edi, Edie, Edita, Editha, Edithe, Ediva, Edy, Edyth, Edytha, Edythe, Eidith, Eidyth, Eidytha, Eyde, Eydie, Eydith

Edlyn OE. "Small noble one."
Edelynn, Edlin, Edlinn, Edlinna, Edlynn

Edmonda (Fem. **Edmund**) OE. "Wealthy defender." A

popular, and sainted, king of the East Angles in the 9th century gave the masculine version of the name enough popularity to survive the Norman Conquest. The feminine variants are unusual.

Edma, Edmée, Edmonde, Edmunda

Edna Heb. "Pleasure, enjoyment." Perhaps arising from the same root as **Eden**. First used in the 18th century, but very popular in the last half of the 19th century, especially in America. Now almost unheard-of. Poet Edna St. Vincent Millay; novelist Edna Ferber.

Eddi, Eddie, Eddna, Eddnah, Eddy, Ednah

Edrea OE. "Wealthy, powerful."

Edra, Eidra, Eydra

Edris (Fem. **Edric**) Anglo-Saxon. "Wealthy, powerful." The masculine version was an Old English name revived slightly in the 19th century; feminine variants are uncommon.

Edrice, Edriss, Edryce, Eidris, Eidriss, Eydris, Edrys, Idrice, Idris, Idrys

Edwardine (Fem. **Edward**) OE. "Wealthy defender." Rare and slightly awkward variant of a steadily well-used masculine name.

Edwarda, Edwardeen, Edwardene, Edwardina, Edwardyne

Edwige Fr. from OG. "Happy battle."

Eduvigis, Edvig, Edvigis, Edwig, Hedvig, Hedwig, Hedwige

Edwina (Fem. **Edwin**) OE. "Wealth/friend." Feminine variant of an Anglo-Saxon name revived in the 19th century, but never hugely popular.

Edina, Edweena, Edwiena, Edwena, Edwine, Edwinna, Edwyna, Edwynne

Effie Gk. "Pleasant speech." Short version of **Euphemia**, used as an independent name starting in the 1860s. Popularity faded after the 1930s.

Efffemie, Effemy Effi, Effy, Efthemia, Ephie, Eppie, Euphemia, Euphemie, Euphie

Egberta (Fem. **Egbert**) OE. "Brilliant sword."

Egbertha, Egbertina, Egbertine, Egbertyna, Ebgertyne

Egidia Latinized feminine form of **Giles** (Gk. "Kid, young goat"). Mostly Scottish use.

Aegidia, Egidiana

Eglantine OF. Poetic-sounding botanical name for the shrub also known as "sweetbrier."

Eglantyne

Eibhlin Ir. Gael. "Shining, brilliant." Form of **Evelyn,** the English phonetic version, or **Helen**. More commonly anglicized as **Eileen** or **Aileen**.

Aibhlin

Eileen Ir. "Shining, brilliant." Form of **Helen**. Irish names were fashionable in England around 1870, and by the 1920s Eileen was one of the most popular girls' names in Britain. Fashion designer Eileen Fisher; actress Eileen Brennan.

Aileen, Ailene, Alene, Aline, Ayleen, Eila, Eilah, Eilean, Eilleen, Eiley, Eily, Ileana, Ileanna, Ileene, Ilene, Iliana, Ilianna, Leana, Lena, Lianna, Lina

Eiluned Welsh. "Idol." Var. **Lynette**.

Eluned

Eir ONorse. "Peacefulness/mercy."

Eira Welsh. "Snow." Mostly 20th-century use; a pretty name for a winter baby.

Eirian Welsh. "Silver." Another modern Welsh name.

Eithne Ir. "Fire." See **Aithne,** feminine version of **Aidan**.

Aine, Aithnea, Eithne, Ena, Ethnah, Ethnea, Ethnee

Ekaterina Slavic Var. of **Catherine** (Gk. "Pure"). Olympic figure skater Ekaterina Gordeeva.

Yekaterina

Elaine OF. "Bright, shining, light." Form of **Helen**. In the King Arthur myths, Elaine is a maiden who desperately loves Lancelot. Tennyson's version of the tale has her dying of this love, but in an earlier telling, she actually has a son—Galahad—by Lancelot. Tennyson's poetry may have contributed to the 19th-century revival of the name. Film director Elaine May.

Alaina, Alayna, Alayne, Allaine, Elaina, Elana, Elane, Elanna, Elaene, Elayne, Ellaina, Ellaine, Ellane, Ellayne, Lainey, Layney

Elata Lat. "Lofty, elevated."

Elberta (Fem. **Elbert**) OE. "Highborn/shining." Var. **Alberta**.

Elbertha, Elberthe

Eldora Sp. "Covered with gold."

Eldorada, Eldoree, Eldoria, Eldoris

Eleanor Possibly a form of **Helen** (Gk. "light") or from a different Greek root meaning "Clemency, mercy." The queen of Henry II of England, Eleanor of Aquitaine, introduced the name to England in the 13th century, and it has been used steadily since, especially in the U.S., under the influence of much-loved First Lady Eleanor Roosevelt. Charles II's mistress Nell Gwynn; Italian actress Eleonora Duse; women's rights activist Eleanor Smeal.

Aleanor, Alenor, Aleonore, Aline, Allinor, Eileen, Elaine, Eleanora, Eleanore, Elen, Elena, Elenor, Elenora, Elenore, Eleonora, Eleonore, Elianora, Elianore, Elienora, Elienore, Elinor, Elinore, Ella, Elladine, Elleanor, Elleanora, Elle, Ellen, Ellene, Ellenora, Ellenore, Elleonor, Elli, Ellie, Ellin, Ellinor, Ellinore, Elly, Ellyn, Elna, Elnora, Elyn, Enora, Heleanor, Heleonor, Helen, Helena, Helene, Helenora, Leanora, Lena, Lenora, Lenore, Leonora, Leonore, Leora, Lina, Nelda, Nell, Nelle, Nelley, Nelli, Nellie, Nelly, Nonnie, Nora, Norah, Norina

Electra Gk. "Shining, bright." Though the name is derived from the same roots as the word "electricity," many people will associate it with the Greek tragedies of the house of Atreus, told by Aeschylus, Euripides, Sophocles, and retold by Eugene O'Neill in the play *Mourning Becomes Electra*. All versions involve incest, murder, and vengeance.

Alectra, Elektra, Elettra, Ellectra, Ellektra, Ilectra

Elfrida OE. "Elf/power." See **Alfreda**. Uncommon.

Alfrida, Alfrieda, Elfie, Elfre, Elfredah, Elfredda, Elfreeda, Elfrida, Elfrieda, Elfryda, Elfrydah, Ellfreda, Elva, Elvah, Freda, Freddi, Freddy, Freeda, Frieda, Friedah, Fryda

Elga Slavic. "Sacred." See **Olga**.
　　Elgiva, Ellga, Helga
Eliane (Fem. **Elias**) Fr. from Heb. "Jehovah is God."
　　Elia, Eliana, Elianna, Eliette, Elice, Eline, Elyette
Elidi Gk. "Gift of the sun."
Elinda Var. **Belinda**.
Eliora Heb. "The Lord is my light."
　　Eleora, Eliorah, Elleora, Elliora
Elise Fr. var. **Elizabeth** (Heb. "Pledged to God").
　　Eliese, Elisa, Elisee, Elize, Elyce, Elyse, Liese, Liesel,
　　Lieselotte, Liesl, Lise, Lison, Lize
Elisheva Heb. "The Lord is my pledge."
　　Eliseva, Elisheba
Elissa Form of **Alice** or **Elizabeth**. First appeared around
　　the 1930s.
　　Alissa, Allissa, Allyssa, Alyssa, Elissia, Ellissa, Elysa,
　　Elyssa, Elyssia, Ilissa, Ilysa, Ilyssa, Lissa, Lissie,
　　Lissy, Lyssa
Elita Lat. "The elect, chosen."
　　Elitta, Ellita, Lita
Eliza Dim. **Elizabeth**. Frequently used in its own right from
　　the 18th century onward. Especially popular in the first
　　decade of the 20th century. Actress Eliza Dushku.
　　Aliza, Alizah, Elizah, Elyza, Elyzza, Liza
Elizabeth Heb. "Pledged to God." One of the ten most pop-
　　ular girls' names in the U.S. for the past dozen years; in
　　the top 5 in Australia, Canada, and Great Britain. Used in
　　full, it has a pleasant, old-fashioned ring, though some re-
　　search attaches a "seductive" connotation to it (perhaps by
　　association with actress Elizabeth Taylor). It is a source of
　　endless diminutives and nicknames. Saint Elizabeth,
　　mother of John the Baptist; poet Elizabeth Barrett Brown-
　　ing; Queens Elizabeth I and II of England; actresses Eliz-
　　abeth Ashley, Elizabeth Montgomery, Elisabeth Shue,
　　Elizabeth Hurley; politician Elizabeth Dole; suffragette
　　Elizabeth Cady Stanton.
　　Alixyveth, Babette, Belita, Bell, Bella, Belle, Bess,
　　Bessie, Bessy, Beth, Betsey, Betsie, Betsy, Bett,

Betta, Bette, Betti, Bettina, Bettine, Betty, Bettye,
Buffy, Elisa, Elisabet, Elisabeth, Elisabetta, Elise,
Elissa, Eliza, Elizabet, Elizabetta, Elizabette,
Elixyveth, Elle, Elliza, Ellsa, Ellse, Ellsee, Ellsey, Ellsi,
Ellspet, Ellyse, Ellyssa, Ellyza, Elsa, Else, Elsee, Elsie,
Elspet, Elspeth, Elsy, Elyse, Elyssa, Elyza, Elyzza,
Elzbieta, Helsa, Ilsa, Ilsc, Isabel, Isabella, Isabelle,
Isobel, Leesa, Leeza, Lib, Libbey, Libbi, Libbie, Libby,
Libbye, Lilibet, Lisa, Lisabeth, Lisbet, Lisbeth, Lisbett,
Lisbetta, Lisbette, Lise, Lisette, Lissa, Lissi, Lissy, Liz,
Liza, Lizabeth, Lizbeth, Lizette, Lizzi, Lizzy, Lusa,
Lysa, Lysbet, Lysbeth, Lysbette, Lyssa, Lyssie, Lyza,
Lyzbet, Lyzbeth, Lyzbette, Lyzette, Ylisabet,
Ylisabette, Ysabel, Ysabella, Yzabelle

Elkana Heb. "God has made." More commonly used by
men, and a man's name in the Old Testament.
Elkanah, Elkanna

Elke Ger. Var. **Alice** (OG. "Noble, nobility"). Possibly in-
troduced to the English-speaking world by actress Elke
Sommer.
Elka, Ellke, Ilka

Ella OG. "All, completely." Also possibly derived from
Alice, Eleanor, Ellen. Common in the Middle Ages and
revived in America in the late 19th century, but now un-
usual. Singer Ella Fitzgerald.
**Alla, Ela, Elladine, Elletta, Ellette, Elley, Elli, Ellie,
Ellina, Elly**

Ellamae Com. form **Ella** and **May**, two very popular 19th-
century names.
Ellamay

Ellen Var. **Helen** (Gk. "Shining, brightness"). Both forms
have been popular, but rarely at the same time. In Amer-
ica Ellen has dominated since the 1950s, but neither ver-
sion is much used now. A diminutive, **Ellie**, is popular in
Scotland. English actress Ellen Terry; American actresses
Ellen Burstyn, Ellen Barkin, Ellen DeGeneres.
**Elan, Elen, Elena, Elene, Eleni, Elenita, Elenyi, Elin,
Ellan, Ellin, Ellene, Ellie, Ellon, Elly, Ellyn, Elon, Elyn**

Ellice (Fem. **Elias**) Gk. "The Lord is God." Also possibly variant of **Alice** or **Ellis**.
Elice

Elma Dim. of names like **Wilhelmina** (Ger. "Will-helmet") or variant of **Alma** (Lat. "soul").
Ellma

Elmina Dim. **Wilhelmina** (OG. "will/helmet"). Mildly popular in the 19th century.
Almeena, Almena, Almina, Elmeena, Elmena

Elmira Arab. "Aristocratic lady." See **Almera**. Also possibly a feminization of **Elmer** (OE "Highborn and renowned").
Allmera, Allmeera, Almeria, Almira, Almyra, Ellmera, Ellmeria, Ellmeera, Elmeeria, Elmera, Elmeria, Elmerya, Elmyrah, Mera, Meera, Mira, Mirah, Myra, Myrah

Eloise Fr. form of **Louise** (OG. "Renowned in battle"). Made famous in the 12th century by the love letters between Heloise and Abelard. Modern parents, though, are more likely to think of the madcap six-year-old denizen of New York's Plaza Hotel who stars in Kay Thompson's books for children.
Aloysia, Eloisa, Elouisa, Elouise, Heloise

Elrica OG. "Ruler over all."

Elsa Dim. **Elizabeth**. Now rare, in spite of the lingering fame of actress Elsa Lanchester.
Else, Elsie, Elssa, Elsy, Ilsa, Ilse

Elsie Var. **Elizabeth** via its Scottish form, **Elspeth**. Independently used since the 18th century, and extremely popular in the U.S. by the late 19th. After the 1920s, its use faded.
Ellsey, Ellsi, Ellsie, Elsea, Elsee, Elsey, Elsi

Elspeth Scot. var. **Elizabeth**. Unusual outside Scotland. Author Elspeth Huxley.
Elsbeth, Elsbet, Elspet, Elspie

Eluned Welsh. "Idol, image." Used mostly in Wales. The French version, **Lynette**, is more common in the U.S.
Elined, Eiluned, Lanet, Lanette, Linet, Linette, Luned, Lynette, Lynnette

Elva Ir. "Noble, bright." Phonetic anglicization of the unusual Irish name **Ailbhe**.

Ailbhe, Elfie, Elvia, Elvie

Elvina (Fem. **Elvin**) OE. "Noble friend" or "elf friend."

**Alveena, Alvina, Alvine, Alvinia, Elvena, Elveena,
Elvene, Elvenia, Elvine, Elvinia, Vina, Vinni, Vinnie,
Vinny**

Elvira Sp. Meaning unclear, possibly a place name. An
Elvira figures in several versions of the story of Don Juan,
as well as other operas. The name seems to be used more
in art than in life, however.

**Ellvira, Elva, Elveera, Elvera, Elvina, Elvire, Elvyra,
Elwira, Lira**

Elysia Lat. From "Elysium," the mythical home of the
blessed, also known as the "Elysian fields." Dates from
the 1940s.

**Aleesyia, Eleese, Eliese, Elise, Elisia, Elyse, Ileesia,
Ilise, Ilysa, Ilysia, Ilyse**

Emeline OG. Possibly "Industrious." Possibly also a variant of **Emily** or **Amelia**. Norman name revived in the 18th
century, now extremely rare despite its numerous variants.

**Emaleen, Emalene, Emaline, Emalyn, Embline,
Emblyn, Emelen, Emelyn, Emiline, Emlyn, Emmalee,
Emmalene, Emmaline, Emmalyn, Emmalynne,
Emmeline, Emmiline, Emylin, Emylynn**

Emerald Jewel name, less common than **Pearl**, **Ruby**, or
the most popular such name, **Diamond**. Occurs most frequently used in its Spanish form, **Esmeralda**. It is the
birthstone for May. English socialite Emerald Cunard.

Emeralda, Emeraldina, Emeraude, Esmeralda

Emily Lat. Clan name. In spite of the similarity of form, it
has a different root from **Amelia**. Naturally, many of the
variants are very close. A hugely popular name in the 19th
century, lost status after 1900, and is now in favor again.
Poet Emily Dickinson; novelist Emily Brontë, etiquette
maven Emily Post; actress Emily Watson.

**Aemiley, Aemilie, Aimil, Amalea, Amalia, Amalie,
Amelia, Amelie, Ameline, Amelita, Amy, Eimile, Em,
Emalee, Emalia, Emelda, Emelea, Emeli, Emelia,**

Emelie, Emelina, Emeline, Emelita, Emelly, Emely, Emelyn, Emelyne, Emera, Emila, Emilea, Emilee, Emiley, Emili, Emilia, Emilie, Emiline, Emilla, Emillea, Emilley, Emillie, Emilly, Emlyn, Emlynn, Emlynne, Emmalee, Emmalie, Emmaline, Emmalyn, Emmalynn, Emmalynne, Emmelee, Emmely, Emmey, Emmi, Emmie, Emmilee, Emmilie, Emmily, Emmlee, Emmy, Emmye, Emyle, Emylee, Milka

Emina Lat. "Eminent."

Emma OG. "Embracing everything." Royal name in medieval England, and hugely popular at the end of the 19th century. Brought back to notice by Emma Peel in the popular TV series "The Avengers," and is now one of the top girls' names in Ireland and Scotland. Still less common in America, but gaining favor. Lady Emma Hamilton, Lord Nelson's mistress; Emma Bovary of *Madame Bovary;* Jane Austen's novel *Emma;* actresses Emma Samms, Emma Thompson.

Em, Ema, Emelina, Emeline, Emelyne, Emmaline, Emmalyn, Emmalynn, Emmalynne, Emme, Emmeleia, Emmeline, Emmelyn, Emmelyne, Emmet, Emmett, Emmette, Emmi, Emmie, Emmot, Emmott, Emmy, Emmye

Emmanuelle (Fem. **Emmanuel**) Heb. "God is among us." Fashion designer Emmanuelle Khanh.

Emanuela, Emanuella, Emanuelle, Emmanuella, Emonualle, Emonualle

Ena Short for names like **Georgina, Regina,** etc. Queen Victoria's granddaughter Princess Victoria Eugenie, who became queen of Spain, was known as Princess Ena.

Eena, Ina

Enid Welsh. "Life, spirit." Name from the King Arthur myths revived mildly in the early 19th century and quite popular in England by the 1920s. Never much used in America. Author Enid Bagnold.

Eanid, Ened, Enedd, Enidd, Enyd, Enydd

Enrica (Fem. **Henry**) It. "Home ruler."

Enricka, Enricketta, Enriqueta, Enriquette

Erica (Fem. **Eric**) Scan. "Ruler forever." Though a staple in

Scandinavia, it wasn't used in the English-speaking world until the late 19th century. It still has a strongly European flair. Writer Erica Jong; singers Erykah Badu, Rickie Lee Jones; actresses Ricki Lake, Erika Christensen.

Aerica, Aericka, Airica, Airicka, Airika, Enrica, Enrika, Eraca, Ericka, Erika, Erricka, Errika, Eryca, Erycka, Eyrica, Rickee, Ricki, Rickie, Ricky, Rikki, Rikky

Erin Ir. Gael. "From the island to the west." Erin is a literary term for Ireland, hence the name's popularity among Irish-descended families. Ironically, it is not much used in Ireland itself.

Aeran, Aerenne, Aerin, Airin, Eire, Eirin, Eirinn, Eiryn, Eirynn, Erina, Erinn, Eryn, Erynn

Erlinda Heb. "Spirited."

Erma Var. **Irma** (OG. "Universal, complete"). Enjoyed a brief period of use from around 1890 to 1940; now almost unknown. Humorist Erma Bombeck.

Ermina, Erminia, Erminie, Irma, Irminia, Irminie, Hermia, Hermine, Herminie, Hermione

Ermine OF. "Weasel." Has come to be synonymous with the trappings of royalty, since the robes of royalty are typically trimmed with the fur and tails of ermine, a variety of weasel that turns white in winter.

Ermin, Ermina, Erminia, Erminne

Erna Var. **Ernestine**. Also possibly derived from an Irish root meaning "to know." Modern use.

Ernaline, Ernalynn

Ernestine (Fem. **Ernest**) OE. "Sincere." Use at the end of the 19th century follows **Ernest**'s enormous popularity for boys at that period. A bit dated now.

Erna, Ernaline, Ernesta, Ernestina, Ernestyna

Erwina (Fem. **Erwin**) OE. "Boar/friend."

Irwina

Esma Var. **Esmé**. Possibly short form of **Esmeralda**.

Esmée Fr. "Esteemed." Originally a male name brought to Scotland by a French cousin of James VI. Now used more for girls, though scarce. J.D. Salinger titled a short story "For Esmé with Love and Squalor."

Esmae, Esmay, Esmé, Ismé

Esmeralda Sp. "Emerald." Jewel name first used in the 1880s, and more common than **Emerald**.

Em, Emmie, Emerald, Emerant, Emeraude, Esma, Esmaralda, Esmarelda, Esmaria, Esmie, Esmiralda, Esmiralde, Esmirelda, Ezmeralda

Esperanza Sp. "Hope."

Esperance, Esperantia

Esta Var. **Esther**.

Estelle OF. "Star." See **Astra, Esther, Stella**. French form of a name apparently coined by Charles Dickens for a character in his 1861 novel *Great Expectations*. Her name is **Estella**, and perhaps because she's such an unhappy creature, Estelle is the more common form of the name. Actresses Estelle Getty, Estelle Parsons.

Essie, Estel, Estele, Estell, Estella, Estrella, Estrellita, Stella, Stelle

Esther Per. "Star." More particularly, the planet Venus. Esther in the Bible was an orphan named Hadassah who became wife of King Ahasuerus under her new name. Her story is told in the Old Testament Book of Esther. In the U.S. the name reached its peak of popularity around 1900, and is now unusual. Swimming actress Esther Williams; cosmetics pioneer Estee Lauder.

Essie, Essy, Esta, Estée, Ester, Ettey, Etti, Ettie, Etty, Hester, Hesther, Hettie, Hetty, Hittie

Etana (Fem. **Ethan**) Heb. "Strength of purpose."

Ethel OE. "Noble." A short form of various old-fashioned names like **Etheldreda**. First appeared on its own in the 1840s, and by the 1870s was very popular. This is one 19th-century name, however, that is unlikely to be revived in the 21st century. Actresses Ethel Barrymore, Ethel Merman.

Ethelda, Ethelin, Ethelinda, Etheline, Ethelyn, Ethelynne, Ethill, Ethille, Ethlin, Ethlyn, Ethlynn, Ethyll

Etheldreda OE. "Noble power." Saint's name from the 7th century, occasionally used in Britain. **Audrey** is the more common modern form.

Ethelinda OG. "Noble serpent." Not a composite, but an

old name revived in the 19th century, along with many variants.

Athelina, Ethelenda, Ethelene, Ethelind, Ethelinde, Etheline, Ethlin, Ethlinda, Etholinda, Ethylind

Etta Feminine diminutive suffix (**Georgette, Henriette**) that has attained the status of an independent name.

Ettie, Etty

Eudocia Gk. "Well thought of."

Docia, Docie, Doxie, Doxy, Eudokia, Eudosia, Eudoxia

Eudora Gk. "Generous gift." Unusual name from Greek mythology (Eudora was a minor goddess) that was somewhat popular at the turn of the 20th century. Writer Eudora Welty.

Dora, Dorey, Dorie, Eudore

Eugenia (Fem. **Eugene**) Gk. "Wellborn." The French form, **Eugenie,** was made famous by Napoleon III's beautiful empress, and has persisted in the European royal houses. Recently used in Britain for the second daughter of the Duke and Duchess of York. Actresses Gena Rowlands, Geena Davis.

Eugenie, Evgenia, Geena, Gena, Gene, Genia, Genie, Gina, Janie, Jeena, Jenna, Jennie

Eulalia Gk. "Sweet-speaking."

Eula, Eulalee, Eulalie, Eulaylia, Eulaylie, Lallie, Lally

Eunice Gk. "Victorious." Biblical name: In the New Testament, Eunice is the mother of Timothy. Occasionally used in the modern era. Philanthropist Eunice Kennedy Shriver.

Eunices, Eunike, Euniss, Unice, Uniss

Euphemia Gk. "Favorable speech." Early Christian name borne by a 4th-century virgin martyr, but more common in its short forms like **Effie** through the 19th century. Rare since the 1930s.

Effam, Effie, Effy, Ephan, Ephie, Eufemia, Euphemie, Euphemia, Euphie, Phemie, Fanny

Eurydice Gk. In mythology, the wife of the musician Orpheus. She was poisoned by a snake, and Orpheus went to the underworld to find her. His music so charmed Hades that he was allowed to bring her back to life, if he could lead her to the upper world without looking at her. He failed, and she returned to Hades.

Euridice, Euridiss

Eustacia (Fem. **Eustace**) Lat. "Giving fruit." The male form was used a bit in the 19th century, but the feminine form is rare.

Eustacie, Stacey, Stacia, Stacie, Stacy

Eva Form of **Eve** (Heb. "Life") More common in Europe. Actress Eva Gabor; dictator Eva Peron.

Eeva, Evita

Evadne Gk. Meaning unclear, but may mean something like "Enjoying good fortune" or "Pleasing one."

Evadney, Evadnie, Evanne

Evangeline Gk. "Good news." Derived from "evangel," the term that came to be used for the Gospels, or the four New Testament accounts of Christ's life. First used in English by Alfred Tennyson in his 1847 poem "Evangeline."

Engie, Eva, Evangelia, Evangelina, Evangelista, Evangeliste, Eve, Vangie, Vangy

Evania Gk. "Peaceful."

Evanne, Evannie, Evanny

Eve Heb. "Life." In the form **Eva,** somewhat popular from the mid-19th century, usually as a shortened version of **Evangeline**. Eve, the French form of the name, is used steadily but not in great numbers. In Ireland the Gaelic form, **Aoife,** is very popular. A clever name for the first girl in a family of boys. Actress Eve Arden; pop musician Eve.

Aoife, Eba, Ebba, Eva, Evaleen, Evelina, Eveline, Evelyn, Evetta, Evette, Evey, Evie, Evita, Evlyn, Evonne, Evvie, Evvy, Evy

Evelina OG. or OF., possibly "Hazelnut." Norman import to Britain, where it was brought to prominence by Fanny Burney's popular novel *Evelina,* in the 18th century. Gradually overwhelmed by **Evelyn**.

Eveleen, Evelene, Eveline, Evelyne

Evelyn OG. Obscure meaning, from the same root as **Evelina**. Not, as it would seem, a combination of **Eve** and

Lynn, but originally a surname and later a boy's name. Its greatest popularity came in the first quarter of the 20th century in both Britain and the U.S. Track star Evelyn Ashford.

Aveline, Evaleen, Evalyn, Evalynn, Evalynne, Eveleen, Evelene, Eveline, Evelyne, Evelynn, Evelynne, Evilyn, Evlin, Evline, Evlyn, Evlynn

Evette Fr. Variant form of **Yvette,** in turn a diminutive of **Yvonne.** Also used as a diminutive for **Eve,** though the roots are different.

Eevette, Evetta, Eyvetta, Eyvette

Evonne Fr. Var. **Yvonne.** Tennis star Evonne Goolagong.

Evon, Eyvonne

 Fabia (Fem. **Fabian**) Lat. clan name. Possibly meaning "One who grows beans."

Fabiana, Fabiane, Fabianna, Fabienne, Fabiola

Fabrizia It. "Works with the hands."

Fabrice, Fabricia, Fabrienne, Fabriqua, Fabritzia

Faida Arab. "Plentiful."

Fayda

Faith ME. "Loyalty." One of the most common of the virtue names used by the Puritans, along with **Hope** and **Charity.** Modern use is sparing. Actress Faith Prince; singer Faith Hill.

Fae, Faithe, Fay, Faye, Fayth, Faythe, Fe

Faline Lat. "Like a cat." Unusual spelling of a familiar term. Second-time parents may recognize this as the name of Bambi's girlfriend in the Disney cartoon.

Faeleen, Fayline, Felina, Feyline

Fallon Ir. Gael. "Descended from a ruler." Surname brought to public notice and some popularity by a character on the TV serial "Dynasty."

Fallan, Fallen

Fanny (Dim. **Frances**) Lat. "From France." This form became extremely popular in the early 19th century and remained a favorite until around 1910, when its inexplicable adoption as a term for the buttocks extinguished it as a first name. Cookbook author Fannie Farmer; author Fannie Flagg; actress Fanny Ardant.

Fan, Fania, Fannee, Fanney, Fannie

Farica (Dim. **Frederica**) OG. "Peaceful ruler."

Faricka, Fericka, Flicka

Farrah ME. "Lovely, pleasant." Unknown as a first name until the enormous fame of actress Farrah Fawcett.

Fara, Farah, Farra

Fatima Arab. Meaning unclear, though Fatima was Mohammed's favorite daughter. According to the Koran, she was one of only four perfect women in the world. Fatima is also the name of Bluebeard's last wife in some versions of that tale.

Fateema, Fateemah, Fatimah, Fatma, Fatmah

Faustine (Fem. **Faust**) Lat. "Fortunate, enjoying good luck." There is some irony to the name, since the Faust of legend sold his soul to the Devil. Two Roman empresses were called Faustina, and the name was common under the Roman Empire, but little used today.

Fausta, Fauste, Faustina

Fawn OF. "Young deer." Names for girl children have been drawn from various segments of the natural world—flowers, gems, seasons, months—but animal names, for some reason, are rarer. Biographer Fawn Brodie.

Faina, Fanya, Faun, Fauna, Faunia, Fawna, Fawne, Fawnia, Fawnya

Fay OF. "Fairy." Or Dim. **Faith**. First used in significant numbers in the 1920s, probably inspired by the fame of actresses Fay Wray and Fay Compton. Actress Faye Dunaway.

Fae, Fay, Faye, Fee, Fey

Fayette OF. "Little fairy."

Fayetta
Fedora Gr. Var. **Theodora** (Gk. "Gift of God"). In this form, also a kind of soft felt hat with a modest brim, much favored by men until the early 1960s.
Fadora
Felda OG. "From the field."
Felicia (Fem. **Felix**) Lat. "Lucky, fortunate, happy." **Felice** was used in Britain until the early 19th century, when it was replaced by Felicia, which has since been supplanted by **Felicity**. None of them is very common. Actress Phylicia Rashad.
Falecia, Faleece, Falicia, Falisha, Falishia, Felice, Feliciana, Felicidad, Felicie, Felicienne, Félicité, Felicity, Felis, Felisa, Felise, Felisha, Feliss, Felita, Feliz, Feliza, Felysse, Filicia, Filisha, Phalicia, Phalisha, Phelicia, Phylicia, Phyllicia, Phyllisha
Fenella Ir. Gael. "White shoulder." Var. **Fionnula**. This is the anglicized form.
Finella, Fynella
Fern OE. "Fern." Also, diminutive of **Fernanda**. Unusual botanical name.
Ferna, Ferne
Fernanda (Fem. **Ferdinand**) OG. Possibly "Peace/courage" or "Voyage/courage." Very rare feminine of an equally rare male name.
Anda, Annda, Ferdinanda, Ferdinande, Fern, Fernande, Fernandina, Fernandine, Nan, Nanda
Fernley OE. Place name. "Fern meadow." In Britain, has been used as a first name since the turn of the century for both sexes. Little heard in the U.S.
Fernlea, Fernlee, Fernleigh, Fernlie, Fernly
Fidelity Lat. "Loyalty." Latin form of **Faith**. In the U.S. use of the word for large financial institutions diminishes its appeal as a proper name.
Fedila, Fidella, Fideia, Fidele, Fidelia, Fidelita, Fidella
Fifi Fr. Dim. **Josephine** (Heb. "Jehovah increases"). The stereotypical name for a French poodle, which would seem to limit its human use.
Fifine

Filia Gk. "Friendship." Currently popular in Greece.
Philia

Filippa Var. **Philippa** (Gk. "Lover of horses").

Filomena It. Var. **Philomena** (Gk. "Loved one").

Fina Sp. Dim. **Josefina** (Heb. "Jehovah increases").

Fiona Ir. Gael. "Fair, pale." Apparently coined by an English author at the turn of the 20th century, and its popularity in Britain has been growing since the 1930s. Rare in the U.S. Musician Fiona Apple.
Fee, Ffion, Ffiona, Ffyona, Fione, Fionna, Fyona

Fionnula Ir. Gael. "White shoulder."
Fenella, Finella, Finola, Fionnuala, Fionnualagh, Nola, Nuala

Flaminia Lat. "Priest."

Flana Ir. Gael. "Russet hair." Author Flannery O'Connor.
Flanagh, Flanna, Flannerey, Flannery

Flavia Lat. "Yellow hair." Originally a Latin clan name, and common enough in the Roman Empire, but never revived in an English-speaking country.
Flavie, Flaviere, Flavyere

Fleur Fr. "Flower." In John Galsworthy's *The Forsyte Saga,* one of the principal characters is called Fleur, which brought the name to some prominence. The BBC TV adaptation of the 1970s also provoked a spate of use.
Fleurette, Fleurine

Flora Lat. "Flower." The name of the Roman goddess of springtime, and of a 9th-century martyred saint. Flora Macdonald was a Scottish heroine who helped Bonnie Prince Charlie escape the English. The name was naturally popular in Scotland, and throughout England in the last half of the 19th century. Now little used.
Fiora, Fiordenni, Fiore, Fiorella, Fiori, Fleur, Flo, Flor, Floralia, Flore, Florella, Florelle, Florentia,Florentina, Florenza, Florenzia, Floria, Florida, Florie, Florine, Floris, Florise, Florrie, Florry, Flory

Florence Lat. "In bloom." Used for both men and women until the 17th century, when it faded from sight. Modern use is almost entirely inspired by the fame of Florence

Nightingale, who was actually named for the Italian city where she was born. Like many names popular in the Victorian era, it fell out of fashion by the 1930s. Athlete Florence "Flo Jo" Griffith Joyner; actress Florence Henderson.

Fiorentina, Fiorenza, Flo, Floellen, Flor, Flora, Florance, Flore, Florenca, Florencia, Florencita, Florentia, Florentina, Florentyna, Florenza, Florenzia, Flori, Floria, Floriane, Floriana, Florie, Florina, Florincia, Florinda, Florine, Floris, Florrance, Florrie, Florry, Florynce, Floss, Flossey, Flossie, Flossy

Flower OF. "Blossom."

Florida Lat. "Flowery." Spanish Var. **Florence**. Spanish explorer Ponce de Leon dubbed the southern state "Florida" for the many flowers he found there. Infrequent current use as a first name probably refers to the state.

Fortune Lat. "Good fate." Garden-variety name in the Roman Empire; Fortuna was the goddess of happiness. Revived somewhat by the Puritans but almost unknown today.

Fortuna, Fortunata

Fran (Dim. **Frances**) Lat. "From France." Used as a given name on its own. Comedienne Fran Drescher; writer Fran Lebowitz.

Frani, Frannee, Franni, Frannie, Franny

Frances (Fem. **Francis**) Lat. "From France." Until the 17th century, **Francis** was used for both sexes. Spelled with an "e," it was a very popular choice in the first quarter of the 20th century, but little used since then. Actresses Fanny Brice, Frances McDormand, Franka Potente.

Fan, Fancey, Fanchette, Fancie, Fancy, Fanechka, Fania, Fanney, Fannie, Fanny, Fanya, Fran, Francee, Franceline, Francene, Francesca, Francess, Francetta, Francette, Francey, Franchesca, Franci, Francie, Francine, Francisca, Franciska, Francoise, Francyne, Frania, Franie, Frank, Franka, Frankie, Franky, Franni, Frannie, Franny, Fransabelle, Fransabella, Franzetta, Franzi, Franziska, Fronia

Freda OG. "Peaceful." Dim. **Alfreda, Frederica,**

Winifred. Most popular at the end of the 19th century, when **Fred** was fashionable for men. As **Frida,** currently quite popular in Spain. Artist Frida Kahlo.

Freada, Freeda, Freida, Frida, Frieda, Frydda

Fredella Com. form **Freda** and **Ella**.

Fredelle

Frederica OG. "Peaceful ruler." Following the popularity of **Frederic,** substantially used in the late 19th century, but now unusual. Opera singer Frederica von Stade.

Farica, Federica, Fred, Fredalena, Freddee, Freddey, Freddi, Freddie, Freddy, Fredericha, Frederickina, Frederine, Frederique, Fredi, Fredia, Fredie, Fredricia, Fredrika, Frerika, Friederike, Rica, Ricki, Rickie, Ricky, Rikki, Rikky

Freya Scan. "Highborn lady." In Norse myth, the goddess of love, corresponding perhaps to the Roman Venus. Friday is named for her. Author Freya Stark.

Fraya

Fritzi (Fem. **Fritz**) OG. "Peaceful ruler." German form of **Frederick**.

Fulvia Lat. "Blond one."

Gabrielle (Fem. **Gabriel**) Heb. "Heroine of God." Used in English-speaking countries for the last ninety years, though the Italian form, **Gabriella,** has been popular since the 1950s. Gabriel is an archangel who appears in Christian, Jewish, and Muslim texts. Tennis player Gabriela Sabatini; fashion designer Gabrielle "Coco" Chanel; volleyball player Gabby Reece.

Gabbe, Gabbi, Gabbie, Gabi, Gabriel, Gabriela, Gabriella, Gabriell, Gabriellen, Gabriellia, Gabrila,

Gabryel, Gabryelle, Gabryella, Gaby, Gabysia, Gavi, Gavra, Gavraila, Gavrielle, Gavrila, Gavrilla, Gavrina

Gada Heb. "Fortunate."

Gaea Gk. "The earth."

Gaia, Gaiea, Gala

Gaetana It. Place name. Gaeta is a region in southern Italy; the Gulf of Gaeta is just north of Naples.

Gaetane

Gail Heb. "My father rejoices." A diminutive of **Abigail** with an unusually strong life of its own, dating from around 1940, with special popularity in the 1950s in the U.S. Authors Gael Greene, Gail Sheehy, Gail Godwin; track star Gail Devers.

Gael, Gahl, Gaila, Gaile, Gaill, Gal, Gale, Gayel, Gayelle, Gayla, Gayle, Gayleen, Gaylene, Gayline, Gayll, Gaylla, Gaylle

Galatea Gk. "White as milk." In Greek myth the sculptor Pygmalion fell in love with his ivory statue of Aphrodite, and prayed to the goddess to bring the statue to life. When his prayer was answered, he married his creation. The myth, via G. B. Shaw's play *Pygmalion,* is the source of the musical *My Fair Lady.*

Galatée, Galathea

Galiena OG. "High one."

Galiana, Galianna, Galliena, Galyena

Galina Rus.Var. **Helen** (Gk. "Shining brightly"). Currently very popular in Russia.

Galya

Gallia Lat. "Gaul." The Latin term for the country that would later be known as France; a name used from time to time for French babies.

Gala, Galla

Galya Heb. "The Lord has redeemed."

Galia, Gallia, Gailya

Gardenia Flower name. The powerfully sweet-smelling flower is named for the 18th-century Scottish naturalist Alexander Garden, who first classified it.

Gardeenia

Garland OF. "Garland, wreath."
Garlande, Garldina

Garnet ME. Jewel name, appropriate for January, since it is the birthstone for that month.
Garnette, Granata, Grenata, Grenatta

Gavrila Var. **Gabrielle** (Heb. "Heroine of God").
Gavrilla, Gavryla, Gavrylla

Gay OF. "Glad, lighthearted." A surname in the Middle Ages, used as a first name very heavily in the mid-20th century. The widespread informal use of the word to mean "homosexual" has limited its current use as a name.
Gae, Gai, Gaye

Gaynor Welsh. "White and smooth, soft." Var. **Guinevere**. Used primarily in Britain.
Gaenor, Gayna, Gayner

Gazella Lat. "Gazelle." Unusual use of the animal name as a given name. Gazelles are traditionally thought of as very graceful creatures.
Gazelle

Gemini Gk. "Twin." Appropriate for either a child born under the sign of Gemini, or for one of a pair of twins.
Gemella, Gemelle, Gemina

Gemma It. "Precious stone." Did not, curiously, come into fashion with other jewel names in the late 19th century, but is slightly popular now. Probably helped along by the 1940 canonization of the Italian Saint Gemma, an ordinary young woman whose religious life included manifestations of the stigmata, or the marks of Christ's wounds.
Jemma, Jemsa

Gene Dim. **Eugenia** (Gk. "Wellborn") or Var. **Jean** (Heb. "The Lord is gracious"). More common for boys; actress Gene Tierney may have pioneered use of this spelling for girls.
Genie

Geneva OF. "Juniper tree." There is considerable confusion about the sources of a constellation of names that include Geneva, **Ginevra**, and **Genevieve**. Use of Geneva may refer to the Swiss city; on the other hand, it may also be a reference to the juniper tree, whose old Dutch name was *genever* (hence "gin," which is flavored with juniper berries). Various forms of Genevieve also overlap.

Gena, Genever, Genevia, Genevra, Genevre, Genovefa, Genoveffa, Genoveva, Ginebra, Ginevra, Ginevre, Janeva, Janevra, Jenovefa, Jineeva, Jineva, Joneva, Jonevah

Genevieve A name whose origin is unclear, but sources suggest possibly OG. "White wave" or Celt. "Race of women." Saint Genevieve, the patroness of Paris, was a 5th-century virgin who defended Paris against the depredations of Attila the Hun, among others. Use in English-speaking countries has tended to simmer along at a low level. Actress Genevieve Bujold.

Gena, Genavieve, Geneva, Geneveeve, Genivieve, Gennie, Genny, Genovera, Genoveva, Gina, Janeva, Jenevieve, Jennie, Jenny

Georgette Fr. from Lat. "Farmer." The French form of **George,** in mild use since the 1940s. A purposely wrinkled fabric called georgette was named after its French creator. Author Georgette Heyer; socialite Georgette Mosbacher.

Georgetta, Georjetta, Jorjetta, Jorjette

Georgia (Fem. **George**) Lat. "Farmer." The preferred feminine of George in the U.S. and currently quite fashionable in England. A long-ago farmer in Connecticut is reputed to have named each of his ten daughters for a state, and presumably Georgia was one of the eldest, along with **Virginia** and **Carolina**. Painter Georgia O'Keefe.

George, Georgeann, Georgeanne, Georgeina, Georgena, Georgene, Georgetta, Georgette, Georgiana, Georgianna, Georgianne, Georgie, Georgienne, Georgina, Georgine, Georgyann, Georgyanne, Georgyana, Giorgia, Giorgina, Giorgyna, Jorgina

Georgina (Fem. **George**) Lat. "farmer." A simpler form than **Georgiana,** which has also been used regularly.

Georgeina, Georgena, Georgene, Georgejean, Georgiana, Georgianna, Georgianne, Georgienne, Georgine, Georgyana, Giorgina

Geraldine (Fem. **Gerald**) OG./Fr. "Spear ruler." Though the form was coined in the 16th century, its real popularity followed the fashion for Gerald, in the mid-19th century through the 1950s. Actresses Geraldine Chaplin, Geraldine Fitzgerald; politician Geraldine Ferraro.

Deena, Dina, Dyna, Geralda, Geraldeen, Geraldene, Geraldina, Geralyn, Geralynne, Gerdene, Gerdine, Geri, Gerianna, Gerianne, Gerilynn, Gerri, Gerrilyn, Gerroldine, Gerry, Giralda, Jeraldeen, Jeraldene, Jeraldine, Jeralee, Jere, Jeri, Jerilene, Jerrie, Jerrileen, Jerroldeen, Jerry

Geranium Flower name, though the name of the flower itself derives from the Greek for "crane."

Gerda ONorse. "Shelter."

Garda, Geerda

Germaine Fr. "From Germany." Use today may reflect admiration for the famous author and feminist Germaine Greer.

Germain, Germana, Germane, Germayn, Germayne, Jarmaine, Jermain, Jermaine, Jermane, Jermayn, Jermayne

Gertrude OG. "Strength of a spear." An old name (there was a 7th-century Saint Gertrude) revived to immense popularity with the late 19th-century fashion for the antique. Became so common that it suffered the corresponding fall from favor, and is now resoundingly out of style. Writer Gertrude Stein; actress Gertrude Lawrence.

Geertruide, Geltruda, Geltrudis, Gerda, Gert, Gerta, Gerte, Gerti, Gertie, Gertina, Gertraud, Gertrud, Gertruda, Gertrudis, Gerty, Traudl, Trude, Trudi, Trudie, Trudy

Ghaliya Arab. "Sweet-smelling."

Ghislaine Fr. Unusual name of unclear origin and meaning.

Gillan, Gislaine

Ghita It. Dim. **Margherita** (Gk. "Pearl").

Geeta, Gita

Giacinta It. "Hyacinth."

Giacintha, Jacinta, Jacintha, Jacynth, Jiacintha, Yacinta, Yacintha

Gianina (Fem. **John**) It. from Heb. "God is gracious." The age-old favorite boy's name has spawned endless variants, both masculine and feminine.

Cinetta, Gianetta, Giannina, Giannine, Ginetta, Ginette, Ginnette, Janina, Janine, Jeannine, Jeeanina

Gilberte (Fem. **Gilbert**) OG. "Shining pledge." French variant of a Norman name that was fairly popular in the north of Britain.

Berta, Bertie, Berty, Gigi, Gilberta, Gilbertha, Gilberthe, Gilbertina, Gilbertine, Gill, Gillie, Gilly

Gilda OE. "Gilded." More scholarly sources trace Gilda to **Ermengilda,** a now obsolete Anglo-Saxon name. Actress Gilda Radner.

Gillian Lat. "Youthful." Anglicization of **Juliana**. A standard name in the Middle Ages in England, and revived for about 40 years in this century, but fading since the sixties. Actress Gillian Anderson. Never widespread in the U.S., though its diminutive, **Jill,** had quite a fashionable spell.

Ghilian, Ghiliane, Ghillian, Gilian, Giliana, Gill, Gillan, Gillianna, Gillianne, Gillie, Gillyanne, Jillian, Jillianne, Jillyan, Jyllian

Gina Dim. **Regina, Angelina**, etc. Also could be considered a feminization of **Gene,** or a variant of **Jean**. Independent use dates from the 1920s, concentrated in the 1950s. Currently fashionable in Spain. Actresses Gina Lollobrigida, Geena Davis, Gena Rowlands.

Geena, Geina, Gena, Ginette, Ginna, Jena, Jeena, Jenna

Ginger Lat. "Ginger." Also can be a diminutive of **Virginia** (Lat. "Virgin"). Not to be confused with the usual botanical names, for it depends almost completely on the fame of actress Ginger Rogers, whose given name was Virginia.

Gingee, Gingie, Jinger

Ginny Dim. **Virginia** (Lat. "Virgin").

Ginnee, Ginnie, Jinnee, Jinnie, Jinny

Gioia It. "Joy." Unusual form in this country.

Gioya, Joya

Giovanna (Fem. **John**) It. from Heb. "God is gracious."

Giovana, Jovana, Jovanna, Jovanne

Giselle OG. "Pledge/hostage." Use may reflect a fondness for the famous 19th-century ballet whose tragic heroine is a peasant girl betrayed by a noble suitor. Model Gisele Bundchen.
Ghisele, Ghisella, Gisela, Gisele, Gisella, Giza, Gizela, Gizella

Gitana Sp. "Gypsy."
Gitane, Gitanna, Jeetanna

Gitta Dim. **Brigitte** (Ir. Gael. "Strength, power").
Gitte

Giulia (Fem. **Giulio**) It. from Lat. "Youthful."
Giula, Giuliana, Giulietta, Giullia, Jiulia, Jiuliana, Jiuliya, Jiyulia, Julia, Juliana, Julie, Juliet, Julietta, Juliette, Jullia, Julliana, Julliane

Giuseppina (Fem. **Giuseppe**) It. from Heb. "The Lord adds."
Giuseppa, Josefina

Giustinia (Fem. **Justin**) It. from Lat. "Just, fair."
Giustina, Justina, Justine, Justiniana

Gladys Welsh. Var. **Claudia** (Lat. "Lame"). Suddenly glamorous in the late 19th century, and used in several Edwardian romantic novels, which further heightened its appeal. By the 1930s, beginning to be dated, and now rare. Singer Gladys Knight.
Glad, Gladdis, Gladdys, Gladi, Gladyss, Gwladys, Gwyladyss

Glenda Welsh. "Fair and good." Mildly popular from the 1930s to the 1960s. Actress Glenda Jackson.
Glennda

Glenna (Fem. **Glenn**) Ir. Gael. "Glen." A glen is a narrow valley between hills. Actresses Glenn Close, Glenne Headley.
Gleana, Glenda, Gleneen, Glenene, Glenine, Glen, Glenn, Glenne, lennene, Glennette, Glennie

Glenys Welsh. "Holy."
Glenice, Glenis, Glennice, Glennis, Glennys

Gloria Lat. "Glory." Apparently coined by playwright George Bernard Shaw, in 1898's *You Never Can Tell;* the form **Gloriana** had earlier been used to refer in flattering fashion to Queen Elizabeth I. The exposure given the name by actress Gloria Swanson was probably crucial to its popularity from the 1920s through the 1960s. Now a bit passé. Writers Gloria Steinem, Gloria Naylor; singer Gloria Estefan.

Glaura, Glaurea, Glora, Glorea, Gloree, Glorey, Gloreya, Glori, Glorie, Gloriana, Gloriane, Glorie, Glorra, Glorria, Glory, Glorya, Gloryan, Gloryanna, Gloryanne

Glynis Welsh. "Small glen." Related to **Glenn** and its variants. Popular in the middle of the 20th century, but mostly in Britain. Actress Glynis Johns.

Glinnis, Glinyce, Glinys, Glinyss, Glynnis

Godiva OE. "God's gift." According to the famous story, the 11th century Lady Godiva rode through the town of Coventry naked, covered only by her long hair. Her motive (generally forgotten) was a pact with her husband, the Earl of Mercia, who relieved the townsfolk of certain taxes after her ride.

Golda OE. "Gold." Use is frequently a tribute to the late Israeli Prime Minister Golda Meir. Actress Goldie Hawn.

Goldarina, Goldarine, Goldee, Goldi, Goldie, Goldina, Goldy, Goldia

Grace Lat. "Grace." Originally had nothing to do with physical grace, but rather with divine favor and mercy. Used in that sense by the Puritans, and taken to America, where it was very fashionable at the turn of the century. Periods of popularity followed in England (in the twenties) and Scotland (through the fifties). Little used now, but ripe for revival. Actress and princess Grace Kelly; singer Grace Jones; choreographer Graciela Daniele.

Engracia, Eugracia, Gracee, Gracey, Gracia, Graciana, Gracie, Graciela, Graciella, Gracija, Gracina, Gracious, Grata, Gratia, Gratiana, Gratiela, Gratiella, Grayce, Grazia, Graziella, Grazina, Graziosa, Grazyna

Grainne Ir. Gael. "Love." Primarily used in Ireland.

Grainnia, Grania

Greer Scot. Dim. **Gregory**. (Lat. "Alert, watchful"). Given fame by actress Greer Garson, whose mother's maiden name it was.

Grier

Gregoria (Fem. **Gregory**) Lat. "Alert, watchful."

Gregoriana, Gregorijana, Gregorina, Gregorine, Gregorya, Gregoryna

Greta Ger. Dim. **Margaret** (Gk. "Pearl"). Most used during the 1930s, clearly inspired by Greta Garbo. Marathon runner Greta Waitz.

Greeta, Gretal, Gretchen, Grete, Gretel, Gretha, Grethe, Grethel, Gretna, Gretta, Grette, Grietje, Gryta

Gretchen Ger. Dim. **Margaret** (Gk. "Pearl"). Used on its own in English-speaking countries in this century.

Griselda OG. "Gray fighting maid." In a famous tale told by both Boccaccio and Chaucer, "Patient Griselda" is a meek wife who submits to numerous trials devised by her husband to test her submissiveness. The name has long since been eclipsed by its short form, **Zelda**.

Chriselda, Gricely, Grisel, Griseldis, Griselly, Grishelda, Grishilde, Grissel, Grizel, Grizelda, Gryselde, Gryzelde, Selda, Zelda

Gudrun Scan. "Battle."

Gudren, Gudrid, Gudrin, Gudrinn, Gudruna, Gudrunn, Gudrunne, Guthrun, Guthrunn, Guthrunne

Guida It. "Guide."

Guinevere Welsh. "White and smooth, soft." The name of King Arthur's ill-fated queen. The most common form today is **Jennifer**.

Gaenna, Gaynor, Genever, Genevieve, Genevra, Geniffer, Geniver, Genivra, Genna, Gennie, Gennifer, Genny, Ginevra, Guenever, Guenevere, Gueniveer, Guenna, Guennola, Guinever, Guinna, Gwen, Gweniver, Gwenn, Gwennie, Gwennola, Gwennora, Gwennore, Gwenny, Gwenora, Gwenore, Gwyn, Gwynn, Gwynna, Gwynne, Janifer, Jen, Jeni, Jenifer, Jennee, Jenni, Jennie, Jennifer, Jenny, Wendee, Wendie, Wendy, Win, Winne, Winnie, Winny

Gulielma (Fem. **Wilhelm**) It. from OG. "will-helmet."

Guglielma

Gunhilda ONorse. "Battle-maid."
   Gunhilde, Gunilda, Gunilla, Gunna, Gunnel, Gunnhilda
Gustava (Fem. **Gustav**) Swed. "Staff of the gods."
   Gustha
Gwen Dim. **Gwendolyn, Guinevere**. Often given as an independent name. Pop singer Gwen Stefani.
   Gwenn, Gwyn, Gwynn
Gwenda Welsh. "Fair and good." Rare since the 1960s, even in Wales.
   Gwennda, Gwynda
Gwendolyn Welsh. "Fair bow." In some legends, Merlin the magician has a wife named Gwendolyn. The old Welsh name was revived in the late 19th century, and is now rare, though its diminutive, **Wendy,** lingers on.
   Guendolen, Guendolin, Guendolinn, Guendolynn, Guenna, Gwen, Gwenda, Gwendaline, Gwendolen, Gwendolene, Gwendolin, Gwendoline, Gwendolynne, Gwenna, Gwenette, Gwenndolen, Gwenni, Gwennie, Gwenny, Gwenyth, Gwyn, Gwyneth, Gwynn, Gwynna, Gwynne, Wendi, Wendie, Wendy, Win, Winne, Wynne
Gwladys Welsh. Var. **Gladys**.
Gwyneth Welsh. "Happiness." Most popular in Wales and Britain in the 1930s and 1940s, but never a strong name in America. Actress Gwyneth Paltrow.
   Gweneth, Gwenith, Gwenyth, Gwineth, Gwinneth, Gwinyth, Gwynith, Gwynna, Gwynne, Gwynneth, Winnie, Winny, Wynne, Wynnie
Gwynn Welsh. "Fair, blessed." Also dim. **Gwendolyn** or **Gwyneth**.
   Gwin, Gwinna, Gwinne, Gwyn, Gwynna, Gwynne
Gypsy OE. The tribe of Romany was originally called "gypsy" because it was thought that they had originated in Egypt. Use of the name, as in the case of Gypsy Rose Lee, is more often as a nickname.
   Gipsee, Gipsey, Gipsy

H

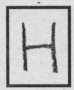

Habibah Arab. "loved one."
  Habiba, Habibi, Haviva, Havivah, Hebiba
Hadria Lat. Place name. "From Adria." Var.
Adrian.
  Hadriana, Hadriane, Hadrianna, Hadrien, Hadrienne
Hagar Heb. "Forsaken." In the Old Testament, Hagar is the
handmaid of Abraham's barren wife Sarah, and Sarah sends
her away when she has a son by Abraham. Though the Pu-
ritans tended to scour the Old Testament for feminine
names, this was not one they popularized, and its sparing
use has dwindled further since early in the 20th century.
  Haggar, Hagir, Hajar
Haidée Gk. "Modest." The name was brought to public
knowledge by Byron, who used it in his poem "Don
Juan." It has never really caught on.
  Jaidee, Hadee, Hyday
Halcyone Gk. "Kingfisher." In ancient myth, the kingfisher
laid its eggs on the sea, and they floated on the water for
the two weeks preceding the winter solstice. During this
time the waves were always calm, hence the expression
"halcyon days" to mean a time of tranquil happiness.
  Halcyon, Halcyona
Haldana ONorse. "Half-Danish." The name takes on real
significance when you consider that in ancient Britain, the
Danes were fierce and frequent invaders.
  Haldane, Haldanna
Haley OE "Hay meadow" variant **Hailey**. This name and
Hallie, in their various spellings, have become very popular recently. Haley and Hailey are entered as different
names on the Social Security Administration's list of pop-
ular names, but combined, they would probably number
just below the top ten.
  Halea, Haleigh, Hailey, Hayley

Halfrida OG. "Peaceful heroine" or "Peaceful home."

Halimah Arab. "Gentle, soft-spoken."
   Haleema, Haleemah, Haleima, Halima, Helima

Halimeda Gk. "Thinking of the sea."
   Halameda, Halette, Hali, Hallie, Meda, Medie

Hallie (Fem. **Henry**) OG "Ruler of the home or estate."
Hallie is considered a form of **Harriet,** as **Hal** is a nickname for **Harry.** Parents probably don't differentiate,
though, between Hallie and the very similar and fashionable **Hailey.** Actress Halle Berry.
   Hali, Halle, Hallee, Halley, Halli

Hana Jap. "Flower." Fashion designer Hanae Mori.
   Hanae, Hanako

Hannah Heb. "Grace." In the Old Testament, Hannah is
the mother of the prophet Samuel. The name was steadily
popular from around 1600 through the 19th century,
peaking around 1800. Hannah has been a top-ten favorite
in the U.S. since the mid-nineties. It is also extremely
fashionable throughout Britain and, as **Hanne,** in Germany. Writer Hannah Arendt; sportscaster Hannah
Storm.
   Ann, Anna, Anne, Annie, Chana, Chanah, Chanha,
   Channach, Channah, Hana, Hanna, Hanne, Hannele,
   Hannelore, Hannie, Hanny, Honna, Nan, Nanney,
   Nannie, Nanny

Happy Eng. "Cheerful, lighthearted." Though it was common enough in the 19th century, **Felicity** or **Hilary** are
now more likely to be used now. Happy does occur as a
nickname.

Haralda ONorse. "Army ruler" or "Army power." This
form was coined during the great 19th-century popularity
of **Harold,** but (as with many feminine variants, like
Arthuretta) never really caught on.
   Halley, Hallie, Hally, Harolda, Haroldene, Haroldina

Harley OE. Place name. "The long field." Familiar to most
people as half of the name of a great motorcycle, the
Harley-Davidson.
   Arlea, Arlee, Arleigh, Arley, Harlea, Harlee, Harleigh,
   Harlie, Harly

Harmony Lat. "Harmony."
    Harmonee, Harmoney, Harmonia, Harmonie
Harriet (Fem. **Henry**) OG. "Ruler of the home or estate."
    An informal version of **Henrietta,** very popular in the
    18th and 19th centuries, and after nearly 100 years of ob-
    scurity, ready for a revival. Avid readers are likely to as-
    sociate the name with the children's book *Harriet the Spy.*
    Author Harriet Beecher Stowe; civil rights leader Harriet
    Tubman.
    Hallee, Halllie, Harrie, Harrietta, Harriett, Harrietta,
    Harriette, Harriot, Harriott, Harriotte, Hatsee,
    Hatsey, Hatsie, Hatsy, Hattie, Hatty
Hayfa Arab. "Slender, well-shaped."
    Haifa
Hayley OE. Place name: "Hay meadow." Other sources
    suggest derivation from a Norse word, *haela,* which
    means "hero." Probably neither meaning nor history con-
    tributes much to the recent popularity of this name, which
    was made famous by actress Hayley Mills in the 1960s,
    and 30 years later, was one of the top 50 names given to
    American girls. Now, along with variant **Haley,** it is still
    extremely popular.
    Haeley, Haelie, Haely, Hailea, Hailee, Haileigh, Haily,
    Haleigh, Halie, Hally, Haylea, Haylee, Hayleigh,
    Hayley
Hazel OE. Tree name. The late 19th-century vogue for
    botanical names tended to concentrate on flowers rather
    than trees; Hazel is an exception. Track star Hazel Clark.
    Hazal, Hazell, Hazelle, Hazle
Heather ME. Flower name. Introduced with other botani-
    cal names in the late 19th century, but really took off in
    the late 20th century, especially in the U.S., where its as-
    sociation with Scotland may have endowed it with an
    upper-class aura. Actress Heather Locklear.
    Heath, Hether
Hebe Gk. "Youth." In Greek legend, Hebe was the goddess
    of youth and also cupbearer to the gods. Her name was
    used mostly in the late 19th century.

Hedda OG. "Warfare." The more common anglicized version of **Hedwig**. Mid-20th-century gossip queen Hedda Hopper.
Heda, Heddi, Heddie, Hedi, Hedvig, Hedvige, Hedwig, Hedwiga, Hedy, Hetta

Hedwig OG. "Warfare, struggle, strife." Almost unknown in English-speaking countries. Actress Hedy Lamarr was born Hedwig Kiesler.
Hadvig, Hadwig, Hedvig, Hedviga, Hedvige, Hedwiga, Hedwige, Hedy

Hedy Gk. "Delightful, sweet," or Heb. "My echo." Use is more likely to reflect the glamorous Hedy Lamarr's popularity.
Heda, Hedia, Hediah, Hedyla

Heidi Dim. **Adelaide** (OG. "Noble, nobility"). Made popular by Johanna Spyri's famous novel of 1881, first in German-speaking countries, later in the U.S. Its surge of popularity in the 1970s may have been influenced by a highly publicized TV production of the late 1960s.
Heida, Heide, Heidey, Heidy, Hydee

Helen Gk. "Light." The most famous Helen is probably Helen of Troy, the daughter of Zeus by Leda. Her phenomenal beauty was, in some versions, the root cause of the Trojan War; hers was "the face that launched a thousand ships." The name has been understandably popular through the ages, and has spawned many variants, of which **Eleanor** is the most common. Writer Helen Keller; actresses Helen Hayes, Helen Hunt, Helen Mirren, Helena Bonham-Carter; publisher Helen Gurley Brown; singer Helen Reddy.
Aileen, Ailene, Aleanor, Alene, Aline, Eileen, Elaina, Elaine, Elana, Elayne, Eleanor, Eleanore, Elena, Eleni, Elenora, Elenore, Eleonora, Elianora, Elinor, Ella, Elladine, Elleanora, Elle, Ellee, Ellen, Ellenora, Ellette, Ellie, Ellin, Elliner, Ellinor, Elly, Ellyn, Galina, Halina, Heleanor, Helenore, Helena, Helenann, Hélène, Helia, Hella, Hellen, Hellena, Hellene, Hellenor, Hellia, Ileana, Ilene, Ilona, Jelena, Lana,

Leanora, Lena, Lenore, Leonora, Leonore, Leora,
Lienor, Lina, Nelda, Nell, Nellette, Nelliana, Nellie,
Nelly, Nonnie, Nora, Yelena

Helga OG. "Holy, sacred." Var. **Olga**.
Helge, Hellga, Hellge

Helice Gk. "Spiral." An unusual name that comes from the same Greek root as helix, or double helix, the shape of the DNA molecule.
Helica, Helike

Helma OG. "Helmet." See **Wilhelmina**.
Hillma, Hilma

Heloise Fr. Var. **Louise** (OG. "Renowned in war"). The 12th-century French philosopher Pierre Abelard fell in love with and seduced his student Heloise. Her uncle and guardian had him emasculated, even though he married Heloise. She became a nun, he a monk.
Aloysia, Eloisa, Eloise, Heloisa, Lois

Helsa Dan. Var. **Elizabeth** (Heb. "Consecrated to God").
Hellsa

Henrietta (Fem. **Henry**) OG. "Ruler of the house." More formal version of **Harriet** that briefly became popular at the turn of the century. A bit of a mouthful for today's parents.
Enrichetta, Enrichette, Enriqueta, Etta, Ettie, Etty,
Hatsie, Hatsy, Hattie, Hatty, Hendrika, Henia, Henie,
Henka, Hennie, Henrie, Henrieta, Henriette, Henrika,
Henryetta, Hetti, Hettie, Yetta, Yettie

Hepzibah Heb. "My delight is in her." Old Testament name widely used by the Puritans, but by the 20th century it had almost died out, in part because of its lack of euphony.
Chepziba, Chepzibah, Eppie, Hefzia, Hefziba,
Hephzia, Hephziba, Hepsie, Hepsibah, Hepzi, Hepzia

Hera Gk. "Queen." In Greek myth, Hera was the wife (and sister) of Zeus, ruler of the gods. She is usually portrayed as a jealous woman who persecutes her husband's numerous mistresses.

Hermione Gk. "Earthly." Very rare. Actress Hermione Gingold.
Erma, Herma, Hermia, Hermina, Hermine, Herminia

Hermosa Sp. "Beautiful."

Hertha OE. "Earth." The name of the German or Scandinavian Earth Mother.
Eartha, Erda, Ertha, Herta

Hesper Gk. "Evening or evening star." The Greeks referred to Italy as Hesperia, since the sun set and the evening star rose there. It is also, fittingly enough, the name of a town in California.
Hespera, Hesperia

Hester Gk. "Star." Var. **Esther**. The most famous Hester is probably the adulteress in Hawthorne's *The Scarlet Letter*, Hester Prynne.
Hesther, Hestia, Hettie, Hetty

Hibernia Lat. Place name for Ireland.

Hibiscus Lat. Botanical name for the plant colloquially known as the marsh mallow.

Hilary Gk. "Cheerful, happy." The name comes from the same root as the word "hilarious." There were a 4th-century saint and a 5th-century pope named Hilary, and the name was used for boys until the 17th century. The late-19th-century revival, though, made it generally a girl's name, which was especially fashionable in the 1950s. Parents can't consider the name now without reference to former First Lady Hillary Clinton. Actress Hilary Swank.
Hilaria, Hilarie, Hillary, Hillery, Hilliary

Hilda OG. "Battle woman." One of the Valkyrie of Teutonic legend was named Hilda. A medieval name with a Victorian revival that lasted through the 1930s. Now unusual.
Hilde, Hildie, Hildy

Hildegarde OG. "Battle stronghold." Rare in English-speaking countries. Opera star Hildegarde Behrens.
Hellee, Hilda, Hildagard, Hildagarde, Hilde, Hildegard, Hildegaard, Hildegunn, Hille

Hildemar OG. "Battle-renowned."
Hildemarr

Hildreth OG. "Battle counselor." Briefly used at the turn of the 20th century in Britain.
Hildred

Hilma Dim. **Wilhelmina** (OG. "Will-helmet").
Halma, Helma

Hinda Heb. "Doe, female deer."
Hynda

Hippolyta Gk. Meaning not entirely clear, but alludes to horses. Very unusual.
Hippolita

Holda OG. "Hidden."
Holde, Holle, Hulda

Hollis OE. Place name. "Near the holly bushes." The usual transference of a masculine to a feminine name may be accelerated in this case because Hollis sounds like **Holly**.
Hollace, Holles, Holless, Holliss, Holyss

Holly OE. Botanical name. First used at the turn of the 20th century and newly popular in the 1960s. Obviously a seasonal favorite most intensively used in December. Actress Holly Hunter; singer Holly Near.
Hollee, Holleigh, Holley, Hollie, Hollye

Honey OE. The word used as a name. May be as a diminutive of **Honora,** but is more likely to be a transference of the endearment.
Honeah, Honee

Honora Lat. "Woman of honor." As **Honour,** used by the Puritans (along with other abstract concepts like **Constance**). **Honoria** was more common in the 18th century. No version of the name is widely used now. Actress Honor Blackman.
Honor, Honorah, Honorata, Honoria, Honorine, Honour, Nora, Norah, Norine, Norry

Hope OE. "Hope." One of the three cardinal virtues, along with Faith and Charity, and probably the one that has survived best as a name, particularly in the U.S. Actress Hope Lange.

Horatia Lat. Clan name, possibly meaning "timekeeper." The name was coined by the 18th-century admiral Lord Horatio Nelson, for his daughter.
Horacia, Horaisha, Horasha

Hortense Lat. Clan name. A related word means "of the

garden." *Hortensia* is the French term for the hydrangea shrub.

Hartencia, Hartinsia, Hortensia, Hortenspa, Hortenxia, Hortinzia, Ortensia

Huberta (Fem. Hubert) OG. "Brilliant mind."

Hubertina, Hubertine, Uberta, Ubertina

Huette (Fem. Hugh) OG. "Mind, intellect." A feminization of a name that has never had a particular vogue.

Huela, Huella, Huetta, Hugette, Hughette, Hughina, Ugetta

Hulda OG. "Loved one." Or Heb. "Mole." Very unusual, occurs in Scandinavian or English-speaking countries.

Huldah, Huldie

Hyacinth Gk. Flower name. There was a 3rd-century saint of this name, which was used for boys as well as girls. In Greek legend, Apollo loved a beautiful youth of the name; the hyacinth flower sprang up from his blood when he died.

Cintha, Cinthia, Cinthie, Cinthy, Giacinta, Giacintia, Hyacintha, Hyacinthe, Hyacinthia, Hyacinthie, Hyacintia, Jacenta, Jacinda, Jacinta, Jacintha, Jacinthe, Jackie, Jacky, Jacynth

Hypatia Gk. "Highest."

Hypacia, Hypasia

I   **Iantha** Gk. "Purple flower." Popular in the later 19th century, possibly influenced by Romantic poets earlier in the century.

Ianthe, Ianthia, Ianthina, Janthia

Ida Meaning unclear: possibly OE. "Prosperous, happy" or OG. "Hardworking." Very fashionable at the turn of the 20th century in America, but little used in modern times.

Eida, Eidah, Idaleen, Idalene, Idalia, Idalina, Idaline, Idalya, Idalyne, Ide, Idelfa, Idelfia, Idell, Idella, Idelle, Idetta, Idette

Idina Var. **Edina** (OE. "From Edinburgh, Scotland").

Iduna ONorse. "Loving one."

Idonia, Idunna

Ieesha Var. **Aisha** (Arab. "Woman"; Swahili. "Life").

Eyeesha, Ieasha, Ieashia, Ieashiah, Ieeshah, Iesha, Yeesha

Ignacia (Fem. **Ignatius**) Meaning unclear, though some sources suggest Lat. "Ardent, burning."

Ignatia, Ignazia, Iniga

Ila OF. Place name: "Island."

Eila, Ilanis, Ilanys, Isla

Ilana Heb. "Tree."

Elana, Elanit, Eleana, Eleanna, Ileana, Ileanna, Iliana, Ilianna, Ilanit

Ilene Modern variant of **Aileen** (Gk. "Light").

Ilean, Ileen, Ileene

Iliana Gk. "Trojan." The poetic name for the ancient city of Troy was "Ilion." **Ileana** has been used by the Greek royal family. Actress Ileanna Douglas.

Ileana, Ileane, Ileanna, Ileanne, Illeanna, Illia, Illiana

Ilka Slavic. "Flattering, hardworking." Writer Ilka Chase.

Ilke, Milka

Ilona Hung. Var. **Helen** (Gk. "Light"). Also carries the connotation of "beautiful," no doubt because of the legendary beauty of Helen of Troy.

Elona, Ellona, Elonna, Illona, Ilone, Ilonka, Ilonna, Yllona, Ylonna

Ilsa Ger. Var. **Elizabeth** (Heb. "Pledged to God"). Mostly limited to Germany, especially in the 19th century.

Ellsa, Elsa, Else, Illsa, Ilsae, Ilsaie, Ilse

Iluminada Sp. "Lit up."

Illuminada, Illuminata, Iluminata, Yluminata

Ima Var. **Emma** (OG. "Embracing everything").

Imelda OG./It. "All-consuming fight." A name occasionally used (especially in Catholic families, after a virgin saint) until the explosive fame of Philippine First Lady Imelda

Marcos. Now it seems slated for a long period of neglect. Actress Imelda Staunton.

Amelda, Himalda, Imalda, Ymelda

Immaculada Sp. "Without stain." A reference to the Immaculate Conception.

Imacolata, Imaculada, Immaculata, Immacolata

Imogen Lat. Some sources claim it means "Last-born," while others suggest "Image," while still another traces it back to "Innocent." Despite Shakespeare's use of the name, it was obscure until the 20th century. Still highly unusual. Actresses Imogene Coca, Imogen Stubbs.

Emogen, Emogene, Imogene, Imogenia, Imogine, Imojean, Imojeen

Ina Lat. Suffix to make male names feminine, as in **Clementina** or **Edwina**. Used independently since the Victorian era. Cookbook author Ina Garten.

Ena, Yna

India Country name. Like any pretty geographic name, could be used by parents who have a special attachment to the country. Model India Hicks.

Indya

Inez Sp. Var. **Agnes** (Lat. "Pure"). Unusual in English-speaking countries, but **Ines** is currently very fashionable in Spain. Designer Inès de la Fressange.

Ines, Inesita, Inessa, Ynes, Ynesita, Ynez

Inga Scan. "Guarded by Ing." Ing, in Norse mythology, was a powerful god of fertility and peace. His name is an element in several modern names like **Ingrid** and **Ingmar**. **Inge** is very popular in Germany. Actress Inger Stevens.

Ingaberg, Ingaborg, Inge, Ingeberg, Ingeborg, Inger, Innga, Inngeborg

Ingrid Scan. "Beautiful." The most popular of the "Ing" names, doubtless because of the fame of Swedish actress Ingrid Bergman.

Inga, Inge, Inger, Ingmar

Inocencia Sp. "Innocence."

Innocencia, Innocenta, Inocenta, Inocentia, Ynocencia

Ioanna Gk. Var. **Hannah** (Heb. "Grace").

Ioana, Ioanah, Ioannah, Joanna, Yohanna

Iola Gk. "Cloud of dawn."
Iole

Iolanthe Gk. "Violet flower." The more common form is the Spanish variant, **Yolanda**. Gilbert and Sullivan's 1882 operetta *Iolanthe* did little to popularize this form.
Iolanda, Iolanta, Iolantha, Jolantha, Jolanthe, Yolantha, Yolanthe, Yolley, Yollie

Iona Gk. Place name. Island off the coast of Scotland, site of an early monastery. Use as a name is mostly Scottish. Orchestra conductor Iona Brown.

Ione Gk. "Violet." Flower name in an exotic, little-used form. Actress Ione Skye.
Ionia, Ionie

Iphigenia Gk. "Sacrifice." In Greek myth, the daughter of Agamemnon. Her father sacrificed her to gain advantage in the Trojan war, though in most versions of the story, she is saved by Artemis.
Efigenia, Ephigenia, Ephigenie, Ifigenia, Iphigeneia, Iphigenie, Genia

Irene Gk. "Peace." Very common under the Roman Empire, but first appeared in English-speaking countries in the mid-19th century. It caught on quickly and was very popular in the first quarter of the 20th century. As **Irina**, fashionable in Russia. Actresses Irene Dunne, Irene Worth.
Arina, Eireen, Eiren, Eirena, Eirene, Erena, Erene, Ira, Ireen, Iren, Irena, Irenea, Irénée, Irenka, Irina, Irine, Iryna, Orina, Oryna, Rena, Rene, Renie, Rina, Yarina

Iris Gk. "Rainbow." Also (and this is probably the source of its popularity) name of a flower. Its use was established and faded with other flower names, from around 1890 to the 1920s. Novelist Iris Murdoch.
Irida, Iridiana, Iridianny, Irisa, Irita

Irma OG. "Universal, complete." Rare now, but somewhat used in the first part of this century.
Erma, Ermengard, Irmina, Irmine, Irmgard, Irmgarde

Irvette (Fem. **Irving**) OE. "Seafriend." Also Scot. place name. A rather awkward transformation of a name that was never immensely popular.
Earvette, Earvina, Ervette, Ervina, Irvina

Isabel Sp. Var. **Elizabeth** (Heb. "Pledged to God"). Most fashionable in the last quarter of the 19th century, though popularity has increased steadily in the last dozen years with the trend toward old-fashioned feminine names. **Belle** and **Bella** are also independently used, probably because of their own attractive meaning ("beautiful") in French and Spanish. Henry James named the heroine of his *Portrait of a Lady* Isabel Archer. Actresses Isabella Rossellini, Isabelle Adjani; fashion designer Isabel Toledo.

Bel, Belia, Belicia, Belita, Bell, Bella, Belle, Bellita, Ib, Ibbie, Isa, Isabeau, Isabele, Isabelita, Isabell, Isabella, Isabelle, Ishbel, Isobel, Isobell, Isobella, Isobelle, Issie, Issy, Izabella, Izabelle, Izzie, Izzy, Sabella, Sabelle, Ysabeau, Ysabel, Ysabella, Ysobel, Yzabelle, Yzobel, Yzobelle

Isadora (Fem. **Isidore**) Lat. "Gift of Isis." Isis was the principal goddess of ancient Egypt, and Isidore was a popular name among the ancient Greeks. The most famous Isadora was, of course, modern dance pioneer Isadora Duncan.

Isidora, Ysadora

Isis Egypt. The supreme goddess of ancient Egypt, Isis ruled with her brother/husband, Osiris, and her son, Horus.

Isla Name of a Scottish river, used in Britain as a first name.

Islay

Isolde Meaning unclear, though some sources offer Welsh "Fair lady." In legend Isolde is an Irish princess loved by Tristan, but she marries his uncle, King Mark. There are many versions of the tale, the most famous of which is probably Wagner's opera *Tristan und Isolde.* Use of this version of the name probably reflects admiration for the opera.

Iseult, Iseut, Isold, Isolda, Isolt, Isolte, Isota, Isotta, Isotte, Yseult, Yseulte, Yseut, Ysolda, Ysolde, Ysotta, Ysotte

Ita Ir. Gael. "Thirst." Name of a 6th-century Irish saint. Rare outside of Ireland.

Ivana (Fem. **Ivan**) Slavic Var. **John** (Heb. "Jehovah is gracious"). Most recently in the news with Ivana Trump, the ex-wife of Donald Trump.
Iva, Ivanka, Ivanna

Ivory Lat. Word used as name, possibly related to the vogue for jewel names in the late 19th century.
Ivoreen, Ivorine

Ivy OE. Botanical name. Most popular in the first quarter of the 20th century. Author Ivy Compton-Burnett.
Ivee, Ivey, Ivie

Jacinda Sp. Var. **Hyacinth** (Gk. Flower name). There was a 3rd-century Saint Hyacinth, and the name was used for boys as well as girls. In Greek legend, Apollo loved a beautiful youth of the name; the hyacinth flower sprang up from his blood when he died.
Giacinda, Giacintha, Giacinthia, Jacenda, Jacenta, Jacey, Jacie, Jacindia, Jacinna, Jacinta, Jacinth, Jacintha, Jacinthe, Jacinthia, Jacy, Jacynth, Jacyntha, Jacynthe, Jacynthia

Jackie Dim., usually of **Jacqueline**. Used as an independent name in the 20th century, most notably by Jacqueline Kennedy Onassis.
Jackee, Jackey, Jacki, Jacky, Jacquey, Jacqui, Jacquie

Jacobina (Fem. **Jacob**) Heb. "He who supplants." **James** is an anglicization of Jacob, and has always been a favorite name in Scotland, which may account for the Scottish use of this feminization.
Jackee, Jackie, Jackobina, Jacky, Jacoba, Jacobetta, Jacobette, Jacobine, Jacobyna, Jakobina, Jakobine

Jacqueline Fr. Dim. **Jacob** (Heb. "he who supplants"). Existed in Britain as early as the 17th century, but used in numbers only from the beginning of the 20th century. Grew quickly, and was quite a favorite by midcentury. In the U.S., parents may have been inspired by the glamorous First Lady Jacqueline Kennedy, who has put an indelible stamp on the name. It is well enough used to be familiar but not fashionable. Actresses Jaclyn Smith, Jacqueline Bisset.

Jacalin, Jacalyn, Jackalin, Jackalinne, Jackelyn, Jacketta, Jackette, Jacki, Jackie, Jacklin, Jacklyn, Jacklynne, Jackqueline, Jacky, Jaclin, Jaclyn, Jacolyn, Jacqualine, Jacqualyn, Jacquel, Jacquelean, Jacquelin, Jacquella, Jacquelle, Jacquelyn, Jacquelynne, Jacquenetta, Jacquenette, Jacquetta, Jacquette, Jacqui, Jacquine, Jaculine, Jaquelin, Jaqueline, Jaquelyn, Jaquith, Zakelina, Zacqueline, Zhakelina, Zhaqueline

Jade Sp. Jewel name, for the semiprecious green stone. Perhaps because the jewel comes from the Orient, the name has a vaguely exotic air. Actress Jada Pinkett.

Jada, Jadra, Jaida, Jayda, Jayde, Jaydra, Zhade

Jadwige Pol. "Safety in battle."

Jadwiga

Jael Heb. "Mountain goat." An Old Testament name that occurred from time to time among the Puritans and again in the 19th century. Now rare.

Jaelle, Jayel, Jayil

Jaffa Heb. "Beautiful." Also a place name: an ancient city that served as the port for Tel Aviv.

Jafit, Joppa

Jaime Sp. Var. **James** (Heb. "He who supplants"). Some parents, however, may prefer to consider it as French for "I love," *J'aime,* in which case they should be prepared to insist on the "Zh-" pronunciation.

Jamee, James, Jamey, Jamie, Jayme, Jaymee

Jamesina (Fem. **James**) Heb. "He who supplants." An old-fashioned form that has been abandoned in favor of the less formal **Jamie,** etc.

Jamesetta, Jamesette

Jamie (Fem. var. **James**) Heb. "He who supplants." Also used as a boy's name, but once a name becomes entrenched as a feminine choice, parents tend to avoid it for their male children. Actresses Jamie Lee Curtis, Jami Gertz.

Jaime, Jaimee, Jaimey, Jaimi, Jaimie, Jaimy, Jama, Jamee, Jamei, Jamese, Jami, Jammie, Jayme, Jaymee, Jaymie

Jamila Arab. "Lovely." Currently popular among Moslem families.

Jameela, Jameila, Jamelia, Jamilah, Jamilla, Jamille, Jamillia

Jan (Fem. **John**) Heb. "The Lord is gracious." Author Jan Morris.

Jana, Janah, Janina, Janine, Jann, Janna, Jannah

Jana (Fem. **John**) Heb. "The Lord is gracious." A Slavic variation of **Jane**. Tennis star Jana Novotna.

Iana, Janaya, Janayah, Janna, Jannah, Yana, Yanna

Jane (Fem. **John**) Heb. "The Lord is gracious." This is the simplest current variant of John (though **Joan** predates it), popular since the 16th century. It has been a tried-and-true standby like **Mary** or **Katherine,** as its number of variants demonstrate. When many women at a time shared the same name, variants sprang up to differentiate them from one another, hence **Janet, Janine, Janelle,** etc. Author Jane Austen; actresses Jane Fonda, Jane Seymour, Jayne Mansfield, Jane Wyman, Janeane Garofalo, Jane Kaczmarek; newscaster Jane Pauley.

Gene, Gianina, Giovanna, Iva, Ivana, Ivancka, Ivanka, Ivanna, Jaine, Jainee, Jan, Jana, Janaya, Janaye, Jandy, Janeczka, Janeen, Janel, Janela, Janelba, Janella, Janelle, Janean, Janeane, Janene, Janerita, Janessa, Janet, Janeta, Janeth, Janetta, Janette, Janey, Jania, Janica, Janice, Janie, Janina, Janine, Janique, Janis, Janise, Janit, Janka, Janna, Jannel, Jannelle, Janney, Janny, Jany, Jayne, Jaynell, Jean, Jeanette, Jeanie, Jeanne, Jeannette, Jeannine, Jenda, Jenella, Jenelle, Jenica, Jeniece, Jeni, Jenie, Jensina, Jensine, Jess, Jinna, Joana, Joanna, Johanna,

Johnetta, Johnna, Johnetta, Jonella, Jonelle, Joni, Jonie, Juana, Juanita, Sheena, Shene, Sinead, Vania, Vanya

Janet The most common diminutive form of **Jane** is Janet, but other forms such as **Janeta** and **Jonet** preceded it. Janet was originally mostly Scots, and was very popular in the 1950s. Like most midcentury favorites, it is now out of style. Actresses Janet Leigh, Janet Gaynor; singer Dame Janet Baker; swimmer Janet Evans; figure skater Janet Lynn.

Gianetta, Janeta, Janeth, Janetta, Janette, Jannet, Jannetta, Janit, Janot, Jenetta, Jenette, Jennet, Jennette, Jinnet, Jinnett, Johnetta, Johnette, Jonette

Janice Var. **Jane**. Coined at the turn of the 20th century, in general circulation by the thirties and popular in the fifties. Like **Janet**, now out of favor. Singer Janis Joplin.

Janess, Janessa, Janesse, Janessia, Janiece, Janique, Janis, Janiss, Jannice, Janyce, Jency, Jenice, Jeniece, Jenise, Jennice

Jasmine Per. "Jasmine flower." Flower name with exotic connotations. The turn-of-the-century vogue for flower names had its source in the English upper class, but was usually confined to temperate-zone specimens. (England's Queen Mother, for instance, had sisters named Rose and Violet Hyacinth.) Jasmine became fashionable a bit later, in the 1930s. Now Jasmine is a steady favorite. Author Jessamyn West; model Yasmeen Ghauri.

Ismenia, Jaslyn, Jaslynn, Jasmin, Jasmina, Jasminda, Jassamayn, Jazan, Jazmin, Jazmon, Jazzmin, Jazzmine, Jazzmon, Jazzmyn, Jazzmynn, Jess, Jessamine, Jessamy, Jessamyn, Jessie, Jessimine, Jessimine, Yasmeen, Yasmin, Yasmina, Yasmine, Yasminia

Jay Lat. "Jaybird." A medieval name that has survived in a small way, especially in the U.S., where it is given to boys and girls alike. Its use may be inspired by a great American jurist, John Jay. Gymnast Jaycie Phelps.

Jae, Jaya, Jaycie, Jaye, Jaylene, Jeh, Jey, Jeyla

Jean Var. **Jane**. Scottish origin, unusual elsewhere until the turn of the 20th century; most popular in the 1930s. Now preferred for boys, probably among this country's francophone populations as it is a French version of **John**. Actresses Jean Arthur, Jean Harlow.

Gene, Genie, Jeana, Jeane, Jeanee, Jeaneen, Jeanelle, Jeanene, Jeanette, Jeanie, Jeanine, Jeanique, Jeanna, Jeanne, Jeanneen, Jeannetta, Jeannette, Jeannie, Jeannine, Jeannique, Jenette, Jenica, Jennet, Jennetta, Jennine

Jeannine (Fem. **John**) Var. **Jean** (Heb. "The Lord is gracious"). Modern usage.

Janine, Jeanine, Jenine, Jannine, Jennine

Jelena Rus. Var. **Helen** (Gk. "Light").

Galina, Yelena

Jemima Heb. "Dove." Old Testament name: Jemima was one of the three beautiful daughters of the persecuted Job. The Puritans brought the name to the U.S., where it is now probably most familiar because of the "Aunt Jemima" brand name for pancake mix and syrup.

Jamima, Jemimah, Jemmimah, Jemmie, Jemmy, Mima, Mimma

Jena Arab. "Little bird."

Jenna

Jenilee Com. form. **Jenny** and **Lee**.

Jenilea, Jennielee, Jennylee

Jenna Dim. **Jennifer** or Var. **Jean** (Heb. "The Lord is gracious.") Made famous by a character on *Dallas,* played by Priscilla Presley. This name is currently quite fashionable, especially since 2000. First Daughter Jenna Bush; actress Jenna Elfman.

Jena

Jennie Dim. **Janet** or **Jennifer**. Given as an independent name since the 19th century. Swedish soprano Jennie Lind; talk show host Jenny Jones.

Jenee, Jennee, Jenney, Jenni, Jenny

Jennifer Welsh. "White and smooth, soft." The modern and most popular form of **Guinevere,** originally a Cornish variant. Its immense 20th-century popularity began in the

1920s and grew to a 1950s peak in Britain. In the U.S. the name reached the number one spot in the early eighties, and is now slipping down the charts. Actresses Jennifer Gray, Jennifer Jones, Jennifer Jason Leigh, Jennifer O'Neill, Jennifer Aniston, Jennifer Connelly, Jennifer Garner, Jennifer Lopez.

Genna, Genni, Gennie, Gennifer, Geniffer, Genniver, Genny, Jen, Jena, Jenefer, Jeni, Jenifer, Jeniffer, Jenn, Jenna, Jennee, Jenni, Jennica, Jonnie, Jennlver, Jenny

Jeremia (Fem. **Jeremiah**) Heb. "The Lord is exalted."

Jeree, Jeremee, Jeremie, Jeri, Jerri, Jerrie, Jerry

Jerrie OG./Fr. "Spear ruler." Dim. **Geraldine**.

Jeree, Jeri, Jerree, Jerrey, Jerri, Jerry, Jery

Jerusha Heb. "Married, a possession."

Jarusha, Jeruscha, Jerushah

Jessica Heb. "He sees." Coined by Shakespeare from the Old Testament Iscah or Jesca. His Jessica was the daughter of Shylock in *The Merchant of Venice*. Popular in the U.S. in the 1970s, and still one of the top ten names in the nation. Also very fashionable in England. Actresses Jessica Lange, Jessica Tandy, Jessica Alba, Jessica Capshaw, Sarah Jessica Parker.

Jess, Jessa, Jessaca, Jessaka, Jessalin, Jessalyn, Jesse, Jesseca, Jessey, Jessie, Jessika, Jessy

Jessie Dim. **Jessica**. Also, in Scotland, a diminutive of **Janet**.

Jess, Jessa, Jesse, Jessey, Jessi, Jessy

Jesusa Sp. Derived from Mary de Jesus, a name for the Virgin Mary.

Jette Dan. "Black as coal." Mostly used in northern Europe.

Yette

Jewel OF. Word as first name. Though the vogue for jewel names occurred at the turn of the 20th century (along with the flower-name fashion), Jewel came into use a little later, in the 1930s. Pop singer Jewel.

Jewell, Jewella, Jewelle

Jezebel Heb. "Pure, virginal." An Old Testament name that carries strong connotations that contradict its meaning: It was used as a term for a "painted lady" or a brazen hussy as portrayed by Bette Davis in the film *Jezebel*.

Jessabell, Jetzabel, Jezabel, Jezabella, Jezebelle, Jezibel, Jezibelle, Jezybell

Jill Dim. **Gillian,** ultimately of **Juliana** (Lat. "Youthful") Jill was popular before the 17th century, and revived to widespread use after the 1920s. Now quite scarce. Actresses Jill St. John, Jill Eikenberry, Jill Ireland; English novelist Jilly Cooper; fashion designer Jil Sander.

Jil, Jilian, Jilana, Jillan, Jillana, Jillane, Jillayne, Jilleen, Jillene, Jilli, Jillian, Jillianne, Jillie, Jilly, Jillyan, Jyl, Jyll

Jillian Var. **Gillian,** Dim. **Juliana.** (Lat. "Youthful")

Jilian, Jiliana, Jilan, Jillana, Jillane, Jilliana, Jillianne, Jillyan, Jillyanna, Jilliyanne

Jimena Sp. "Heard."

Jinny Dim. **Virginia** or Var. **Jenny.** Mostly 19th-century use in this form.

Jinna, Jinnee, Jinni, Jinnie

Jinx Lat. "Spell."

Jinxx, Jynx

Jo Dim. **Joan, Josephine,** etc. Often used in combination, as in Jo Ann, Betty Jo. The second daughter in Louisa May Alcott's *Little Women* was called Jo, short for Josephine. The usage hasn't caught on widely.

Joakima (Fem. **Joachim**) Heb. "God will judge."

Joaquina, Joaquine

Joan (Fem. **John**) Heb. "The Lord is gracious." The medieval feminine version of John; Jeanne d'Arc's first name, for instance, was translated as Joan, **Jeanne**'s popular English equivalent. It was neglected for **Jane** by the 17th century. A brief intense revival occurred early in the 20th century for a score of years, but Joan is again widely neglected. Actresses Joan Crawford, Joan Collins; singer Joan Baez; comedienne Joan Rivers; musician Joni Mitchell; marathon runner Joan Benoit.

Joane, Joanie, Joannie, Jone, Jonee, Joni

Joanna Var. **Jane** or **Joan**. Its 19th-century use increased with the revival of Joan, and continued to grow until around 1950 in the U.S. **Joanne,** the French form, was hugely popular in Britain in the 1970s. Actresses Joanna Lumley, Joanne Woodward; author Joanne (J.K.) Rowling.

Jo, Joana, Joann, Jo Ann, Joanne, Jo Anne, Joeann, Johanna, Johannah

Jobeth Com. form **Jo** and **Beth**. Unusual, found mostly in the 1950s. Actress JoBeth Williams.

Joby (Fem. **Job**) Heb. "Persecuted." Unusual version of an Old Testament name widely used by the Puritans and their descendants well into the 19th century.

Jobey, Jobi, Jobie, Jobina, Jobyna

Jocasta It. "Lighthearted." In spite of its pleasant meaning, the name is little used because of its history. In Greek myth, Jocasta is the mother of Oedipus; he later unwittingly marries her, unleashing a series of gruesome tragedies. Interior design writer Jocasta Innes.

Jokasta

Jocelyn Derivation unclear; possibly Old German, possibly Lat. "Cheerful." It was a man's name in the Middle Ages, revived as a girl's name in the early 20th century. Cellist Jocelyn DuPré.

Jocelin, Joceline, Jocelinda, Jocelyne, Josaline, Joscelin, Josceline, Joscelyn, Joselina, Joseline, Joselyn, Joselyne, Josiline, Josline, Jossline, Josselyn, Josslyn, Joycelin

Jocosa Lat. "Joking."

Giocosa

Jody Dim. **Joan, Judith**. Used mostly since the 1950s in the U.S.; in the Canadian top ten in the 1970s. Actress Jodie Foster.

Jodee, Jodey, Jodi, Jodie

Joelle (Fem. **Joel**) Heb. "Jehovah is the Lord." Probably popularized by a vogue for combined forms beginning with "Jo," like **Joanne** and **Jolene**. Reached its peak in the 1960s. Actress Joely Richardson.

Joela, Joelin, Joell, Joella, Joelliane, Joellin, Joelly, Joely, Joelynn, Joetta, Jowella, Jowelle

Johanna (Fem. **Johann**) Ger. Var. **John** (Heb. "the Lord is gracious"). A European-sounding choice among the numerous feminizations of John.

Giovanna, Joanna, JoeHannah, Johana, Johannah, Jovanna

Johnna (Fem. **John**) Heb. "The Lord is gracious." May also be considered a contraction of **Johanna**.

Giana, Gianna, Giovanna, Jana, Janna, Johna, Johnetta, Johnette, Jovanna

Joie Fr. Var. **Joy**. Actress Joie Lee.

Joi

Jolan Gk. "Violet flower." This is a Middle-European form of **Iolanthe**. The most popular form in the U.S. is **Yolanda**.

Jola, Jolaine, Jolande, Jolanne, Jolanta, Jolantha, Yolanne

Jolene Com. form **Jo** and **-lene**. In the 1940s names ending in "-lene" (**Darlene, Marlene,** etc.) began to be fashionable, and a form beginning with "Jo" was a natural result. These names are now little used.

Joeline, Joeleen, Jolean, Joleen, Jolena, Jolina, Joline, Jolyn, Jolyna, Jolyne, Jolynn

Jolie Fr. "Pretty." Used mainly since the 1960s.

Joely, Jolee, Joley, Joli, Joliet, Jolietta, Joliette, Joly

Jonquil Flower name. Unlike most flower names, this one did not appear until the 1940s, and its two decades of popularity were mostly limited to Britain. The jonquil is a variety of narcissus closely related to a daffodil.

Jordan Heb. "Descend." Named after the River Jordan. First used in the Middle Ages by Crusaders returning from the Holy Land. Revived slightly in the 19th century, mostly for boys. It is still very well used for boy babies.

Jardena, Johrdan, Jordain, Jordana, Jordane, Jordanka, Jordanna, Jorden, Jordena, Jordenn, Jordie, Jordin, Jordyn, Jorey, Jori, Jorie, Jorrdan, Jorry, Jourdan

Josephine (Fem. **Joseph**) Heb. "Jehovah increases." Napoleon's famous Empress Josephine's real name was

Marie Josephe (for the parents of Jesus), but Josephine
was used as a diminutive. It did not become fashionable
until the mid-19th century, and has never caught on
widely in the U.S. Cabaret star Josephine Baker.
**Fifi, Fifine, Fina, Finetta, Finette, Guiseppina, Jo,
Joette, Joey, Joline, Josana, Josanna, Josanne,
Josee, Josefa, Josefena, Josefene, Josefina, Josefine,
Josepha, Josephe, Josephene, Josephina, Josephyna,
Josephyne, Josetta, Josette, Josey, Josiane,
Josianna, Josianne, Josie, Josy, Jozsa**

Jovita Lat. "Made glad."
Giovita

Joy Lat. "Joy." Used in the Middle Ages and sparingly by
the Puritans, then revived at the turn of the 20th century.
Unusual after the height of its popularity in the 1950s.
**Gioia, Gioya, Jioia, Jioya, Joi, Joice, Joie, Joya,
Joyann, Joye**

Joyce Lat. "Joyous." Used in the Middle Ages, but nearly
died out until the early years of the 20th century, when it
had a spurt of immense popularity, especially in Britain.
Advice columnist Dr. Joyce Brothers; writer Joyce Carol
Oates.
Joice, Joycelyn, Joyse, Joyous

Juanita Sp. Var. Joan.
**Janita, Juana, Juniata, Junita, Juwaneeta, Juwanita,
Nita, Wahnita, Wahnna, Wanna, Waneeta, Wanita**

Judith Heb. "Jewish." Old Testament name overlooked by
the Puritans in their quest for girls' names, but fashion-
able from the 1920s through the 1950s. In the Apoc-
rypha, Judith is a Jewish heroine who decapitates the
Assyrian general Holofernes and shows his head to the
Hebrew army, inciting them to victory. Actress Dame Ju-
dith Anderson; movie critic Judith Crist; chess champion
Judit Polgar.
**Giuditta, Jodie, Jody, Judee, Judi, Judie, Judit,
Judita, Judite, Juditha, Judithe, Judy, Judye, Jutta**

Judy Dim. **Judith**. Dates back to the 18th century, but its
true popularity follows that of Judith in the 20th century.
Jody is another frequently used diminutive. Actresses

Judy Garland, Judy Holliday, Dame Judi Dench; singer Judy Collins.

Judee, Judey, Judi, Judie, Judye

Julia (Fem. **Julius**) Lat. Clan name. "Youthful." Along with **Juliana,** used among the early Christians, but it was rare in the Middle Ages. Since the 1700s it has gone mildly in and out of fashion without ever being a tremendous favorite. **Julie,** in this century, has been much more popular but in the last ten years the the European form with the "-a" ending has soared to very frequent use. Chef Julia Child; opera star Julia Migenes; actresses Julia Ormond, Julia Roberts, Julia Louis-Dreyfus, Julia Stiles.

Giulia, Giuliana, Giulianna, Giulianne, Giulietta, Jiulia, Joleta, Joletta, Jolette, Julee, Juley, Juli, Juliaeta, Juliaetta, Juliana, Juliane, Juliann, Julianne, Julie, Julienne, Juliet, Julieta, Julietta, Juliette, Julina, Juline, Julinka, Juliska, Julissa, Julita, Julitta, Julyana, Julyanna, Julyet, Julyetta, Julyette, Julyne, Yulia, Yuliya

Juliana (Fem. **Julian** Lat. clan name. "Youthful." Appeared in the early Christian era, and medieval use contracted it to **Gillian** (and from there to **Jill**). Although a royal name in the Netherlands, it is unusual now, possibly seeming too stately. Contracted forms like **Liana** may eclipse it. Actresses Julianne Phillips, Julianne Moore, Julianna Margulies.

Giuliane, Giulianne, Juliane, Julianna, Julianne, Julieanna, Julieanne, Juline, Julinda, Julyana, Julyane, Julyanna, Julyanne

Julie Fr. Dim. **Julia** (Lat. Clan name. "Youthful"). Imported from France in the 1920s and fashionable very quickly, especially in the 1970s. It had earlier taken root on the Continent, as evidenced by Strindberg's 1888 tragedy *Miss Julie.* Actresses Julie Andrews, Julie Harris, Julie Walters, Julie Kavner; cookbook author Julee Rosso; pop singer Julee Cruise.

Jooley, Joolie, Julee, Juley, Julienne, Jullee, Jullie, July, Jully

Juliet Lat. Clan name. "Youthful." Dim. **Julia**. Can scarcely be used without reference to Shakespeare's famous tragic heroine. Girls named Juliet can expect a certain amount of teasing about Romeo. Dancer Juliet Prowse; actresses Juliet Stevenson, Juliette Lewis.

Giulietta, Juliaetta, Julieta, Juliett, Julietta, Juliette, Julyet, Julette

June Month used as name, dating from the 20th century but most popular in the 1950s. Scarcely seen today. Actress June Allyson.

Junella, Junelle, Junette, Junia, Juniata, Junieta, Junina, Junine, Junya, Jyune

Juno Lat. "Queen of heaven." Juno was the Roman equivalent of Hera in classical mythology: Jupiter's wife, and the gods' queen. Not widely used in any era; in modern times the adjective "Junoesque" has come to be used for tall women with curvy figures, possibly because of the way Juno is often portrayed in Old Master paintings.

Juneau, Juneaux, Junot

Justine Lat. "Fair, righteous." **Justina** was the original form, but the French version took over in the 1960s, probably aided by Lawrence Durrell's famous novel *Justine*. Actress Justine Bateman.

Giustina, Justa, Justeen, Justene, Justie, Justina, Justinn, Justy, Justyna, Justyne

K

Kadenza Lat. "With rhythm." Modern variant of Cadence.

Cadenza, Kadena, Kadence

Kaitlin Var. **Caitlin**, Irish form of **Catherine** (Gk. "Pure"). A name as popular as Catherine has produced endless variations over the years, and recently

Caitlin and its variants have become just as popular as the more familiar form.

Caitlin, Caitlyn, Kaitlyn, Katelyn, Katelynn, Katelynne, Kathlin, Kathlinne, Kathlyn

Kala Var. Kali.

Kali Sanskrit. "Black one."

Kalli

Kalila Arab. "Beloved."

Cailey, Cailie, Caylie, Kailey, Kalie, Kalilah, Kayllie, Kaly, Kaylee, Kylila, Kylilah

Kalliope Gk. Myth name. Calliope was the muse of epic poetry. Many of the "C" names that come from the Greek are spelled with a "K" in their original form.

Kallyope

Kallista Gk. "Most beautiful."

Cala, Calesta, Calista, Callie, Cally, Kala, Kalesta, Kalista, Kalli, Kallie, Kally, Kallysta

Kama Sanskrit. "Love," Heb. "Ripe."

Kamilah Arab. "Perfect."

Kamila, Kamilla, Kamillah

Kamilla European var. **Camilla**. Some sources trace Camilla to the young girls who assisted at pagan religious ceremonies.

Camilla, Cammie, Kamella, Kamila, Kamilka, Kamilla, Kamille, Kamyla, Kemilla, Milla, Millie

Kandace Var. Candace (Lat. "Glowing white"). Historically the name was the ancient title of the queens of Ethiopia before the 4th century. Not much used before the middle of the 20th century.

Candie, Candy, Dacie, Kandice, Kandiss, Kandy

Kara Var. **Cara** (Lat. "Dear one"). Principally used from the 1970s onward

Cara, Carina, Carita, Karina, Karine, Karita, Karrah, Karrie

Karen Dan. Var. **Katherine** (Gk. "Pure"). Took hold in the 1930s in English-speaking countries, and blossomed to great popularity in the 1950s and 1960s. Unusual today. Writer Karen Blixen (Isaak Dinesen); singer Karen Carpenter; actress Karen Allen.

Caren, Carin, Caron, Caronn, Carren, Carrin, Carron, Carryn, Caryn, Carynn, Carynne, Kari, Karin, Karna, Karon, Karryn, Karyn, Kerran, Kerrin, Kerron, Kerrynn, Keryn, Kerynne, Taran, Taren, Taryn

Karimah Arab. "Giving."

Kareema, Kareemah, Kareima, Karima

Karla Var. **Carla** (OG. "Man"). One of the endless names that derive from **Charles**. Fans of John Le Carré's novels will remember that George Smiley's Russian nemesis used the code name Karla.

Karlah, Karlla, Karrla

Karlotta Ger. Var. **Charlotte** (Fr. from OG. "Man").

Karlota, Karlotte, Lotta, Lottee, Lottey, Lottie

Karma Hindi. "Destiny, spiritual force." A New Age name if ever there was one.

Karolina Slavic. Var. **Caroline** (Lat. "Little and womanly").

Karaline, Karalyn, Karalynna, Karalynne, Karla, Karleen, Karlen, Karlena, Karlene, Karli, Karlie, Karlina, Karlinka, Karolina, Karoline, Karolinka, Karolyn, Karolyna, Karolyne, Karolynn, Karolynne, Leena, Lina, Lyna

Kasmira (Fem. **Casimir**) Old Slavic. "Bringing peace." Very unusual.

Kassandra Var. **Cassandra**. (Gk. Possibly Fem. Alexander).

Kate Dim. **Katherine**. Long-standing independent name, especially popular in the late 19th century. Writer Kate Chopin; actresses Kate Capshaw, Kate Jackson, Kate Nelligan, Kate Hudson, Kate Beckinsale, Kate Winslet; German artist Kaethe Kollwitz; designer Kate Spade; model Kate Moss.

Cait, Caitie, Cate, Catee, Catey, Catie, Kaethe, Kait, Kaite, Kaitlin, Katee, Katey, Kathe, Kati, Katie

Katherine Gk. "Pure." One of the oldest recorded names, with roots in Greek antiquity. Almost every Western country has its own form of the name, and phonetic variations are endless. It has been borne by such illustrious women as Saint Catherine of Alexandria, the early martyr who was tortured on a spiked wheel; Empress Catherine the

Great of Russia; and three of Henry VIII's six wives. It is currently very popular as **Katharina, Katja** or **Katya** in Northern Europe, albeit displaced by **Caitlin** in England and Scotland. It is still a standard among American girls' names. Actresses Catherine Oxenberg, Catherine Deneuve, Katharine Hepburn, Catherine Zeta-Jones; skater Katarina Witt.

Cait, Caitlin, Caitlinn, Caitrin, Caitrine, Caitriona, Caitrionagh, Caity, Caren, Cari, Carin, Caron, Caronne, Carren, Carri, Carrin, Carron, Caryn, Carynn, Cass, Cassey, Cassi, Cassie, Cat, Cataleen, Cataleena, Catalin, Catalina, Cataline, Catarina, Catarine, Cate, Cateline, Caterina, Cathaleen, Cathaline, Catharin, Catharina, Catharine, Catharyna, Catharyne, Cathee, Cathelina, Catherine, Catherina, Catheryn, Cathie, Cathirin, Cathiryn, Cathleen, Cathline, Cathlyne, Cathrine, Cathrinn, Cathryn, Cathrynn, Cathy, Cathye, Cati, Catie, Catina, Catlaina, Catreen, Catreina, Catrin, Catrina, Catrine, Catriona, Catrionagh, Catryna, Caty, Cay, Caye, Ekaterina, Kaatje, Kait, Kaitee, Kaitie, Kaitlin, Kaitlinn, Kaitrin, Kaitrine, Kaitrinn, Kaitrinna, Kaitriona, Kaity, Karen, Karena, Kari, Karin, Karon, Karri, Karrin, Karyn, Karynn, Kasia, Kasienka, Kasja, Kaska, Kasya, Kass, Kassi, Kassia, Kassie, Kas, Kat, Kata, Kataleen, Katalin, Katalina, Katarina, Katchen, Kate, Katee, Katell, Katelle, Katenka, Katerina, Katey, Katha, Katharine, Katharyn, Kathee, Kathelina, Katheline, Katherin, Katherina, Katheryn, Katheryne, Kathi, Kathie, Kathileen, Kathirin, Kathiryn, Kathirynn, Kathleen, Kathlene, Kathleyn, Kathline, Kathlyne, Kathrene, Kathrine, Kathrinna, Kathryn, Kathryne, Kathy, Kathyrine, Kati, Katie, Katica, Katina, Katinka, Katka, Katla, Katlaina, Katleen, Katline, Katoushka, Katouska, Katrena, Katrien, Katrina, Katrine, Katriona, Katrionagh, Katryna, Katushka, Katuska, Katy, Katya, Kay, Kaye, Kit, Kittey, Kitti, Kittie, Kitty, Rina, Trina, Trinchen, Trine, Trinette, Yekaterin, Yekaterina

Kathleen Ir. Var **Katherine** (Gk. "Pure"). Its use outside of Ireland began in the 1840s, and may have been influenced by the great wave of Irish emigration sparked by the potato famines of those years. U.S. popularity peaked in the 1950s. Actress Kathleen Turner.

Cathaleen, Cathaline, Cathleen, Kaitlin, Kaitlinn, Katha, Kathaleen, Kathaleya, Kathaleyna, Kathaline, Kathelina, Katheline, Kathleyn, Kathlin, Kathline, Kathlyn, Kathlyne, Kathyline, Katleen, Katlin, Katline, Katlyne

Kathy Diminutive, usually of **Katherine**. Rarely used as a given name by itself. TV host Kathie Lee Gifford; actress Kathy Najimy.

Cathie, Cathy, Kathee, Kathey, Kathie

Katrina Var. **Katherine** (Gk. "Pure"). Appealing for its European sound. Actress Katrin Cartlidge.

Caitrionagh, Catreena, Catreina, Catrina, Catriona, Catrionagh, Kaitrina, Kaitrona, Katreena, Katreina, Katriona, Katrionagh, Katryna, Ketreina, Ketrina, Ketryna, Kotrijna, Kotryna

Kay Dim. **Katherine**. First appeared at the turn of the 20th century, but widespread in the middle of the century. Actress Kaye Ballard; author Kay Thompson.

Caye, Kai, Kaye

Kayla Modern variant of **Katherine** (Gk. "Pure") or Dim. **Michaela** (Heb. "Who is like the Lord?"). After being very fashionable in the 1980s, still steadily used.

Cayla, Caylie, Kaela, Kaila, Kaylyn

Keely Ir. Var. **Kelly** ("Battle maid"). Actress Keeley Shaye Smith.

Kealey, Kealy, Keeley, Keeli, Keelia, Keelie, Keighley, Keighly, Keili, Keilie, Keyley, Keylie, Keylley, Keyllie

Keisha Modern name, possibly formed as a short version of **Lakeisha**, which, in turn, may be a variant of **Aisha** (Arab. "Woman"). Very popular with African-American families.

Keasha, Keesha, Keeshah, Keicia, Keishah, Keshia, Kicia

Kelila Heb. "Crowned."
   Kayla, Kayle, Kaylee, Kelula, Kelulah, Kelulla, Kyla, Kyle

Kelly Ir. Gael. "Battle maid." Originally a very common Irish last name, and very popular as a girl's first name from about the 1950s, peaking in the 1970s in America. Actresses Kelly McGillis, Kelly Preston, Kelly Ripa.
   Kellee, Kelley, Kelli, Kellie, Kellina

Kelsey OE. Place name, incorporating a word particle that means "island." Mostly recent usage, for boys as well as girls.
   Kelcey, Kelcie, Kelcy, Kellsey, Kellsie, Kelsea, Kelsee, Kelseigh, Kelsi, Kelsy

Kendra Origin unclear: Some sources suggest OE, "Knowing," while one proposes a modern combination of **Ken** and **Sandra**. Modern, in any case.
   Kendrah, Kenna, Kindra, Kinna

Kenya Place name used as first name.
   Kenia, Kennya

Kerensa Cornish. "Love." Unusual name that has spread a bit from Cornwall since the 1970s, but still of limited popularity.
   Karensa, Karenza, Kerenza

Kerry Ir. Place name: Kerry is a county in southwestern Ireland. Also, according to some sources, Ir. Gael. "Darkhaired." Actress Keri Russell.
   Keree, Keri, Kerrey, Kerri, Kerria, Kerridana, Kerrie

Ketura Heb. "Incense." Old Testament name: Keturah was Abraham's second wife. Revived by the Puritans and used with some steadiness through the 19th century.
   Katura, Keturah

Kezia Heb. "Cassia." Cassia is the generic name for a variety of trees and shrubs, one of which produces cinnamon. One of the three daughters of Job (along with Jemima; though their existence is mentioned in the Old Testament, their names are apocryphal). The name was adopted by the Puritans and brought to the U.S. in the 18th century, when it was popular. Use has declined gradually since then.

Kazia, Kessie, Kessy, Ketzia, Ketziah, Keziah, Kezzie, Kissie, Kizzie, Kizzy

Kiana Modern name of unclear origin.

Kia, Kiah, Kianna, Quiana, Quianna

Kim Dim. **Kimberly**. Used as an independent name from the mid-20th century, influenced by the careers of actresses Kim Novak and Kim Basinger. Actress Kim Cattrall.

Kimana, Kimm, Kym, Kymme

Kimberly OE. Place name. The "-y" suffix indicates a meadow. *The Facts on File Dictionary of First Names* traces the masculine use of the name to the Boer War, when many English soldiers were fighting in the South African town of Kimberley. It was used for girls after 1940 and became a great favorite in the 1960s and 1970s. Judge Kimba Wood.

Kim, Kimba, Kimber, Kimberlee, Kimberleigh, Kimberley, Kimberli, Kimberlie, Kimberlyn, Kimblyn, Kimm, Kimmie, Kimmy, Kym, Kymberleigh, Kymberley, Kymmberly, Kymbra, Kymbrely

Kineta Gk. "Active one." From the same root as "kinetic."

Kinetta

Kinneret Heb. "Harp." Also a place name in Israel.

Kira Var. **Kyra** (Gk. "Lady").

Keera, Kiera, Kierra, Kiria, Kiriah, Kirya, Kirra

Kirsten Scan. Var. **Christine** (Gk. "Christian"). Used generally from 1940, though the Scots had adopted this form long ago (possibly because of their geographical proximity to Scandinavia). Actresses Kirstie Alley, Kirsten Dunst.

Keerstin, Keirstin, Kersten, Kerstin, Kiersten, Kierstin, Kierstynn, Kirsteen, Kirsti, Kirstie, Kirstin, Kirsty, Kirstynn, Kjerstin, Kristyn, Krystin

Kitty Dim. **Katherine** (Gk. "Pure"). Used independently before the 16th century and during the 18th and 19th. In the intervening 200 years it was a slang term for a woman of dubious morals. Author Kitty Kelley.

Kit, Kittee, Kittey

Kizzy Var. **Keziah** (Heb. "Cassia"). Adopted enthusiastically by parents after it was publicized in Alex Haley's *Roots* as a traditional African name. Spoilsport scholars, however, point out that **Keziah** and its variants were common slave names as early as the 18th century.

Kissie, Kizzie

Klara Hung. Var. **Clara** (Lat. "Bright").

Klari, Klarice, Klarika, Klarissa, Klarisza, Klaryssa

Klaudia Pol. Var. **Claudia** (Lat. "Lame").

Klementina Var. **Clementia** (Lat. "Mild, giving mercy").
Clemence, Clementine, Klementijna, Klementine, Klementyna

Klotild Hung. Var. **Clothide** (Ger. "Renowned battle").
Klothild, Klothilda, Klothilde, Klotilda, Klotilde

Konstanze Ger. Var. **Constance** (Lat. "Steadfastness").
Constancia, Constantijna, Constantina, Konstance, Konstantia, Konstantijna, Konstantina, Kosta, Kostatina, Kostya, Tina, Stanze

Kora Gk. "Maiden." Though some sources trace the name to classical myth, its modern form was probably coined by American writer James Fenimore Cooper in *The Last of the Mohicans* (1826). It grew in popularity through the 19th century, but now its variant forms are more often used. The "K-" spelling is a particularly modern twist.
Cora, Corabel, Corabella, Corabelle, Corabellita, Corella, Corena, Coretta, Corey, Cori, Corilla, Corrie, Corry, Coryna, Korabell, Koree, Koreen, Korella, Korena, Korenda, Korette, Korey, Korilla, Korina, Korinna, Korinne, Korissa, Korrina, Korrine, Korynna, Koryssa

Kornelia Var. **Cornelia** (Lat. "Like a horn").
Cornelia, Kornelija, Kornelya

Kristen Com. form **Kirsten** and **Kristina,** var. **Christine** (Gk. "Anointed, Christian.") Looks Scandinavian, but isn't. Popular in the last 50 years, along with similar forms like **Kristin** and **Kristine.** Actresses Kristin Scott Thomas, Kristin Davis.
Khristin, Krissie, Krissy, Krista, Kristan, Kristeen, Kristel, Kristelle, Kristi, Kristijna, Kristin, Kristina,

Kristine, Kristyn, Kristyna, Krisztina, Krysia, Krysta, Krystyna

Krystal Var. **Crystal** (Gk. "Ice") Transferred use of the word, mostly modern, and increasing since the 1950s. The "K" spelling is a recent variation, perhaps prompted by the *Dynasty* character Krystle Carrington.

Cristalle, Cristel, Crysta, Khristalle, Khristel, Khrystle, Khrystalle, Kristle, Krystal, Krystaline, Krystalle, Krystalline, Krystle

Kyle Scot. Place name. "Narrow spit of land." Well-traveled parents may have crossed the Kyle of Lochalsh to reach the Isle of Skye. Traditionally used more often for boys than for girls.

Kyall, Kyel

Kylie Fem. **Kyle**. Pop singer Kylie Minogue.

Keyely, Kilea, Kiley, Kylee, Kyley

Kynthia Gk. Var. **Cynthia** (Gk. "From Mount Cynthos").

Kyra Gk. "Lady." A contraction of *Kyria,* the Greek title of respect for a woman. Ballerina Kyra Nichols; actress Kyra Sedgwick.

Kaira, Keera, Keira, Kira, Kyreena, Kyrha, Kyria, Kyrra

Lacey OF. Place name of obscure meaning, used as a boy's name in the 19th century and increasingly for girls today. Country singer Lacy J. Dalton.

Lace, Lacee, Laci, Lacie, Lacy, Laicee, Laicey, Laisey

Ladonna Modern elaboration of **Donna** (It. "Lady").

LeDonna

Lainey Dim. **Elaine** (OF. "Bright, shining, light").

Laney

Laila Arab. "Night." See **Leila**. Usually taken to indicate dark hair or a dark complexion. Actress Laila Robbins.

Laela, Lailah, Lailie, Laily, Laleh, Layla, Laylah

Lakeisha Popular modern name made up of elements in vogue in the 1980s, the fashionable "La-" prefix attached to **Aisha** (Arab. "Woman"). There are numerous forms, most of them phonetic variations.

Lakeesha, Lakecia, Laketia, Lakeysha, Lakicia, Lakisha, Lakitia, Lekeesha, Lekeisha, Lekisha

Lalage Gk. "Babbler, prattler." Extremely unusual, though it occurs in literature.

Lalia

Lallie Dim. **Lalage** (Gk. "Babbler, prattler"). More common than its source, though still rare. Journalist Lally Weymouth.

Lalia, Lally

Lana Var. **Helen** (Gk. "Light") or **Alanna** (Gael. "Rock" or "Comely"). Made famous by actress Lana Turner (whose real name was **Judy**), but not widely used.

Lanae, Lanette, Lanna, Lanny

Lane ME. Place name. More common for boys than for girls, though still unusual for both. This is the kind of name that is likely to be a mother's maiden name transferred to a first name.

Laine, Lainey, Laney, Lanie, Layne

Lani Haw. "Sky."

Lara Unclear origin. Some sources suggest Lat. "Famous"; others trace the name to the Greek **Larissa**. Parents may be reminded of the famous "Lara's Theme" from the 1965 film *Dr. Zhivago*. Actress Lara Flynn Boyle.

Larina, Larra

Laraine Var. **Lorraine** (Fr. "From Lorraine"). Actress Laraine Newman.

Laraene, Larayne, Lareine, Larina, Larine

Lareina Sp. "The queen." Compares to **Leroy** (Fr. "The king"). Uncommon.

Larayna, Larayne, Lareine, Larena, Larrayna, Larreina

Larissa Gk. "Lighthearted." From the same root as **Hilary**.

Unusual, even in times like the 18th century, when more elaborate names were the norm. Currently popular in Russia.

Larisa, Laryssa, Lerissa, Lissa, Lorissa, Lyssa

Lark ME. Nature name, used since the 1950s mostly in the U.S. Larks are usually thought of as playful, lighthearted songbirds.

Lassie ME. "Little girl." "Lass" is a Scottish and Northern English term for a girl, but the association for most parents is more likely to be a highly intelligent collie as seen on a popular TV series in the 1960s and again in the 1990s.

Lassey

Latanya Modern combined form: the "La-" prefix added to **Tanya**.

Latania, Latanja, Latonia, Latonya

Latifah Arab. "Gentle, pleasant." Singer/actress Queen Latifah.

Lateefa, Lateefah, Lateifa, Lateiffa, Latifa, Latiffa

Latisha Var. **Letitia** (Lat. "Happiness").

Laticia, Latitia, Letisha, Letticia, Lettisha

Latoya One of the most famous of the modern "La-" names, probably because of Latoya Jackson's renown. Derivation and meaning are mysterious.

Latoyah, Latoia, Latoyla, Letoya

Latrice Modern combined form: **Patricia** (Lat. "Noble") with the "La-" prefix.

Latrecia, Latreece, Latreese, Latreshia, Latricia, Leatrice, Letreece, Letrice

Laudomia It. "Praise to the house."

Laura Lat. "Laurel." In classical times, a crown made from the leaves of the bay laurel was given to heroes or victors. Two famous Lauras are the unknown woman to whom the poet Petrarch addressed his sonnets, and the heroine of the 1940s film *Laura*. The greatest popularity of the name came at the mid- to late 19th century, and it has remained quite a steady favorite ever since. A series of children's books were written by and about Laura Ingalls Wilder of

Little House on the Prairie fame. Actresses Laura Dern, Laura Linney; singer Laura Branigan; First Lady Laura Bush.

Laranca, Larea, Lari, Lauralee, Laure, Laureen, Laurel, Laurella, Lauren, Laurena, Laurence, Laurene, Laurentia, Laurentine, Laurestine, Lauretha, Lauretta, Laurette, Lauri, Lauriane, Laurianne, Laurice, Lauricia, Laurie, Laurina, Laurinda, Laurine, Laurnea, Lavra, Lawra, Lollie, Lolly, Lora, Loree, Loreen, Loren, Lorena, Lorene, Lorenza, Loretta, Lorette, Lorey, Lori, Lorie, Lorinda, Lorine, Lorita, Lorna, Lorretta, Lorrette, Lorri, Lorrie, Lorry, Lory

Laurel Lat. "Laurel tree." Nature name whose popularity has coasted on the coattails of **Laura,** especially in the 20th century.

Laural, Lauralle, Laurell, Loralle, Lorel, Lorelle

Lauren Var. **Laura** or feminization of **Lawrence.** Introduced to the public by Lauren Bacall, and immediately popular probably because the streamlined "modern" character of the name struck a chord in the 1940s. It might be fading from sight by now, but has been given extended popularity by the influential designer Ralph Lauren (né Ralph Lifshitz), who has endowed it with fashionable associations. Popular in the U.S. and throughout Great Britain. Model Lauren Hutton; First Daughter Lauren Bush; basketball player Lauren Jackson.

Laren, Larentia, Larentina, Larenzina, Larren, Laryn, Larryn, Larrynn, Larsina, Larsine, Laurence, Laurin, Lauryn, Laurynn, Loren, Lorena, Lorene, Lorenn, Lorenza, Lorin, Loryn, Lorne, Lorren, Lorrin, Lorrynn, Lourenca, Lourence, Lowran, Lowrenn, Lowrynn, L'Wren

Laveda Lat. "Cleansed."

Lavella, Lavelle, Laveta, Lavetta, Lavette

Laverne Lat. Classical goddess of minor criminals, though the parents who made this name mildly popular in the 20th century probably didn't know that. It sounds enough like the romance languages' word for "green" (*vert, verde*) to have acquired misplaced connotations of green trees or springtime.

Laverine, Lavern, Laverna, Laverrne, Leverne, Loverna, Verne

Lavinia Lat. "Women of Rome." Classical name. Revived in the Renaissance, again used in the 18th century, rather neglected for the last 200 years:

Lavena, Lavenia, Lavina, Lavinie, Levenia, Levinia, Livinia, Louvenia, Louvinia, Lovina, Lovinia, Luvena, Luvenia, Luvinia, Vinnie

Lavonne Modern combined form, probably "La -" attached to **Yvonne** (OF. "Yew wood"). Popular somewhat earlier (1950s–1980s) than most of the other "La-" names.

Lavonda, Lavonna, Lahvonne, Levonne, Levonda

Leah Heb. "Weary." Old Testament name: Leah was the wife of Jacob, married to him by a ruse in the place of her sister Rachel. Follows the typical usage pattern of the Old Testament names: revived by the Puritans, and still used with considerable steadiness. The form **Léa** is currently popular in France. Actress Lea Thompson.

Lea, Lee, Leia, Leigh

Leala OF. "Loyal."

Lealia, Lealie

Leandra (Fem. **Leander**) Gk. "Lion man." A spurt of use in the 1960s and 1970s has faded.

Leanda, Leiandra, Leodora, Leoine, Leoline, Leonelle

Leanne Com. form **Lee** and **Ann**. Singer LeAnn Rimes.

Leana, Leeann, Leanna, Lee-Ann, Leianne, Leyanne, Leigh-Anne, Leighanna, Lianne

Leatrice Com. form **Lee** and **Beatrice**.

Leda Gk., possibly Dim. **Letitia** (Lat. "Joy, gladness"). In classical myth Leda was visited by Jupiter in the form of a swan, and produced four children, among them the beautiful Helen of Troy.

Leida, Leta, Lida

Lee OE. Place name: "Pasture or meadow." One of the few truly unisex names. Usually a name becomes exclusively feminine once it is used for girls, like **Ashley** or **Leslie**.

The tenacious masculine hold on Lee may have been helped by tough-guy actor Lee Marvin. U.S. use seems to have been sparked by admiration for Confederate General Robert E. Lee. Peaked in the 1950s. Actress Lee Remick; Princess Lee Radziwill.

Lea, Leigh

Leila Arab. "Night." Used by authors in the early 19th century for exotic female characters, and more widely by American parents later in the century. American pronunciation of the first syllable varies, as the different spellings make clear.

Layla, Leela, Leelah, Leilah, Leilia, Lela, Lelah, Lelia, Leyla, Lila, Lilah

Leilani Haw. "Flower from heaven."

Lelia Lat. Clan name of unknown meaning, used in Britain and the U.S. in the late 19th century.

Leelia, Lilia

Lemuela (fem. **Lemuel**) Heb. "Devoted to God." Feminization of a name that was mildly popular in the 19th century.

Lemuelah, Lemuella, Lemuellah

Lena Lat. Diminutive of names like **Helena, Caroline, Marlene**. Independent use dates from the mid-19th century. Actress Lena Olin; singer Lena Horne; director Lina Wertmuller.

Leena, Leina, Lina

Lenis Lat. "Mild, soft, silky." Very rare.

Lene, Leneta, Lenice, Lenita, Lennice, Lenos

Lenna (Fem. **Leonard**) OG. "Lion's strength."

Lenda, Leonarda

Lenore Gk. "Light." Var. **Eleanor**.

Lenor, Lenora, Lenorah, Lenorr, Lenorra, Lenorre, Leonora, Leonore

Leoda OG. "Of the people."

Leota

Leona (Fem. **Leon**) Lat. "Lion." American version; **Léonie** is more popular in Europe. Use since the 1940s has grown, but the notorious Leona Helmsley has probably put a stop to its popularity. Singer Leontyne Price.

Leeona, Leeowna, Leoine, Leola, Leone, Leonelle, Leonia, Leonie, Leontine, Leontyne, Leowna

Leonarda (Fem. **Leonard**) OG. "Lion's strength."

Lenarda, Lenda, Lennarda, Leonarde

Léonie (Fem. **Leon**) Lat. "Lion." The French form of the name, more common in Britain than Leona.

Leoline, Leone, Leoni, Leonine, Leontine

Leonora Gk. "Light." Var. **Eleanor**. Name used for the heroine of three major operas (*Fidelio, Il Trovatore,* and *La Favorita*), but like many literary names, uncommon in real life.

Leanor, Leanora, Leanore, Lenora, Lenore, Leonore, ora, Norah

Leopoldine (Fem. **Leopold**) OG. "Bold people."

Leopolda, Leopoldina

Leora Gk. "Light." Dim. **Eleanor**.

Leeora, Liora

Leslie Scot. Gael. Place name. Some sources suggest, "The gray castle." Became a last name, then (in the 18th century) a first name used for boys and girls. Boys' use has been tied to admiration for actor Leslie Howard, and is more common in Britain. Not much used now. Actresses Lesley-Ann Down, Lesley Ann Warren.

Leslea, Leslee, Lesleigh, Lesley, Lesli, Lesly, Lezlee, Lezley, Lezlie

Leta Lat. "Glad, joyful." Classical name mildly revived at the turn of the 20th century.

Leeta, Lita

Letha Gk. "Forgetfulness." In Greek myth, a river in Hades that causes the dead to forget their lives on earth.

Leitha, Leithia, Lethe, Lethia

Letitia Lat. "Joy, gladness." In medieval England, the form was **Lettice**, which survived into the 20th century. (The name's resemblance to the principal ingredient of salad cannot have promoted its use.) Current use, which is rare, is usually of the Latinized form, Letitia. Etiquette expert Letitia Baldrige.

Laetitia, Laetizia, Latashia, Latia, Latisha, Leda, Leta, Letha, Letice, Leticia, Leticja, Letisha, Letizia, Letta, Lettice, Lettie, Lettitia, Letty, Letycja, Tish, Tisha

Levana Lat. "To rise." In Roman mythology, the goddess of newborn babies, whose fathers accepted them as legitimate in a ceremony involving lifting the infant from the ground.
Levania, Levanna, Levona, Livana, Livanna

Levina Lat. "Lightning bolt."

Lewana Heb. "Shining white one: the moon."
Levana, Levanna, Lewanna, Livana

Lexia Dim. Alexandra (Gk. "Defender of mankind").
Lexa, Lexie, Lexina, Lexine, Lexya

Leya Sp. "The law."

Liana Fr. "To twine around." Liana is the name of a vine common to tropical rain forests. Can also be a diminutive of Italianate names like **Ceciliana** or **Silviana**.
Leana, Leiana, Liahna, Liane, Lianna, Lianne

Liane Diminutive of French variants like **Juliane, Lilliane**. Also a spelling variant of **Lee-Ann**.
Leeanne, Leeahnne, Liahne, Lianne

Libby Dim. Elizabeth (Heb. "Pledged to God").
Lib, Libbee, Libbey, Libbie, Libet, Liby, Lilibet, Lilibeth

Liberty ME. "Freedom." Unusual, but occurs in "revolutionary" times like the 1970s.

Lida Slavic. "Loved by the people."
Leida, Lidah, Lyda

Liese Dim. Elizabeth (Heb. "Pledged to God"). Mostly found in Germany.
Liesa, Liesel, Liesl

Lieselotte Com. form Liese (Heb. "Pledged to God") and Charlotte (Fr. "Little womanly one").

Lila Arab. "Night." Can be a diminutive of **Delilah** (Heb. "Lovelorn, seductive"). Philanthropist Lila Acheson Wallace.
Layla, Leila, Lilah, Lyla, Lylah

Lilac Flower name. Not very common.
Lilach

Lilias Scot. Var. Lillian (Lat. "Lily").
Lilas, Lillas, Lillias

Lilibet Dim. Elizabeth (Heb. "Pledged to God"). The unlikely pet name of Her Majesty Queen Elizabeth II of England.

Lilibeth, Lillibet, Lilybet

Lilith Arab. "Ghost, night demon." One Old Testament translation refers to her as "the night hag." She was supposed to descend on sleepers and suck their blood. Connotations of the name are so fearsome that it is rarely used.

Lillis

Lillian Lat. "Lily." Very common variation of the flower name, flourishing at the turn of the 19th/20th centuries. Actress Lillian Gish and First Mother Lillian Carter were born during the name's peak of fashion, which faded after the 1930s. Pretty as it is, it carries a rather dated aura. Writer Lillian Hellman.

Lila, Lili, Lilia, Lilian, Liliana, Liliane, Lilias, Lilli, Lillia, Lillianne, Lillie, Lilly, Lillyan, Lillyanne, Lily, Lilyan, Lilyann

Lily Lat. Flower name. Possibly because the lily plays such a large part in Christian iconography, this has been one of the most popular of the flower names and has produced many variants. The "-y" ending, usually thought of as feminine, has probably also boosted its use, though it has not been popular since 1900. Ripe for a revival among parents with a taste for nostalgia. **Lilia** is currently well used in Russia. Actresses Lillie Langtry, Lily Taylor, Lily Tomlin, LeeLee Sobieski.

Leelee, Lil, Lila, Lilas, Lili, Lilia, Lilian, Liliana, Liliane, Lilias, Lilie, Lilla, Lilley, Lilli, Lillia, Lillianne, Lillie, Lillika, Lillita, Lilly, Liliosa, Lily, Lilyan, Lilyanne

Lina Diminutive of names ending with "-line," like **Caroline, Helena, Marlene**. Var. **Lena**. Given as an independent name from the 1850s.

Leena, Leina

Linda Sp. "Pretty." Though the name existed as a particle of other English names (**Belinda, Melinda**) by the time of its great vogue in the 20th century (late 1930s to 1960s), it was probably interpreted as "pretty." Rather neglected now. First daughter Lynda Bird Johnson; actresses Linda

Evans, Linda Hunt; singer Linda Ronstadt; journalist Linda Ellerbee; fashion designer Lindka Cierach.

Lin, Lindee, Lindey, Lindi, Lindie, Lindira, Lindka, Lindy, Linn, Lynda, Lynde, Lyndy, Lyn, Lynn, Lynne, Lynnda, Lynndie

Lindsay OE. Place name: "Island of linden trees." Originally a surname, used for boys until the middle of this century, but quite popular as a girl's name in the '80s and '90s. Use has tapered off. Actress Lindsay Wagner.

Lind, Lindsea, Lindsee, Lindseigh, Lindsey, Lindsy, Linsay, Linsey, Linsie, Linzi, Linzy, Linzee, Linzy, Lyndsay, Lyndsey, Lyndsie, Lynnsey, Lynndsie, Lynnzey, Lynsey, Lynzey, Lynzi, Lynzy

Linette Welsh. "Idol" or OF. "Linnet" (a small bird). In historical terms, probably a variant of **Lynette,** which is not, surprisingly enough, a form of **Lynn.** These names and their variations were most popular from the 1940s into the 1960s.

Lenette, Lanette, Linet, Linnet, Linnetta, Lonette, Lynette, Lynnet, Lynnette*

Linnea Scan. "Lime or linden tree" is the meaning given by most sources, but an informal network of people named Linnea trace the name to a mountain flower growing in northern climates that botanist Carl Linnaeus named for himself. A popular series of children's books by Christian Bjork featuring a character named Linnea has given the name greater exposure.

Linea, Linnaea, Lynea, Lynnea

Lisa Dim. **Elizabeth** (Heb. "pledged to God"). Used in numbers only since the 1950s, and reached the U.S. top ten in the 1970s. Actresses Lisa Bonet, Lisa Kudrow; talk show host Leeza Gibbons; basketball player Lisa Leslie.

Leesa, Leeza, Liesa, Liesebet, Lise, Liseta, Lisetta, Lisette, Liszka

Lissa Dim. **Melissa** (Gk. "Bee"). May also be considered a variation of **Lisa.** Unusual.

Lissette, Lyssa

Livia Dim. **Olivia** (Lat. "Olive"). Though the historical connotations of Olivia should concern peace and harmony, in the modern era it is hard not to think of the little green morsel at the bottom of a martini glass. Joyce fans, on a higher plane, may use the name to pay homage to the character Anna Livia Plurabelle from *Finnegan's Wake.*

Livija, Livvy, Livy, Livya, Lyvia

Liza Diminutive of **Elizabeth** and more particularly of **Eliza**. The vogue for **Lisa** gave Liza some reflected popularity, but the immense fame of entertainer Liza Minnelli must account for a great deal of its use.

Litsea, Litzea, Liz, Lizette, Lizzie, Lyza

Loelia Var. **Leila** (Arab. "Night"). Unusual form used occasionally at the turn of the 20th century.

Lois Var. **Louise** (OG. "Renowned in battle" though some sources suggest Gk. "Better"). Also, surprisingly enough, a biblical name. Use peaked early in the 20th century. Superman's consort Lois Lane.

Lola Dim. **Dolores** (Sp. "Sorrows"). The most famous Lola has been the 19th-century courtesan Lola Montez, which has given the name a slightly racy aura. It is fairly well used regardless.

Loela, Lolla

Lolita Dim. **Lola** (Sp. "Sorrows"). Made famous by Vladimir Nabokov's 1958 novel about a 12-year-old nymphet and her much older admirer, Humbert Humbert.

Lona Var. **Leona** (Lat. "Lion"). Uncommon. Actress Loni Anderson.

Lonee, Lonie, Lonna, Lonnie

Lora Var. **Laura** (Lat. "Laurel"). Not, as it might seem, a modern phonetic variant, but a throwback to the 14th century, when this was the usual spelling of the name.

Lorabelle, Loree, Lorenna, Lorey, Lori, Loribelle, Lorra, Lorree, Lorrie, Lory, Lowra

Lorelei Ger. Place name. Derives from the name of a dangerous rock jutting into the Rhine. Though popularly supposed to be an old myth, the tale of a siren perched on the rock to lure ships to destruction actually dates from a novel of 1801. The name, however, carries connotations of risky allure.

Laurelei, Laurelie, Loralee, Loralie, Loralyn, Lorilee, Lorilyn, Lura, Lurette, Lurleen, Lurlene, Lurline

Lorelle Dim. **Laura** or **Laurel** (Lat. "Laurel tree").
Laurelle, Lorrella, Lowrelle

Lorenza (Fem. **Lorenzo**) Lat. "From Laurentium." Very unusual in English-speaking countries, being primarily an Italian name.
Laurenca, Laurenza

Loretta Dim. **Laura** (Lat. "Laurel"). A name that cropped up with the 19th-century taste for elaboration, and became famous with actress Loretta Young. Country singer Loretta Lynn; actress Loretta Swit.
Laretta, Larretta, Lauretta, Laurette, Leretta, Lorretta, Lowretta

Lori Dim. **Laura** (Lat. "Laurel"). Unlike Lora, this is a modern spelling and was very popular in the 1960s. The rage for the "-i" ending on names has diminished considerably since then.
Loree, Lorri

Lorna Scot. Place name converted into a female name for the 19th-century romantic novel *Lorna Doone*. Used occasionally, but to most North Americans, it is probably the name of a cookie. Entertainer Lorna Luft.
Lorrna

Lorraine Fr. "From Lorraine." Lorraine is an area in eastern France, but this is not just your average place name: It was often used for Joan of Arc (who was from Lorraine), and for the style of quiche with bacon and gruyere cheese. It can also be considered an elaboration of **Lora**. Was well used from the 1930s, and in the U.S. its vogue peaked in the 1940s. Rare now. Actress Laraine Newman.
Laraine, Larayne, Laurraine, Leraine, Lerayne, Lorain, Loraine, Lori, Lorine, Lorrayne

Lottie Dim. **Charlotte** (Fr. "Little, womanly"). Mostly 19th-century use. Singer Lotte Lenya.
Lotta, Lotte, Lotie, Lotti, Lotty

Lotus Gk. "Lotus flower." The name signifies different plants in several different cultures: The Egyptians consider it a kind of water lily, while to the Greeks it is a shrub. It also has great significance in the Indian religions and in Homeric legend, where eating the lotus causes people to forget their homes and families and long for a life of idleness.

Lou Dim. **Louise**. Used mostly in America, and in combined forms such as **Louann, Mary Lou, Louella**, etc.
Louanna, Louanne, Louella, Lu, Loulou

Louise (Fem. **Louis**) OG. "Renowned in battle." Actually a French (and more euphonious) version of **Ludwig**. **Louisa** was the preferred form in the 18th and 19th centuries, eclipsed by Louise at the turn of the century. Currently very unusual in the U.S. Author Louisa May Alcott; actresses Louise Brooks, Louise Lasser.
Aloisa, Aloise, Aloysia, Eloisa, Eloise, Heloisa, Heloise, Lois, Loise, Lola, Lolita, Lou, Louisa, Louisetta, Louisette, Louisina, Louisiana, Louisiane, Louisine, Louiza, Lovisa, Lowise, Loyise, Lu, Ludovica, Ludovika, Ludwiga, Luisa, Luise, Lujza, Lujzika, Lula, Lulita, Lulu

Love OE. "Love." Unromantically enough, probably not the name of the emotion but a transferred surname. Singer Courtney Love.
Loveday, Lovey

Luana OG. Com. form **Louise** and **Anne**. One of many possible phonetic versions of the name.
Lewanna, Lou-Ann, Louanna, Louanne, Luane, Luann, Luannah, Luannie, Luwana

Lucerne Lat. "Lamp." Also the name of a city in Switzerland; parents have occasionally named children for the cities where they were born—or, in the modern era of frankness, conceived.
Lucerna

Lucetta Dim. **Lucy** (Lat. "Light"). Mostly 19th century, now very unusual.
Loucetta, Loucette, Lucette

Lucia It. Var. **Lucy** (Lat. "Light"). Uncommon form in English-speaking countries. Ballet patron Lucia Chase.

Lucille Fr. Var. **Lucy** (Lat. "Light"). As **Lucilla,** used by the Romans and revived in the 19th century. Lucille came into use at the turn of the 20th century, and its considerable popularity (roughly 1940–1960) seems to have been inspired by comedienne Lucille Ball.

Loucille, Luseele, Lusile, Lucila, Lucile, Lucilla, Lucyle

Lucinda var. **Lucy** (Lat. "light"). Popular along with the other "-inda" names of the 18th century (**Clarinda, Belinda**), and boosted by the fondness for **Lucille**.

Cindy, Loucinda, Lusinda

Lucita Sp. Dim. **Lucy** (Lat. "light"). Also an allusion to the Virgin Mary as Santa Maria de Luz.

Lusita, Luzita

Lucretia Lat. Clan name of uncertain meaning, though some sources suggest "wealth." The famous story of the rape of Lucretia concerns a Roman matron who, having been raped, stabbed herself rather than live with her shame.

Loucrecia, Loucresha, Loucretia, Loucrezia, Lucrece, Lucrecia, Lucreecia, Lucreisha, Lucreesha, Lucresha, Lucrezia*

Lucy Lat. "Light." The vernacular form of **Lucia,** and more widely used in modern times, peaking in the U.S. at the turn of the century. The 4th-century martyr Saint Lucy, patroness of sight, is often depicted with a pair of eyes in a dish, though her martyrdom did not involve being blinded. The Lucy in Charles Schulz's much-loved "Peanuts" comic strip is the prototypical bossy little girl. For a pretty name with few negative connotations, it is surprisingly little-used in the U.S., though very popular in England. Actress Lucy Liu.

Lou, Loulou, Lu, Luce, Lucetta, Lucette, Luci, Lucia, Luciana, Lucida, Lucie, Lucienne, Lucile, Lucilia, Lucilla, Lucille, Lucina, Lucinda, Lucine, Lucita, Lucyna, Lucyja, Lucza, Lusita, Luz, Luzija

Ludmilla Slavic. "Beloved of the people."

Ludmila, Lyuba, Lyudmila

Luella OE. Com. form **Louise** (OG. "Renowned in battle") and **Ella** (OG. "All"). Can also be said to come from **Lucy**; it's often not possible to trace a name's roots accurately. Columnist Louella Parsons.

Loella, Lou, Louella, Lu, Luelle, Lula, Lulu

Lulu Dim. **Louise** (OG. "Renowned in battle"). Fashion designer Lulu Guinness.

Luna Lat. "Moon."

Luneth, Lunetta, Lunette, Lunneta

Lupe Sp. Allusion to the Virgin Mary as she miraculously appeared to a peasant boy in Guadalupe, Mexico.

Lupelina

Lurleen Modern variant of **Lorelei** (Ger. place name).

Lura, Lurette, Lurlene, Lurline

Luz Sp. "Light." Another name for the Virgin Mary: Santa Maria de Luz.

Lydia Gk. "From Lydia." Lydia was an area of Asia famous for its two rich kings, Midas and Croesus. The name (biblical in origin) was used heavily in the 18th and 19th centuries, less so in the 20th. Cookbook author Lydie Marshall.

Lidia, Lidie, Lidija, Lyda, Lydie

Lynette Welsh. "Idol." Though it looks like a modern elaboration of **Lynn,** this is actually a French version of the Welsh **Eiluned,** and was popularized by the English poet Tennyson. However, its use (middling, since the 1940s) has certainly depended on the appeal of Lynn.

Lanette, Linett, Linette, Lynett, Lynetta

Lynn Dim. **Linda** (Sp. "Pretty"). This is one of those names that, along with its variations, is so popular as to virtually swamp its source. Most used in the 20th century. Actress Lynn Redgrave.

Lin, Linell, Linn, Linnell, Lyn, Lynae, Lyndel, Lyndell, Lynelle, Lynette, Lynna, Lynne, Lynell, Lynnelle, Lynnett, Lynette

Mab Ir. Gael. "Joy, hilarity." Welsh. "Baby." In old English, Welsh, and Irish stories, Queen Mab is monarch of the fairies.
Mave, Mavis, Meave

Mabel Dim. **Amabel** (Lat. "Lovable"). Very popular at the turn of the 20th century, but uncommon now, perhaps because it has the air of being a period artifact. Singer Mabel Mercer.
Amabel, Amable, Amaybel, Amaybelle, Amayble, Mab, Mabelle, Mable, Maible, Maybel, Maybelle, Mayble

Madeline Gk. Place name: Magdala was a town on the Sea of Galilee, the home of Saint Mary Magdalen, whom Jesus healed and who was present at his crucifixion. **Magdalen** was the common form in the Middle Ages, but the "g" was dropped, leaving Madeline as the standard form. The French version, **Madeleine,** became more popular in the 1930s, but the name, pretty as it is, has never been a standard. Many people may be familiar with this name from Ludwig Bemelmans's French schoolgirl Madeline in her wide-brimmed hat, from the children's books. Actresses Madeline Kahn, Madeleine Stowe.
Dalanna, Dalenna, Lena, Lina, Lynn, Mada, Madalaina, Madaleine, Madalena, Madalyn, Maddalena, Maddie, Maddy, Madel, Madelaine, Madelayne, Madeleine, Madelena, Madelene, Madelina, Madella, Madelle, Madelon, Madge, Madlen, Madlin, Madlyn, Mady, Madzia, Magda, Magdala, Magdalen, Magdalena, Magdalene, Magdalina, Magdaline, Magdalini, Magdeleine, Magdelina, Magdolna, Maidel, Maighdlin, Mala, Malena, Malina, Marleah, Marleen, Marlen, Marlena, Marlene, Marline, Marlyne, Maud, Maude

Madge Dim. **Madeline, Margaret** (Gk. "Pearl").

Madison OE. "Son of the mighty warrior." Another obscure masculine name that has crossed over into fashionable use for girls. It has been in the top ten names for American girls since 1997, but in 1993 was ranked no higher than 78th.
Maddie, Maddison, Madisen, Madisson

Madonna Lat. "My lady." Used mostly by devout Catholic families, like the parents of rock star Madonna Louise Ciccone. Her global fame coupled with some of her more racy public personas make her an unlikely role model for parents.
Madona

Madra Sp. "Mother."

Maeve Ir. Gael. Possibly "Delicate, fragile." Name of a 1st-century queen of Ireland, and used mostly in that country.

Magda Ger. Var. **Madeline** (Gk. "from Magdala") or **Maida** (OE. "Maiden").

Maggie Dim. **Margaret** (Gk. "Pearl"). Used as an independent name in the late 19th century. Although babies are more likely to be given the full name these days, Maggie is precisely the kind of nostalgic-sounding nickname that appeals to today's parents. Dance impresario Maguy Marin; actresses Maggie Smith, Maggie Gyllenhall.
Magali, Maggey, Maggi, Maggy, Magli, Maguy

Magnilda OG. "Strong in warfare."
Magnhilde

Magnolia Lat. Flower name. The tree was named after 17th-century French botanist Pierre Magnol. Because of the tree's popularity on old southern plantations, the name is redolent of Dixie.
Maggie, Maggy, Nola

Mahala Heb. "Tender affection." Old Testament name that was well used in the 19th century. Singer Mahalia Jackson is keeping it alive today.
Mahalah, Mahalath, Mahalia, Mahaliah, Mahalla, Mahelia, Mehalia

Maia Gk. "Mother." In Greek myth, a nymph who became mother of Hermes; also the Roman goddess of the springtime, for whom the month of May is named. Uma Thurman and Ethan Hawke named their daughter Maya. Writer Maya Angelou.

Maaja, Maiah, Maj, Maja, May, Maya, Mayah, Moia, Moja, Moya, Mya

Maida OE. "Maiden." Used with some frequency in the 19th century, often in the diminutive form **Maidie**.

Maddie, Maddy, Mady, Magda, Maidel, Maidie, Mayda, Maydena, Maydey

Maisie Dim. **Margaret** (Gk. "Pearl"). Originally a Scottish variation by way of **Margery**, it became more widespread early in the 20th century. Literary parents may be reminded of Henry James's novel *What Maisie Knew*.

Maisey, Maisy, Maizie, Mazey, Mazie

Majesta Lat. "Majesty."

Majidah Arab. "Splendid."

Majida

Malka Heb. "Queen."

Malcah, Malkah, Malke, Malkia, Malkie, Milcah, Milka, Milke

Mallory OF. "Unhappy, unlucky." Literally, *malheureux.* Originally a nickname, transferred to a last name and thus to a first name. Used for boys as well.

Mallary, Mallerey, Malloreigh, Mallorey, Mallorie, Malorey, Malorie, Malory

Malva Gk. "Slender, delicate." Also a flower name.

Melva, Melvina

Malvina Literary name invented by a romantic poet of the 18th century: It may come from the Gaelic words for "smooth brow." Sculptor Malvina Hoffman.

Mal, Malva, Malvie, Maveena, Mavina, Mel, Melva, Melvie, Melvina, Melvine

Mamie Dim. **Margaret** (Gk. "Pearl") or **Mary** (Heb. "Bitter"). First Lady Mamie Eisenhower.

Maime, Mame, Mayme

Manda Dim. **Amanda** (Lat. "Much-loved").

Mandee, Mandie, Mandy

Mandisa South African. "Sweet."

Mandy Dim. **Amanda** (Lat. "Much-loved"). Popular in Great Britain a generation ago. Pop singer Mandy Moore.
Mandee, Mandie

Mansi Hopi. "Plucked flower."

Manuela (Fem. **Emmanuel**) Sp. from Heb. "The Lord is among us."
Manuelita

Mara Heb. "Bitter." In the Old Testament, Naomi says, "Call me Mara, for the Almighty has dealt very bitterly with me." This is widely considered to be the root of that all-time favorite, **Mary**.
Mahra, Marah, Maralina, Maraline, Mari, Marra

Marcella (Fem. **Marcellus**) Lat. "Warlike." First cropped up at the turn of the 20th century. Very unusual.
Marcela, Marcele, Marcelle, Marcellina, Marcelline, Marchella, Marchelle, Marcie, Marcile, Marcilee, Marcille, Marcy, Maricel, Marquita, Marsalina, Marsella, Marselle, Marsellonia, Marshella, Marsiella

Marcene (Fem. **Mark**) Lat. "Warlike." An American variant that occurred in the 1940s and 1950s, following on the popularity of **Marcia**.
Marceen, Marcena, Marcenia, Marceyne, Marcina

Marcia (Fem. **Mark**) Lat. "Warlike." Used in Imperial Rome and not revived until the late 19th century. It gradually became a great favorite in the middle of the 20th century, but was passé by the 1970s. Actress Marsha Mason.
Marcelia, Marcene, Marchita, Marci, Marciane, Marcie, Marcile, Marcille, Marcilyn, Marcilynn, Marcina, Marcita, Marcy, Marquita, Marsha, Marseea, Marsia, Martia

Marcy Dim. **Marcella** (Lat. "Warlike").
Marcee, Marcey, Marci, Marcie, Marsee, Marsey

Mare Ir. Var. **Mary** (Heb. "Bitter"). Actress Mare Winningham.
Mair, Maire

Marelda OG. "Renowned battle maid."
Marilda, Marrelda

Margaret Gk. "Pearl." One of the standard female names of the Western world. In the Middle Ages the virgin martyr Saint Margaret (swallowed by a dragon) was hugely popular, keeping the name current. An 11th-century queen of Scotland was also a saint, and the name is especially common in Scotland. It has been neck and neck with **Mary** from the 17th century until the 1970s, when more novel names have moved to the forefront. Britain's Princess Margaret and Prime Minister Margaret Thatcher; actresses Margaret Sullavan, Marg Helgenberger; anthropologist Margaret Mead; writer Margaret Mitchell.
Greta, Gretal, Gretchen, Gretel, Grethel, Gretta, Grette, Gretl, Madge, Mag, Maggi, Maggle, Maggy, Maiga, Maighread, Mairead, Maisie, Maisy, Malgorzata, Marcheta, Marchieta, Marga, Margalit, Margalo, Margareta, Margarete, Margaretha, Margarethe, Margaretta, Margarette, Margarida, Margarit, Margarita, Margarite, Margaruite, Marge, Marged, Margeret, Margeretta, Margerie, Margerita, Margery, Marget, Margette, Margey, Marghanita, Margharita, Margherita, Marghretta, Margie, Margies, Margisia, Margit, Margize, Margo, Margot, Margred, Margret, Margreth, Margrett, Margrid, Marguarette, Marguarita, Marguerita, Marguerite, Marguita, Margy, Marjery, Marjey, Marji, Marjie, Marjorey, Marjorie, Marjory, Marketa, Marketta, Markie, Markita, Marquetta, Meg, Megan, Meggi, Meggie, Meggy, Meghan, Meta, Metta, Mette, Meyta, Peg, Pegeen, Peggie, Peggy, Rita

Margery Fr. Dim. **Margaret**. Imported to England in the 12th century and steadily used there until a late-19th-century revival that lasted into the 1930s, usually as **Marjorie**. Because it is unusual but not outlandish, a good candidate for revival. Novelists Margery Allingham, Margery Sharp.
Marchery, Marge, Margeree, Margerey, Margerie, Margey, Margi, Margie, Margy, Marje, Marjerie, Marjery, Marjie, Marjorey, Marjori, Marjorie, Marjory, Marjy

Margo Fr. Dim. **Margaret**. Another import that never matched the popularity of **Margery**. Actress Margaux Hemingway changed the spelling of her name to match that of a famous Bordeaux wine, Chateau Margaux. Ballet star Dame Margot Fonteyn.
Margaux, Margot

Marguerite Fr. Var. **Margaret**. Also botanical, the French name for a daisy, and popular at the same time (late 19th century to mid-20th) as that flower name. French writers Marguerite Duras, Marguerite Yourcenar.
Margarite, Margaruite, Marghanita, Margherita, Margherite, Marguerita, Margurite

Maria Lat. Var. **Mary** (Heb. "Bitter"). Launched in English-speaking countries in the 18th century as a welcome alternative to the all-too-common Mary. Faded after some 200 years, but revived in the middle of the 20th century, particularly after the popularity of *West Side Story,* with its famous ballad "Maria." This version is now slightly more popular than the Anglo Mary. Singer Maria Muldaur; TV journalist Maria Shriver.
Mariah, Marie, Marja, Marya, Mayra, Mayria, Moraiah, Moriah

Marian Fr. com. form **Mary** (Heb. "Bitter") and **Ann** (Heb. "Grace"). Var. **Mary**. Actually an anglicization of **Marion**. Common in the Middle Ages, and after a period of neglect, revived in the early Victorian era when medieval history was very popular. Singer Marian Anderson; Robin Hood's love interest Maid Marian; track star Marion Jones.
Mariam, Mariana, Mariane, Marion, Maryann, Maryanne

Marianne Fr. Com. form **Marie** (Heb. "Bitter") and **Anne** (Heb. "Grace"). Like **Annemarie,** combines the names of the Virgin Mary and her mother, thus appealing powerfully to Catholic families. In English-speaking countries **Mary Ann** is the standard form, though Marianne has had moments of fashion, in the early 19th and mid-20th centuries. Marianne is the name of the official symbol who personifies the spirit of France, while Mary Ann

Evans was the real name of Victorian novelist George Eliot.

Mariana, Mariane, Mariann, Marianna, Maryann, Maryanna

Maribel Com. form **Mary** (Heb. "Bitter") and **Belle** (Fr. "Beautiful"). This is a modern name.

Maribelle, Marybelle, Meribel, Meribella, Meribelle

Marie Fr. Var. **Mary** (Heb. "Bitter"). Also the earliest English spelling of the name, revived in the 19th century, and in the 1970s nearly as popular as Mary. Now much less in vogue. Scientist Marie Curie; singer Marie Osmond.

Maree

Mariel Dutch. Var. **Mary** (Heb. "Bitter"). Actress Mariel Hemingway.

Marella, Marelle, Marial, Marieke, Mariela, Mariele, Mariella, Marielle, Mariet, Marijke, Marilla

Marietta Fr. Dim. **Mary** (Heb. "Bitter") via **Marie**. Current since the mid-19th century. Philanthropist Marietta Tree.

Maretta, Mariet, Mariette, Maryetta

Marigold Flower name. The golden yellow flower, whose name is a combination of **Mary** and "gold." It cropped up in the 20th century, a bit later than the 19th-century craze for flower names.

Maragold, Marrigold

Marika Dutch. Var. **Mary** (Heb. "Bitter").

Marieke, Marijke, Marike, Mariska, Mariske, Maryk, Maryka

Marilyn Dim. **Mary** (Heb. "Bitter"). Possibly also a combination of Mary and **Ellen** (Gk. "Light"). In any case, a modern name promoted by show business, not in the person of Marilyn Monroe (whose career in the 1950s paralleled the name's decline), but by an earlier star, Marilyn Miller. As is often the case with modern names, there are numerous phonetic variations. Author Marilyn French; opera star Marilyn Horne.

Maralin, Maralynn, Marelyn, Marilee, Marilin, Marillyn, Marilynne, Marralynn, Marrilin, Marrilyn, Marylin, Marylyn

Marina Lat. "From the sea." As in "marine." Also possibly, in the distant mists of time, related to the Latin god of war, Mars. Currently popular in Russia.

Mareina, Marena, Marine, Marinell, Marinella, Marinna, Marna, Marne, Marnetta, Marnette, Marni, Marnie

Marion Fr. Dim. **Mary** (Heb. "Bitter"). Though it was turned into **Marian** when it arrived in Britain in the Middle Ages, this form was revived as well in the 19th century and is now just as common. It is occasionally used for boys as well. Track star Marion Jones.

Marian, Maryon, Maryonn

Maris Lat. "Of the sea." Comes from the phrase *stella maris,* or "star of the sea," which refers to the Virgin Mary.

Marisa, Marise, Marissa, Marisse, Marris, Marys, Maryse, Meris

Marisa Var. **Maris, Marissa**. Somewhat eclipsed by Marissa. Actresses Marisa Berenson, Marisa Tomei.

Mareesa, Mareisa, Marysia, Moreisa, Morisa, Morysa

Marisol Com. form **Mary** (Heb. "Bitter") and *sol* (Sp. "Sun"). A modern name particularly favored in Puerto Rico.

Marissa Var. **Maris** (Lat. "Of the sea").

Maressa, Marisa, Marisse, Marrissa, Merissa, Meryssa, Morissa

Marjolaine Fr. "Marjoram." Unusual botanical name.

Marjorie Var. **Margery.** Dim. **Margaret** (Gk. "Pearl"). Imported to England in the 12th century as Margery, and steadily used there until a late-19th-century revival that lasted into the 1930s. This is currently the most common form, though the name is infrequently given.

Marcharie, Marge, Margeree, Margerey, Margerie, Margery, Margey, Margi, Margie, Margy, Marje, Marjerie, Marjery, Marjie, Marjorey, Marjori, Marjory, Marjy

Marla Var. **Marlene**. Appeared in the 1940s, but hard to find since the 1970s. Actress Marla Gibbs.

Marlah, Marlla

Marlene Com. form **Mary** (Heb. "Bitter") and **Magdalene**

(Gk. "From Magdala"). Marlene Dietrich introduced the name in the 1920s, and it was widespread by the 1940s, but is now rare. Actresses Marlee Matlin, Marley Shelton.

Marla, Marlaina, Marlane, Marlayne, Marlea, Marlee, Marleen, Marlen, Marlena, Marley, Marlie, Marlin, Marline, Marlyn, Marlynne, Marna

Marlo Modern name, possibly a variation of the last name Marlow, or a diminutive of **Marlene**. Briefly popular in the 1970s, perhaps following the TV career of actress Marlo Thomas.

Marlon, Marlow, Marlowe

Marmara Gk. "Sparkling, shining."

Marmee

Marna Origin disputed. May be a diminutive of **Marina** or of **Marlene**.

Marne, Marney, Marni, Marnia, Marnie, Marnja, Marnya

Marsha Var. **Marcia**. The less common form in America.

Marsia, Marsita, Martia

Martha Aramaic. "Lady." In the New Testament, Martha is the woman who bustles around resentfully getting dinner ready while her sister Mary listens to Jesus. She is patron saint of the helping professions. The name has been very widely used since the Puritans revived it, though it is less common in the last 40 years. First Lady Martha Washington; dancer Martha Graham; Martha "Calamity" Jane Burke; actress Martha Plimpton.

Maarva, Marfa, Mariet, Marit, Mart, Marta, Martella, Martelle, Marth, Marthe, Marthena, Marthine, Marthini, Marti, Martie, Martina, Martita, Martta, Marty, Martynne, Martyne, Marva, Mata, Matti, Mattie, Pat, Pattie

Martina (Fem. **Martin**) Lat. "Warlike." Tennis stars Martina Navratilova, Martina Hingis.

Marta, Marteena, Marteina, Martie, Martine, Marty, Tina, Tine

Marvel OF. "Something to marvel at."

Maravilla, Maraville, Marivel, Marivella, Marivelle, Marva, Marvela, Marvele, Marvella, Marvelle

Mary Heb. Though "bitter, bitterness" is the most commonly accepted meaning, the *Facts on File Dictionary of First Names* disputes this. "Rebellious" is also sometimes suggested. Mary is the Greek version of **Miriam**. Although until the Middle Ages it was considered too sacred to use, it gradually became the most common female name. The numerous variants, both English and foreign, cropped up as a result of the name's great popularity. In the modern era it is frequently combined with other names (**Mary Jo, Mary Lou, Mary Beth**). Ironically, the name once thought of as completely commonplace is now quite unusual among young children. Actresses Mary Pickford, Mary Martin, Mary Stuart Masterson; Queens Marie Antoinette and Mary of Scots; artist Mary Cassatt; writer Mary Shelley; political strategist Mary Matalin; pop singer Mary J. Blige.

Mair, Marie, Mal, Malia, Mallie, Mame, Mamie, Manette, Manon, Manya, Mara, Marabel, Marabelle, Mare, Maree, Marella, Marelle, Maren, Maretta, Marette, Maria, Mariam, Marian, Mariann, Marianna, Marianne, Marice, Maridel, Marie, Mariel, Mariella, Marielle, Marietta, Mariette, Marilee, Marilin, Marilla, Marilyn, Marin, Marion, Mariquilla, Mariquita, Mariska, Marita, Maritsa, Maritza, Marja, Marje, Marla, Marlo, Marya, Maryann, Maryanne, Marylin, Marysa, Maryse, Marysia, Masha, Maura, Maure, Maureen, Maurene, Maurine, Maurise, Maurita, Maurizia, Mavra, May, Mayme, aymie, Mayra, Mayria, Meridel, Meriel, Mimi, Minette, Minnie, Minny, Miriam, Mitzi, Moira, Moire, Moll, Mollie, Molly, Morag, Moya, Muire, Murial, Muriel, Murielle, Poll, Polly

Matilda OG. "Battle-mighty." William the Conqueror's wife took the name to Britain in the 11th century, when it was pronounced "Maud." It was revived in the 18th century, but faded again in the 19th, and was never a real favorite in the U.S. Most parents know it only from the famous Australian song "Waltzing Matilda."

Mafalda, Maffalda, Maitilde, Maltilda, Maltilde, Mat,

Matelda, Mathilda, Mathilde, Matilde, Matti, Mattie,
Matty, Maud, Maude, Maudie, Tilda, Tilde, Tildie,
Tildy, Tilli, Tillie, Tilly

Mattea (Fem. Matthew) Heb. "Gift of God."

Mathea, Mathia, Matthea, Matthia, Mattia

Maud Var. Matilda. Although a common enough name
after the Middle Ages, its period of real popularity was
1840–1910, especially in Britain. Now rare. Actress
Maude Adams.

Maude, Maudie

Maura Ir. Var. Mary (Heb. "Bitter").

Moira, Mora, Morah

Maureen Ir. Var. Mary (Heb. "Bitter"). Popular in the baby
boom era, but to today's parents, this is a name for a previous generation. Actresses Maureen O'Sullivan, Maureen O'Hara.

Maura, Maurene, Maurine, Maurise, Maurita,
Maurizia, Mavra, Moira, Mora, Moreen, Morena,
Morene, Moria, Morine

Mauve Fr. "Mallow plant." The petals of the mallow are
purple, hence the use of this word for a color.

Malva

Mavis Fr. "Thrush." Popular mostly in Britain from the turn
of the 20th century into the thirties.

Maxine Lat. "Greatest." A modern name that had its moment from the fifties through the seventies.

Massima, Max, Maxeen, Maxena, Maxence, Maxene,
Maxie, Maxime, Maxina, Maxy

May Several possible sources: a medieval form of **Matthew**
(Mayhew), a nickname form of **Mary,** or an anglicization
of **Maia**. It was very fashionable in the U.S. in the 1870s,
some 50 years before month names (April and June) became current. Actress Mae West; writer Maya Angelou;
poet May Sarton.

Mae, Maia, Maj, Mala, Maya, Mayana, Maye, Mei

Mead OE. Place name: "Meadow." This is more common as
a last name.

Meade

Meara Ir. Gael. "Jollity."

Medea Gk. "Ruling." Since the Medea of Greek myth was a witch who left a trail of dead bodies behind her (including those of her two children), the name has gruesome connotations and is rarely used.

Madora, Medeia, Media, Medora, Medorah

Meg Dim. **Margaret** (Gk. "Pearl"). Rarely given as an independent name. Actresses Meg Tilly, Meg Ryan.

Megan Welsh. Dim. **Margaret** (Gk. "Pearl"). Fairly widespread in the 20th century, and surged into popularity in the early '90s, when it hit the top ten in the U.S. Extremely popular in Great Britain. Actress Megan Mullaly.

Maegan, Meagan, Meaghan, Meg, Megen, Meggi, Meggie, Meggy, Meghan, Meghann, Meghanne, Meighan

Mehitabel Heb. "Benefited by God." Old Testament name rarely used, except by writer Don Marquis in his tales of the great friends *archy and mehitabel,* a cockroach and a cat.

Mehetabel, Mehitabelle, Hetty, Hitty

Meira Heb. "Light."

Melanie Gk. "Black, dark-skinned." Uncommon until the publication of *Gone With the Wind,* whose Melanie Wilkes launched it into fashion. Scarlett, though the more memorable character, did not inspire parents in the same way. Actresses Melanie Mayron, Mclanie Griffith.

Malaney, Malanie, Mel, Mela, Melaina, Melaine, Melainey, Melaney, Melani, Melania, Melanney, Melannie, Melantha, Melany, Mella, Mellanie, Melli, Mellie, Melloney, Melly, Meloni, Melonie, Melonnie, Melony, Milena

Melantha Gk. "Dark flower."

Mallantha

Melba Name coined in honor of the Australian operatic soprano Nellie Melba (the dessert peach Melba and thin Melba toast was also named after her). She, in turn, took her name from her hometown, Melbourne. Actress Melba Moore.

Malva, Mellba, Melva

Melina Gk. "Honey." Use was mostly 19th century. Actress Melina Mercouri.

Melibella, Melibelle, Malina, Mallina, Meleana, Meleena, Mellina

Melinda Lat. "Honey." Names ending in "-inda" (**Belinda, Clarinda**) were very fashionable in the 18th century, when this name was coined. It became more widespread in the 19th century, but is still far from common.

Linda, Lindy, Linnie, Lynda, Maillie, Malina, Malinda, Malinde, Mallie, Mally, Malynda, Mandy, Melina, Melinde, Meline, Mellinda, Melynda

Meliora Lat. "Better." Unusual Roman name used by the Puritans, but now rare.

Melisande Fr. Var. Melissa.

Lisandra, Malisande, Malissande, Malyssandre, Melesande, Melisandra, Melisandre, Melissande, Melissandre, Mellisande, Melysande, Melyssandre

Melissa Gk. "Bee." A name that existed in ancient Greece and occurred steadily through the 19th century, but had no real vogue in English-speaking countries until the 1970s. Now somewhat neglected. Singer Melissa Manchester; actress Melissa Gilbert; dancer Molissa Fenley.

Lissa, Malissa, Mallissa, Mel, Melesa, Melessa, Melicent, Melicia, Melisa, Melisande, Melise, Melisenda, Melisent, Melisha, Melisse, Melita, Melitta, Mellicent, Mellie, Mellisa, Melly, Melosa, Milli, Millicent, Millie, Millisent, Millissent, Milly, isha, Missie, Missy

Melita Gk. "Honey."

Malita, Malitta, Melida, Melitta, Melyta

Melody Gk. "Song." Though it occurred as early as the 13th century, common usage didn't develop until the 1940s, and didn't endure.

Melodee, Melodey, Melodia, Melodie

Melvina Celt. "Chieftain." A variation of **Malvina**, itself a literary name coined in the 18th century. **Melva** is the most common variant, but all forms are rare.

Malvina, Melva, Melvena

Mercedes Sp. "Mercies." Refers to Santa Maria de las Mercedes, or Our Lady of the Mercies. Mostly Catholic use. Actresses Mercedes McCambridge, Mercedes Ruehl.
Merced, Mercede, Mercedez

Mercia OE. Place name: Refers to the English Kingdom of Mercia, which comprised much of central England in the 6th through 9th centuries. The name has been used mostly in the 20th century.

Mercy ME. "Mercy." One of the names of virtues that were so popular among the Puritans (who, since they were very pious but couldn't use saints' names, were often hard put to find appropriate names for their children).
Mercey, Merci, Mercie, Mersey

Meredith Old Welsh. "Great ruler." Occasionally used for boys, especially in Wales. Elsewhere a girl's name, used with some frequency. Actress Meredith Baxter; newscaster Meredith Vieira.
Meradith, Meredithe, Meredyth, Meridith, Merridie, Merry

Meriel Var. **Muriel** (Ir. Gael. "Sea-bright").
Merial, Merielle, Meriol, Merrill, Meryl

Merle Fr. "Blackbird." Use probably inspired by actress Merle Oberon, whose middle name it was. Little used recently.
Merl, Merla, Merlina, Merline, Merola, Meryl, Myrle, Myrleen, Myrlene, Myrline

Merry OE. "Lighthearted, happy." Also dim. **Meredith, Mercy.** May also be considered a variant of its homonym, **Mary.**
Marrilee, Marylea, Marylee, Merree, Merri, Merrie, Merrielle, Merrile, Merrilee, Merrili, Merrily

Meryl Var. **Muriel** via **Meriel.** Strictly a 20th-century name, which in the U.S. is strongly associated with actress Meryl Streep.
Meral, Merel, Merrall, Merrell, Merril, Merrill, Merryl, Meryle, Meryll

Messina Lat. "Middle." Also a place name: Messina is a town in Sicily.
Massina, Mussina

Meta Ger. Dim. **Margaret** (Gk. "Pearl"). Use is mostly German.

Mia It. "Mine." Probably owes much of its use to the career of actress Mia Farrow. Soccer player Mia Hamm; model Mia Tyler.
Mea, Meya

Michaela (Fem. **Michael**) Heb. "Who is like the Lord?" The most common feminine form of Michael is the French **Michelle,** but Michaela gained ground briefly in the 1990s. Actress Michael Learned.
Macaela, MacKayla, Makayla, Makyla, Mechaela, Meeskaela, Mekea, Micaela, Michal, Michael, Michaelina, Michaeline, Michaila, Michalin, Michele, Michelina, Micheline, Michelle, Mickee, Mickie, Miguela, Miguelina, Miguelita, Mahalya, Mihaila, Mihalia, Mihaliya, Mikaela, Mikhaila, Mikhayla, Mishaela, Mishaila, Miskaela

Michelle (Fem. **Michael**) Fr. var. Heb. "Who is like the Lord?" Spelled with one or two *l*s, fashionable right from its 1940s appearance in English-speaking countries. The Beatles' famous song "Michelle" gave the name even more of a boost, putting it on some top-ten lists in the 1970s. Now past its prime. Actresses Michelle Pfeiffer, Sara Michelle Gellar; figure skater Michelle Kwan.
Chelle, Machelle, Mashelle, M'chelle, Mechelle, Meechelle, Meshella, Mia, Micaela, Michaela, Michaelina, Michaeline, Michaella, Michal, Michele, Michelina, Micheline, Michell, Micki, Mickie, Midge, Miguela, Miguelita, Mikaela, Miquela, Misha, Mishaelle, Mishelle, M'shell, Mychelle, Myshell, Myshella

Michiko Jap. "The righteous way." The name of the first commoner ever to become empress of Japan.
Michee, Michi

Mignon Fr. "Cute." First used as a name by the German poet Goethe, and has spread from literary to real-life use, but not with great frequency. Opera singer Mignon Dunne.

Mignonette, Mignonne, Mingnon, Minyonne,
Minyonette

Milada Czech. "My love."

Milagros Sp. "Miracles."

Mila, Milagritos, Miligrosa

Mildred OE. "Gentle strength." An Anglo-Saxon name that
was revived in the 17th century, but its real popularity
came in the U.S. from 1900–1930. By the time of the
1945 film *Mildred Pierce,* it was already slightly dated.

Mildrid, Millie, Milly

Millicent OG. "Highborn power." Norman name that has
been used mostly in Britain, at its most fashionable
around 1900, but never a standard. U.S. Congresswoman
Millicent Fenwick.

Lissa, Mel, Melicent, Melisande, Melisenda, Mellicent,
Mellie, Mellisent, Melly, Milicent, Milissent, Millie,
Millisent, Milly, Milzie, Missie

Mimi Dim. **Mary, Miriam,** etc. First used by parents after
the appearance of Puccini's famous opera *La Bohème*
whose tragic heroine is named Mimi. Actress Mimi
Rogers.

Meemee, Mim

Mindy Dim. **Melinda** (Lat. "Honey").

Mindee, Mindie

Minerva The name of the Roman goddess of wisdom.
Those great revivalists the Victorians brought it back for
their daughters, but by the Jazz Age it was obsolete.

Min, Minette, Minnie, Myna

Minna Dim. **Wilhelmina** (OG. "Will-helmet"). Most common at the turn of the 20th century. **Mina** is currently
well-used in Germany.

Min, Mina, Minetta, Minette, Minne, Minnie, Minny

Minnie Dim. **Mary, Wilhelmina**. Enjoyed a great vogue as
an independent name around the 1870s for no very clear
reason. Most parents now will associate it with Mickey
Mouse's girlfriend. Actress Minnie Driver.

Minnee

Minta Dim. **Araminta**. An 18th-century literary name.

Minty

Mira Lat. "Admirable." Dim. **Miranda** or var. **Myra,** although it is usually pronounced with a short *i*. In Spanish *mira* spelled this way means, "Look!" The name was most used in the 19th century. Fashion designer Myrène de Premonville.

Mireille, Mirella, Mirelle, Mireya, Mirielle, Mirilla, Mirra, Myra, Myrella, Myréne, Myrilla

Mirabel Lat. "Wonderful." In this case the "-bel" ending does not mean "beautiful," though the variations often spell it "-belle." In fact, it was at one period a man's name. Very rare.

Meribel, Meribelle, Mira, Mirabella, Mirabelle

Miranda Lat. "Admirable." Another name contributed to us by Shakespeare, this time directly from the Latin: He used it for the heroine of *The Tempest.* Use has been steadily slight until the early 90s when it had a brief flare of popularity, since extinguished. Actress Miranda Richardson.

Maranda, Meranda, Mira, Miran, Mirandah, Mireille, Mirella, Mirra, Mirranda, Myra, Myranda, Myrella, Myrilla, Myrrilla, Randa, Randi, Randie, Randy

Miriam Heb. Possibly "Bitter" or "Rebellious." This is the source of **Mary,** which is its Latin form, and its translation is not quite clear, though "bitter" is very widely accepted. Overlooked by the Puritan fervor for Old Testament names, but revived in the 18th century and quite common for some 250 years, peaking around 1900 in the U.S. Now unusual. Singer Miriam Makeba.

Mariam, Maryam, Meriam, Meryam, Mimi, Mirham, Mirjam, Mirjana, Mirriam, Miryam, Mitzi, Mitzie, Miyana, Miyanna

Missy Dim. **Melissa** or **Millicent**. Pop singer Missy Elliott.

Missie

Misty OE. "Mist." Briefly popular in the U.S. in the middle of the 20th century.

Mysti

Mitzi Ger. Var. **Mary** (Heb. "Bitter"). Actress Mitzi Gaynor.

Mitzee, Mitzie

Modesty Lat. "Modesty." As **Modesta,** used by the Ro-

mans, but very rare ever since, even during the Puritan
craze for virtue names.

Modesta, Modestia, Modestina, Modestine

Moira Ir. Var. **Mary** (Hcb. "Bitter"). Dancer Moira Shearer.

Moire, Moyra

Molly Dim. **Mary** (Heb. "Bitter"). Not Irish, in spite of the
famous song "Cockles and Mussels" about Dublin's
"sweet Molly Malone." Since a "moll" has meant, at various times, a prostitute or a gangster's girlfriend, the name
has had long periods of disuse, but now that these slang
terms are obsolete, the name has found its way into the top
100 in the U.S. Actress Molly Ringwald; author Mollie
Hardwick.

Moll, Mollee, Molley, Mollie, Molly

Mona Ir. Gael. "Aristocratic." Spread from Ireland in the
mid-19th century. Never widespread, but common enough
not to be outlandish.

Moina, Monah, Monna, Moyna

Monica Possibly Lat. "Adviser" or "Nun." Established by
Saint Monica, the mother of Saint Augustine, and favored
by Catholic families.

**Mona, Monca, Monicka, Monika, Monike, Moniqua,
Monique, Monnica**

Morela Pol. "Apricot."

Morgan Different sources give different meanings, including Welsh "Great and bright" and OE. "Bright or white
sea dweller." Morgan is most common in Wales as both a
first and a last name, for both sexes. The current trend
toward unisex names suggests that the feminizations are
in for a spell of disuse. Actress Morgan Fairchild.

**Morgana, Morgance, Morgane, Morganica, Morganne,
Morgen, Morgin**

Moriah Heb. "The Lord is my teacher." May also be arrived
at as a variant of **Mariah/Maria/Mary**.

Moraia, Moraiah

Moselle (Fem. **Moses**) Heb. Possibly "Savior." Also a variety of delicately sweet white wine.

Mosella, Mosette, Moiselle, Moisella

Mouna Arab. "Wish, desire."
Mounia, Muna, Munira

Muriel Ir. Gael. "Sea-bright." Some names, like this one, seem rooted in a certain period (in this case the first half of the 20th century), but Muriel actually dates back to the Middle Ages. Perhaps the children of the 21st century will eventually find it nostalgic enough to use for *their* children. Novelist Muriel Spark.
Merial, Meriel, Merrill, Muireall, Murial, Muriella, Murielle

Musetta Middle French. "Little bagpipe." "Musette" came to be the term for a dance tune that employed the musette, an instrument fashionable in the 18th century.
Musette

Musidora Gk. "Gift of the Muses."

Myra (Fem. **Myron**) Lat. "Scented oil." Literary name coined in the early 17th century, but real-life use dates from the 19th century. Harpsichordist Dame Myra Hess; author Maira Kalman.
Maira, Mira, Myree

Myrna Ir. Gael. "Tender, beloved." The era of the name's popularity, the 1930s and 1940s, spans the career of actress Myrna Loy.
Meirna, Merna, Mirna, Moina, Morna, Moyna, Muirna

Myrtle Botanical name. The myrtle is a dark green shrub with pink or white blossoms. The name first appeared in the 1850s, before the true vogue for flower names, but it became more popular along with those other names in the 1880s. Now dated.
Mertice, Mertis, Mertle, Mirtle, Myrta, Myrtia, Myrtice, Myrtie, Myrtis

Naavah Heb. "Lovely."
   Nava, Navit
Nabila Arab. "Highborn."
   Nabeela, Nabilah

Nadette OG. "Bear/courageous." Dim. **Bernadette**.

Nadia Rus. "Hope." **Nada** appeared in English-speaking countries at the turn of the 20th century, but Nadia had taken root by the 1960s. Though not outlandish, it has a pleasantly foreign sound. Currently fashionable in Russia. Gymnast Nadia Comaneci; poet Nadezhda Mandelstam.
   Nada, Nadege, Nadejda, Nadezhda, Nadie, Nadija, Nadiya, Nadja, Nady, Nadya, Nadyenka, Nadzia, Nata, Natka

Nadine Fr. Var. **Nadia**. Author Nadine Gordimer.
   Nadeen, Nadena, Nadene, Nadie, Nadina, Nadyna, Nadyne, Naydeen

Naida Gk. "Water nymph."
   Naia, Naiad, Naiada, Nayad, Niada, Nyad, Nyada

Nan Var. **Ann** (Heb. "Grace"). At its most common in the 18th century, but now occurs most often as a nickname for Ann. Its diminutives (**Nana, Nanny**) have come to mean "grandmother" or "person who looks after children."
   Nana, Nance, Nanci, Nancie, Nancy, Nanella, Nanelle, Nanette, Nania, Nanine, Nanna, Nannette, Nannie, Nanny, Nanon, Nettie, Ninon

Nancy Var. **Ann** (Heb. "Grace"). Also originally a nickname whose use as a given name began at roughly the same time as **Nan,** in the 18th century. Nancy, however, took root more firmly (perhaps because it had not acquired any other meanings) and was very popular in the U.S. in the middle of the 20th century. First Lady Nancy Reagan; skater Nancy Kerrigan; writer Nancy Mitford.
   Nainsey, Nainsi, Nance, Nancee, Nanci, Nancie,

**Nancsi, Nanice, Nanncey, Nanncy, Nannie, Nanny,
Nansee, Nansey**

Nanette Fr. Dim. Nan.

Nannette, Nettie, Netty, Ninon

Naomi Heb: "Pleasant." Old Testament name; the mother-
in-law of Ruth, who, after her sons died, said, "Do not call
me Naomi, call me Mara, for the Almighty has dealt very
bitterly with me." Naomi came into English-speaking use
not with the Puritan revival of biblical names, but in the
18th century. Actress Naomi Watts.

**Naoma, Naomia, Naomie, Nayomi, Navit, Noami,
Noémi, Noémie**

Narcissa Gk. "Daffodil." Not actually a flower name, but
the unusual feminine version of the masculine (and
equally unusual) **Narcisse,** which comes from the legend
of the beautiful Greek youth who became enamored of his
own reflection—hence "narcissism."

Narcisa, Narcisse, Narcyssa, Narkissa, Narsissa

Narda Lat. "Scented ointment."

Nastasia Gk. "Resurrection." Dim. **Anastasia.** Actress
Nastassja Kinski.

**Nastassia, Nastassija, Nastassja, Nastassiya,
Nastassya**

Nasya Heb. "The Lord's miracle."

Nasia

Natalie Lat. "Birth day." More specifically, the Lord's
birthday, or Christmas. This is probably the most common
of all the Christmas names, and certainly the only one that
is used for babies born at other times of the year (unlike
Noel). Though there was a 4th-century Saint Natalia, this
Frenchified form did not crop up until the late 19th century. Actresses Natalie Wood, Natalie Portman; singer Natalie Cole.

**Nat, Nata, Natala, Natalee, Natalene, Natalia, Natalja,
Natalina, Nataline, Nataly, Nataliya, Natalya, Natasha,
Natelie, Nately, Nathalia, Nathalie, Nathaliely,
Nathalija, Natilie, Natividad, Nattilie, Nattie, Nettie,
Talia, Talya, Tasha**

Natasha Rus. Var. **Natalie.** Actress Natasha Richardson.

Nastaliya, Nastalya, Natacha, Natascha, Natashenka, Natosha, Natucha

Nathania (Fem. **Nathan**) Heb. "A gift or given of God."

Natividad Sp. "Christmas." See **Natalie**.

Neala (Fem. **Neal**) Gael. "Champion." Unusual feminization of the male name that was quite popular in the middle of the 20th century.

Neale, Nealla, Neila, Neile, Neilla, Neille

Neda (Fem. **Edward**) OE. "Wealthy defender" via the nickname **Ned,** or Rus. "Born on Sunday." In any case, very unusual.

Nedda, Neddie, Nedi

Neila Heb. "Closing, locking."

Neilla

Nell Dim. **Helen, Eleanor** (Gk. "Light"). Used sparingly as an independent name, though some of its variants like **Nellie** have had periods of popularity. Charles II's mistress Nell Gwynn; opera star Nellie Melba.

Nel, Nella, Nellene, Nellie, Nellwen, Nellwin, Nellwyn, Nelly

Neola Gk. "Young one." Comes from the same root as the widely used prefix "neo-."

Nerine Gk. "Sea nymph."

Narine, Narice, Narissa, Nerice, Nerida, Nerina, Nerissa, Neryssa

Nessie Dim. **Agnes** (Gk. "Lamb"). Also the name of the Loch Ness Monster, which might limit its appeal.

Nesha, Nessa, Nessia, Nessya, Nesta, Neta, Netia

Nettie Diminutive of "-ette" names like **Henrietta** or **Nanette**. Use as an independent name mostly around the turn of the 20th century.

Netta, Netty

Neva Sp. "Snowy." Nevada, which means "covered with snow," is one of the American state names (like Florida) that adapts nicely to use as a girl's name. Actress Neve Campbell.

Nevada, Nevara, Neve, Nieves

Nicole (fem. **Nicholas**) Gk. "Victory of the people." **Nicola,** the Italian form, is more common in Britain (though its vogue peaked there in the 1970s). This French version has been more popular in other English-speaking countries, reaching the top ten in the U.S. in the 1980s. Singer Nicolette Larson; actress Nicole Kidman.

Cola, Colette, Cosetta, Cosette, Nichelle, Nichola, Nicholassa, Nichole, Nicholette, Nicholl, Nicholle, Nicia, Nicki, Nickola, Nickole, Nicky, Nico, Nicola, Nicolasa, Nicolea, Nicolene, Nicoleen, Nicolette, Nicolie, Nicolina, Nicoline, Nicolla, Nicolle, Nika, Niki, Nikita, Nikki, Nikky, Niko, Nikola, Nikole, Nikoleta, Nikoletta, Nikolia, Niquole, Niquolle, Nychole, Nycholl, Nykia, Nycole, Nykole, Nykolia, Nyquole, Nyquolle

Nike Gk. "Victory." Also, and more commonly to most Americans, the name of a very popular athletic shoe.
Nika

Nikki Var. Nicole. Used mostly in the 1960s.
Nickie, Nicky, Niki, Nikkey, Nikky

Nina Sp. "Girl." Dim. **Ann** (Heb. "grace") History buffs will remember that Nina was the name of one of Christopher Columbus's three ships. The name is rather uncommon. Ballerina Dame Ninette de Valois.
Neena, Neina, Nenna, Neneh, Ninacska, Nineta, Ninete, Ninetta, Ninette, Ninnette, Ninon, Ninochka, Ninoska, Ninotchka, Nyna

Niobe Gk. "Fern." In myth, Niobe was a boastful queen of Thebes whose children were all killed as a reprimand for her arrogance. In her resulting misery she asked Zeus to turn her to stone. In art she is usually depicted weeping.

Nita Sp. Dim. **Juanita, Anita**, etc. Unusual.

Nixie OG. "Water sprite." Usually beautiful and antagonistic to men, unlike pixies, which, though mischievous, are content to share the world with humans.

Noel Fr. "Christmas." Though used since the Middle Ages for both boys and girls, it is more common for the latter.
Noela, Noeleen, Noelene, Noeline, Noeliz, Noella, Noelle, Noelleen, Noelynn, Nowel, Noweleen, Nowell

Nola Dim. **Finola** (Gael. "White shoulder"). Related to **Nuala** but not, as many parents think, to **Nolan**.

Nowla
Noleta Lat. "Unwilling."
　Nolita
Nona Lat. "Ninth." Although it was originally used for a
　family's ninth baby, it would hardly have survived to this
　day if parents had not been willing to overlook its mean-
　ing.
　Nonah, Noni, Nonie, Nonna, Nonnah
Nora Dim. **Eleanor** (Gk. "Light") or **Honora** (Lat.
　"Woman of honor"). Used independently, especially for
　the half century around 1900. Well-read parents will re-
　member Nora as the heroine of Ibsen's *A Doll's House;*
　she sets a discouraging precedent, however. Writer Nora
　Ephron; pop singer Norah Jones.
　Norah, Norella, Norelle
Norberta (fem. **Norbert**) OG. "Renowned northerner."
Noreen Ir. Dim. **Nora.** Originated in Ireland.
　Norene, Norina, Norine
Norma Lat. "Pattern." From the same root that gave us
　"normal" or "the norm." Launched by Bellini's 1831
　opera of the same name, and boosted in the 1920s by pop-
　ular actress Norma Shearer. Out of fashion for the last
　couple of generations. Fashion designer Norma Kamali.
　Norm, Normie, Normina
Novia Lat. "New"; Sp. "Girlfriend."
　Nova
Nuala Dim. **Fionnula** (Ir. Gael. "White shoulder"). Irish
　writer Nuala O'Faolain.
　Nola, Noola, Nualla, Nula
Nunzia It. "Messenger." See **Annunciata**.
　Nunciata
Nur Arab. "Light." The Arabic name adopted by the former
　Queen of Jordan, an American woman known as Lisa Ha-
　laby until she married the King.
　Noor, Nour, Noura, Nureen, Nurine
Nydia Lat. "Nest." Also Sp. from Gk. "Graceful."
　Nidia, Needia
Nyx Gk. "Night."
　Nix, Nixe

Octavia Lat. "Eighth." Used most often in the Victorian era of large families.
Octaviana, Octavianne, Octavie, Octiana, Octoviana, Ottavia, Tavia, Tavie, Tavy

Odele Derivation disputed. Some sources relate it to either German "Rich" or Greek "Song," but *The Facts on File Dictionary of First Names* claims that it derives from an Old English place name: "Woad hill." Woad is a blue dye reputedly used by the ancient Druids in their religious rites.
Odela, Odelet, Odelette, Odelina, Odeline, Odell, Odella, Odelle, Udele, Udelia, Udilia

Odelia Heb. "I will praise the Lord." Possibly also related to **Odele**.
Oda, Odeelia, Odele, Odelinda, Odella, Odellia, Odilia, Udele, Udelia, Udilia

Odessa Gk. "Long voyage." As in "odyssey," more specifically Homer's epic poem about the wandering Odysseus. The Russian port of Odessa was supposedly named to honor *The Odyssey*.
Odissa, Odyssa, Odyssia

Odette Fr. from Ger. "Wealthy." In the famous ballet *Swan Lake,* the same ballerina usually dances as both Odette, the good swan, and Odile, the evil black swan. Folk singer Odetta.
Odetta

Odile Fr. Var. **Otthild** (OG. "Prospers in battle"). Related to **Odette** and also to **Odelia**. For balletomanes, the malevolent alter ego of Odette.
Odila, Odilia, Odolia, Udelia, Udile, Udilia

Olena Rus. var. **Helen** (Gk. "Light").
Alena, Elena, Lena, Lenya, Olinia, Olinija, Olenya, Olina, Olinia, Olinija

Olesia Gk. "Man's defender."
  Ola
Olethea Var. **Alethea** (Gk. "Truth").
  Oleta
Olga Rus. "Holy." The Russian form of **Helga,** and perhaps more common than Helga in English-speaking countries. The Russian Saint Olga was a princess from Kiev and a 10th-century Christian convert; the name was favored in the ill-fated Russian imperial family. Gymnast Olga Korbut.
  Elga, Helga, Ola, Olenka, Olia
Oliana Polynesian. "Oleander."
  Oleana, Olianna
Olinda Lat. "Scented."
Olivia Lat. "Olive tree." The most common form of the name today, though **Olive** had a flurry of popularity with other nature names at the turn of the 20th century. It would be hard to use Olive today given the fame of Popeye's scrawny girlfriend, Olive Oyl. This form, though, is speeding up popularity charts. Also very popular in England. Actresses Olivia de Havilland, Olivia Hussey; singer Olivia Newton-John.
  Liv, Liva, Livia, Livvie, Livvy, Olia, Oliff, Oliffe, Oliva, Olive, Oliveea, Olivet, Olivette, Olivija, Olivine, Olivya, Ollie, Olva
Olwen Welsh. "White footprint." Along with **Bronwen,** one of the best known Welsh-language first names. Nevertheless, it is very unusual outside Wales.
  Olwenn, Olwin, Olwyn, Olwynne
Olympia Gk. "From Mount Olympus," the home of the gods. Slightly more common in Europe, where it may avoid the faintly commercial connotation of the Olympic Games. Actress Olympia Dukakis; Senator Olympia Snowe.
  Olimpe, Olimpia, Olimpiada, Olimpiana, Olypme, Olympie
Oma Arab. "Leader." Infrequent use.
Omega Gk. "Last." It would seem to be tempting fate to use this name for a youngest child.

Ondine Lat. "Little wave." In myth, Undine is the spirit of the waters. Edith Wharton created a heroine in *The Custom of the Country* who was named Undine for the hair curling tonic that had made her father rich.
Ondina, Ondyne, Undine

Oneida Native American. "Long awaited." In the U.S. probably most familiar as a brand of silverware, which was originally manufactured by a utopian colony that was disbanded in the 19th century because its residents practiced polygamy.
Onida, Onyda

Onella Gk. "Light."

Onora Var. **Honoria** (Lat. "Honor").
Onnora, Onoria, Onorine, Ornora

Oona Ir. Var. **Una** (Lat. "Unity").
Oonagh, Una

Opal Sanskrit. "Gem." One of the less common of the jewel names.
Opalina, Opaline, Opall

Ophelia Gk. "Help." Most famously, the young girl in *Hamlet* who goes mad. Mostly used in the late 19th century, but its connotations are far from happy.
Availia, Filia, Ofelia, Ofilia, Ophélie, Ophelya, Ophilia, Ovalia, Ovelia, Phelia, Ubelia, Uvelia

Ora Lat. "Prayer." Homonym for **Aura,** which means "Gold" or "Breeze."
Orabel, Orabelle, Orareeana, Orarariana, Orra

Oralee Heb. "My light."
Orali, Oralit, Orlee

Oralie Fr. Var. **Aurelia** (Lat. "Golden").
Aurelie, Oralee, Oralia, Orelie, Oriel, Orielda, Orielle, Orlena, Orlene

Orane Fr. "Rising." From the same Latin source as **Oriana.**
Orania, Oriane

Orela Lat. "Announcement from the gods." Related to "oracle."
Orelda, Orella, Orilla

Oriana Lat. "Dawning." From the same root as **Aurora.** Italian journalist Orianna Falacci.

Oria, Oriane, Orianna

Oriole Lat. "Golden." Most commonly the name of a bird with golden markings, or the name of the Baltimore baseball team.

Auriel, Oreolle, Oriel, Oriella, Oriola, Oriolle

Orpah Heb. "A fawn." Old Testament name rarely used. Talk show star Oprah Winfrey's unusual name is the result of a misspelling of this name.

Afra, Aphra, Ofrit, Ophrah, Oprah, Orpa

Orquidea Sp. "Orchid."

Orsa Var. **Ursula** (Lat. "Bear").

Orsalina, Orsaline, Orsel, Orselina, Orseline, Orsola, Orssa, Ursa

Orszebet Hung. Var. **Elizabeth** (Heb. "devoted to God").

Ortensia It. Var. **Hortense** (Lat. clan name).

Ortensa, Ortensija, Ortensya

Otthild OG. "Prospers in battle." **Odile** is perhaps the most common form.

Otthilda Ottila, Ottilia, Ottilie, Ottiline, Ottoline, Otylia

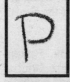

Page Fr. A young boy in training as a personal assistant to a knight. Usually a transferred surname, possibly indicating an ancestor who was a page. Use as a girl's name is quite recent.

Padget, Padgett, Paget, Pagett, Paige, Payge

Pallas Gk. "Wisdom." Another name for the Greek deity Athena, goddess of wisdom.

Paladia, Palladia, Palles

Palma Lat. "Palm tree." Also a place name used in several countries, no doubt to indicate locales where palm trees grew.

Pallma, Pallmirah, Pallmyra, Palmeda, Palmeeda, Palmer, Palmira, Palmyra

Paloma Sp. "Dove." Little known until the recent fame of designer Paloma Picasso, daughter of the artist.

Palloma, Palometa, Palomita, Peloma

Pamela Gk. "All honey." Literary name coined at the end of the 16th century, growing gradually more common until a distinct vogue in the 1950s and 1960s. Likely to be neglected by the current generation of parents, precisely because it was popular among their elders. Actresses Pam Dawber, Pamela Reed, Pamela Anderson; tennis star Pam Shriver.

Pam, Pama, Pamala, Pamalla, Pamelia, Pamelina, Pamelin, Pamelina, Pamella, Pamelyn, Pamelynne, Pamilla, Pammela, Pammie, Pammy, Permelia

Pandora Gk. "All gifted." In Greek myth Pandora was the first woman, endowed with gifts by all the gods. She is famous for the box that was her dowry; it contained all the world's evils, which flew out when the box was opened. One of the more common of the Greek names in English-speaking countries, but still highly unusual.

Dora, Doura, Panndora, Pandorra, Pandoura

Panphila Gk. "All loving." A pleasant notion, though the name might require a lot of explanation.

Panfila, Panfyla, Panphyla

Pansy Flower name from the late 19th century: the name of the flower originally came from the French word for thought, *pensée,* possibly because the petals of the flower are thought to resemble wise little faces.

Pansey, Pansie

Panthea Gk. "All the gods." An early Middle Eastern queen was named Panthea, but the name is more familiar from its close relative "pantheon," which means a temple to all gods.

Pantheia, Pantheya, Panthia

Paquita Sp. Dim. **Frances** (Lat. "From France") via **Paco.**

Paris Place name: the capital city of France.

Parris, Parrish

Parker OE "Park keeper." Occupational name turned last

name, borrowed for a girl's first name. Actress Parker Posey.

Parthenia Gk. "Virginal." Used most often at the turn of the 20th century, when the attributes of the virgin were particularly highly valued.

Partheenia, Parthenie, Parthinia, Pathina, Pathinia

Pat Dim. **Patricia**. Used as an independent name, but neglected with the recent leaning toward the nostalgic and elaborate.

Patience Virtue name. One of the more popular of the 16th-century names, though eclipsed in the 20th century by **Hope**. Patience, after all, is not a very modern virtue.

Paciencia, Patient, Patienzia, Pazienza

Patricia (Fem. **Patrick**) Lat. "Noble, patrician." Obscure until it was used for one of Queen Victoria's granddaughters, which launched its enormous popularity for close to fifty years. It has now returned to near-neglect. In Spain, however, it is a favorite. Singers Patti LaBelle, Patsy Cline, Pat Benatar; choreographer Trisha Brown; actresses Patty Duke, Patricia Neal, Patricia Arquette; First Lady Pat Nixon; Congresswoman Pat Schroeder.

Pat, Patreece, Patreice, Patrica, Patrice, Patricka, Patrizia, Patsy, Patte, Pattee, Pattey, Patti, Pattie, Patty, Tricia, Trish, Trisha

Paula (Fem. **Paul**) Lat. "Small." Roman name that cropped up in English-speaking countries in this century and was rather well used in the Baby Boom era. Actress Paulette Godard; singer Paula Abdul.

Paola, Paolina, Paule, Pauletta, Paulette, Paulie, Paulina, Pauline, Paulita, Paulla, Paullette, Pauly, Pavia, Pavla, Pola, Polina, Pollie, Polly

Pauline (Fem. **Paul**) Fr. from Lat. "Small." Popular earlier than **Paula**, having peaked at the turn of the 20th century in the U.S. Model Paulina Porizkova.

Pauleen, Paulina, Polline, Paulyne

Paz Sp. "Peace."

Pazia Heb. "Golden."

Paza, Pazit

Peace ME. Word used as a name. Though not strictly a

virtue name, this is the kind of abstract quality celebrated
by the Puritans in their choice of names.

Pearl Lat. "Pearl." Probably the most common of the jewel
names, though of course it is not a gemstone. The Greek
form, **Margaret,** is far more widespread and has been
used for centuries, while Pearl only appeared in the late
Victorian era. Writer Pearl S. Buck; singer Pearl Bailey.
**Pearla, Pearle, Pearleen, Pearlette, Pearline, Perl,
Perla, Perle, Perlette, Perley, Perline, Perlline**

Peggy Dim. **Margaret** (Gk. "Pearl.") Used as an independent name since the 18th century, and parents who choose
it today probably do so without thinking of Margaret. Its
greatest vogue came in the first third of the 20th century.
Skater Peggy Fleming; singer Peggy Lee; actress Peggy
Lipton.
Peg, Pegeen, Pegg, Peggie

Pelagia Gk. "Ocean, sea."
**Palasha, Pasha, Pelage, Pelageia, Pelageya, Pelagie,
Pellagia**

Penelope Gk. "Bobbin worker." The bobbin probably
refers to part of the equipment for weaving, since the
Penelope of Greek myth was the wife of Odysseus. To put
off the many suitors who courted her when it seemed that
the wandering Odysseus must be dead, she told them she
couldn't marry until she finished the tapestry she was
weaving. She would work all day and unravel her work at
night, hoping that her husband would come home. The
name was most popular in the middle of the 20th century,
in Britain. Model Penelope Tree; parenting expert Penelope Leach; actresses Penelope Ann Miller, Penelope
Cruz.
**Pen, Penelopa, Penina, Penna, Pennelope, Penney,
Pennie, Penny**

Peninah Heb. "Pearl."
Pnina

Penny Dim. **Penelope** (Gk. "Bobbin worker"). Given as an
independent name mostly in the 20th century.
Penee, Pennee, Penney, Pennie

Peony Unusual flower name.

Pepita Sp. Dim. **Joseph** (Heb. "Jehovah increases") via **Pepe**.

Pepa, Peppie, Peppy, Peta

Perdita Lat. "Lost." Coined by Shakespeare, and rarely used since his day.

Perfecta Sp. "Perfect, flawless." A daunting name to give any child.

Pernella (Fem. **Peter**) Fr. from Gk. "Rock."

Parnella, Pernelle, Pernilla, Pernille

Perry Fr. "Pear tree." Or Dim. **Peregrine** (Lat. "Voyager"). Originally a boy's name and common as a last name, but also used in America as a girl's name. The masculine names with "-y" or "-ie" endings (**Leslie,** for instance) seem more susceptible to feminine appropriation, which is irreversible. Author Perri Klass.

Perrey, Perri, Perrie

Persis Lat. "From Persia."

Perssis, Persys

Petra (Fem. **Peter**) Gk. "Rock." The simplest feminization of a name that seems to resist being feminized: but not for want of trying, as the variants below demonstrate.

Pella, Pernilla, Pernille, Perrine, Pet, Peta, Peterina, Peternella, Petria, Petrina, Petrine, Petronela, Petronella, Petronelle, Petronia, Petronija, Petronilla, Petronille, Petrova, Petrovna, Piera, Pierette, Pierrette, Pietra

Petula Derivation unclear: may be a version of **Peter,** may come from a Latin word meaning "to seek." The name might even be an adaptation of the flower name **Petunia**. Its use is based entirely on the fame of singer Petula Clark.

Petulah

Petunia Flower name, for the rather humble trumpet-shaped flower with white or bright pink blossoms.

Phaedra Gk. "Bright." In Greek myth, the daughter of King Minos, who was married to the hero Theseus and fell in love with her stepson Hippolytus. When he spurned her advances, she committed suicide. One of those pretty Greek names with a not-so-pretty history.

Faydra, Phaedre, Phaidra, Phedra, Phèdre

Pheodora (Fem. **Theodore**) Rus. from Gk. "Gift of God."
  Fedora, Feodora, Fyedora

Philana Gk. "Loving mankind."
  Filania, Filanna, Phila, Philena, Philene, Philina,
  Philine, Phillane, Phillina

Philantha Gk. "Lover of flowers."
  Filanthia, Philanthia, Philanthie

Philiberta OE. "Very brilliant." Feminine of **Filbert,**
  which is the unusual modern form of **Philibert,** an Anglo-
  Saxon saint's name.
  Filberta, Filiberta, Philberta, Philberthe

Philippa (Fem. **Philip**) Gk. "Horse lover." Another unusual
  feminization, though it was used somewhat in the 19th
  century. Something of a curiosity today.
  Felipa, Filipa, Filipina, Filippa, Flip, Pelipa, Pelippa,
  Phil, Philipa, Philippe, Philippine, Phillie, Phillipa,
  Phillipina, Philly, Pippa, Pippie, Pippie, Pippy

Philomena Gk. "Loved one." Name of a saint worshiped
  enthusiastically, especially in Italy, in the 19th and 20th
  centuries. However, her cult was based on nothing more
  than a set of bones discovered in Rome in 1802, which
  linked up very vaguely with a Roman inscription. It was
  assumed that she was a virgin martyr, and many miracles
  were attributed to Saint Philomena after a shrine was established to her. But in 1961, after archaeologists proved
  the bones in the shrine could not have been those of a
  young girl, her veneration was forbidden by Rome.
  Filimena, Filomena, Filomene, Filumena, Philomène,
  Philomina

Phoebe Gk. "Shining, brilliant." One of the epithets of
  Apollo, the sun god, was Phoebus Apollo, referring to the
  fact that he brought light. A Phoebe appears in the New
  Testament, but the name didn't gain ground until the 18th
  century. Reached a peak in the last part of the 19th cen-
  tury, now pleasantly old-fashioned and ripe for revival.
  Singers Phoebe Legere, Phoebe Snow.
  Febe, Pheabe, Phebe, Pheby, Phoebey, Phoeboe

Phyllida Var. **Phyllis** (Gk. "Leafy bough"). Rare name that

appeared in the 16th century; mostly literary use. Actress Phyllida Law.
Fillida, Phillida, Phillyda

Phyllis Gk. "Leafy bough." Name of a mythological woman, taken up by generations of poets to stand for the idealized country lass. Parents applied it to babies increasingly through the 19th century, but it died out after the 1930s. Poet Phyllis McGinley; comedienne Phyllis Diller.
Filis, Fillis, Fillys, Fyllis, Philis, Phillis, Philys, Phylis, Phyllida, Phyllie, Phylliss, Phyllys

Pia Lat. "Pious." More common in Europe than in English-speaking countries. Singer/actress Pia Zadora.

Piedad Sp. "Piety, devotion."

Pilar Sp. "Pillar." An allusion to the Virgin Mary, in her role as a "pillar" of the Church. Used mostly by Spanish-speaking parents.

Piper OE. Occupational name: "Pipe player." Transferred to last name, and occasionally used as a first name, probably inspired, however indirectly, by actress Piper Laurie.

Pippa Dim. **Philippa** (Gk. "Lover of horses"). Almost exclusively British use.
Pippy

Placidia Lat. "Calm, tranquil." From the word that gives us "placid." It seems a bit dangerous, however, to make predictions about a baby's temperament at birth.
Placida, Plasida

Polly Var. **Molly,** Dim. **Mary** (Heb. "Bitter"). Independent name, used especially in the 19th century. Never as common as Molly, for no discernible reason. Actress Polly Bergen.
Poll, Pollee, Polley, Polli, Pollie

Pomona Lat. "Apple." The Roman goddess of fruit trees.

Poppy Lat. Flower name that reached its peak in the 1920s.

Portia Lat. Clan name, obscure meaning. The heroine of Shakespeare's *Merchant of Venice,* an enterprising woman who disguises herself as a lawyer to save her husband's life. In spite of this worthy prototype, the name is uncommon. Actress Portia de Rossi.

Prima Lat. "First."
  Primalia, Primetta, Primina, Priminia
Primavera It. "Spring." Pretty name for a spring baby.
Primrose ME. "First rose." The primrose does not actually
  belong to the rose family, but it is one of the flowers that
  blooms early in spring. A 19th-century flower name.
  Primarosa, Primorosa, Primula
Priscilla Lat. "Ancient." New Testament name and common in the early Christian era, then revived strongly by
  the Puritans. After generations of neglect, it was taken up
  in the 19th century, but has been scarce since the last half
  of the 20th century, possibly because the most natural
  nickname is "Prissy." Actress Priscilla Presley.
  **Cilla, Pris, Prisca, Priscella, Prisilla, Prissie, Prissy,
  Prysilla**
Prudence Lat. "Caution, discretion." Virtue name most
  common in the 19th century after its first popularity in the
  16th and 17th centuries. Use now is mostly British.
  Pru, Prudencia, Prudie, Prudy, Prue
Prunella Lat. "Small plum." Actress Prunella Scales.
  Prunelle
Psyche Gk. "Breath" and, by extension, life or soul. In
  myth Psyche was a mortal girl whom Cupid loved. In
  post-Freudian times someone's psyche is his innermost
  soul or mind.
Purity ME. The word as name; a virtue name comparable
  to **Chastity**.
  Pureza

Queen OE. "Queen."
   Quanda, Queena, Queenette, Queenie
Querida Sp. "Dear, beloved."
   Quinn Ir. Gael. Meaning unknown. Very common Irish last name, occasionally transferred to first-name status, though less often for girls. Actress Quinn Cummings.
Quin
Quincey OF. Place name: "Estate of the fifth son." Last name of a prominent Massachusetts family whose name is borne by a town and by the 6th U.S. President, John Quincy Adams.
   Quinci, Quincie, Quincy, Quinsy
Quintana Place name: Quintana Roo is a state on the east coast of Mexico.
Quintina Lat. "Fifth."
   Quentina, Quintana, Quintessa, Quintona,
   Quintonette, Quintonice

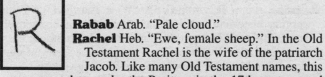

Rabab Arab. "Pale cloud."
Rachel Heb. "Ewe, female sheep." In the Old Testament Rachel is the wife of the patriarch Jacob. Like many Old Testament names, this one was taken up by the Puritans in the 17th century and remained current but not fashionable until parents of the late sixties and seventies used it in great numbers. Still

very popular into the 1990s, now less of a favorite in the U.S. but extremely fashionable in Scotland and Ireland. Actresses Raquel Welch, Rachel Ward, Rachel Griffiths; author Rachel Carson.

Rachael, Racheal, Rachelce, Rachele, Racheli, Rachelle, Rachil, Rae, Raechell, Rahel, Rahil, Rakel, Raquel, Raquela, Raquella, Raquelle, Ray, Raychel, Raychelle, Rashell, Rashelle, Rechell, Shell, Shelley, Shellie, Shelly

Radmilla Slavic. "Industrious for the people."

Radilla, Radinka, Radmila, Redmilla

Rae Dim. **Rachel** (Heb. "Ewe"). Used independently in modern times. Actress Rae Dawn Chong.

Raeann, Raelaine, Raeleen, Raelene, Ray, Raye, Rayette, Raylene, Raylina, Rayma, Rayna, Raynelle, Rayona

Rafa Arab. "Well-being, prosperity."

Rafah

Ragnild Teut. "All-knowing power."

Ragnhild, Ragnhilda, Ragnhilde, Ragnilda, Ranillda, Reinheld, Renilda, Renilde, Reynilda, Reynilde

Raina Var. **Regina** (Lat. "Queen") or fem. **Ray** (OG. "Wise guardian"). Modern name of several possible origins, including allusion to the wet stuff that falls out of the sky. Like many names that have appeared in this century, it has numerous variations, none of which is clearly a favorite.

Raenah, Raene, Rainah, Raine, Rainey, Rainelle, Rainy, Raleine, Raya, Rayann, Rayette, Rayleine, Raylene, Raylina, Rayline, Rayna, Rayne, Rayney, Raynelle, Raynetta, Reyna, Reyney

Ramona (Fem. **Raymond**) Sp. "Wise guardian." A 19th-century historical novel of the same title was immensely successful, and brought the name to wide attention, but it is scarce now. Character in a very popular series of children's books of the same name by Beverly Cleary.

Mona, Ramoena, Ramohna, Ramonda, Ramonde, Ramonna, Ramowna, Romona, Romonda, Romonde

Randy Dim. **Miranda** (Lat. "Admirable"). Mostly U.S. use.
   Randa, Randee, Randelle, Randene, Randi, Randie
Rani Sanskrit. "Queen."
   **Raine, Rana, Ranee, Rania, Ranice, Ranique, Ranit,
   Rayna, Raynell**
Ranita Heb. "Song."
   Ranice, Ranit, Ranite, Ranith, Ranitra, Ranitta
Raphaela (Fem. **Raphael**) Heb. "God heals." The femi-
   nization is very unusual in English-speaking countries,
   though Italian parents use it with some frequency. Author
   Raffaella Barker.
   **Rafa, Rafaela, Rafaelia, Rafaella, Raffaela, Raffaele,
   Raffaella, Rafella, Rafelle, Raphaella, Raphaelle,
   Raphayella, Raphella, Refaella, Refella, Rephaela,
   Rephayelle**
Rashida (Fem. **Rashid**) Turkish. "Righteous, rightly ad-
   vised."
   Rasheda, Rasheeda, Rasheida, Rashidah, Rashyda
Raven Name of the large black bird that is closely related
   to the crow. A fanciful name for a black-haired or dark-
   skinned baby. Actress Raven Symone.
   Ravenne, Rayven, Rayvinn
Reba Dim. **Rebecca**. Singer Reba McEntire.
   Reyba, Rheba
Rebecca Heb. "Joined." A prominent Old Testament name;
   Rebecca is the wife of Isaac and mother of Jacob and
   Esau. Predictably, the name was taken up by the Puritans
   and remained fairly common through the 19th century.
   Subsequent revivals (in the thirties in the U.S., in the late
   sixties in Britain) may have been prompted by literary and
   cinematic use of the name, especially in the novel and film
   Rebecca. Philanthropist Rebekah Harkness; author Re-
   becca West; actress Rebecca De Mornay.
   **Becca, Becka, Beckee, Beckey, Beckie, Becky, Bekka,
   Bekki, Bekkie, Reba, Rebeca, Rebecka, Rebeka,
   Rebekah, Rebekkah, Rebeque, Ree, Reeba, Rheba,
   Revekka, Ribecca, Riva, Rivah, Rivalee, Reveka,
   Revekah, Rivekka, Rivi, Rivka, Rivkah, Rivy**

Regan Ir. Celt. "Son of the small ruler." Use for girls may hark back to Shakespeare's play *King Lear*, but the king's daughter of that name is so cruel that this seems unlikely.
Reghan

Regina Lat. "Queen." Cropped up at the end of the Victorian era, possibly encouraged by the fact that Her Majesty was often known as Victoria Regina. It may also be used as an allusion to the Virgin Mary, Regina Coelis ("Queen of the Heavens"). Nightclub founder Régine; track star Regina Jacobs.
Gina, Raina, Raina, Raine, Regan, Reggi, Reggie, Régine, Reginette, Reginia, Reginna, Reina, Reine, Reinetta, Reinette, Reyna, Rina, Riona, Rionagh

Remedios Sp. "Help, remedy." Currently popular in South America.

Remy Fr. "From Rheims." Champagne, and the fine brandies made from champagne, are the principal product of Rheims, a town in central France.
Remi, Remie, Remmy, Rhemy

Rena Heb. "Melody" or Dim. **Irene** (Gk. "Peace").
Reena, Rina

Renata Lat. "Reborn." The Latin (and less popular) form of **Renée**. It was used in this guise by the Puritans. Author Renata Adler.
Ranae, Ranay, Renae, Renate, René, Renée, Renelle, Renetta, Renette, Renie, Renisa, Renita, Renise, Rennae, Rennay, Rennie

Rene Dim. **Irene** (Gk. "Peace"). Used on its own, primarily around the turn of the 20th century.
Reney, Renie, Rennie

Renée Fr. "Reborn." The French form of **Renata,** more common (though not really widespread) in modern times. Tennis star Renée Richards; actresses Renee Russo, Renée Zellwegger.
Ranae, Ranay, Ranée, Renae, René, Renell, Renelle, Renie, Rennie, Renny, Rhinaye, Rrenae

Renita Lat. "Resistant." Has come into use since the 1980s.
Reneeta, Renyta

Reseda Latin term for a flower more commonly known as mignonette.

Reta Var. **Rita,** Dim. **Margaret** (Gk. "Pearl").
Reda, Reeda, Reeta, Rheta, Rhetta

Rexana It is possible to translate this name by its parts, *rex* being Latin for "king," and *anna* a variant of the Hebrew word for "grace." Or it may be a feminization of **Rex,** or a variant of **Roxane.**
Rexanne, Rexanna, Rexalla, Rexella, Rexetta, Rexina, Rexine

Rhea Gk. "Earth." In Greek myth, Rhea was an earth-mother who bore Zeus, Demeter, Hera, and Poseidon, among other gods. Actress Rhea Perlman.
Rea, Rhia, Ria

Rheta Gk. "A speaker, eloquent." From the same root as the word "rhetoric."

Rhiannon Welsh. "Witch, goddess."
Rhianna, Rhianon, Rianon, Riannon

Rhoda Gk. "Rose," Lat. "From Rhodes." Rhodes is a Greek island originally named for its roses. The name is found in the New Testament, and was used mostly in the 18th and 19th centuries.
Rhodeia, Rhodia, Rhodie, Rhody, Roda, Rodi, Rodie, Rodina

Rhodanthe Gk. "Rose blossom."
Rhodante

Rhona ONorse. "Rough island." A form of **Rona** more common in Britain.
Rhona, Roana

Rhonda Welsh place name: The Rhondda Valley is a significant landmark in southern Wales, named for the river that runs through it. (In Welsh, the name means "noisy.") The most likely cultural association in the U.S. is with the Beach Boys' song, "Help Me, Rhonda!"
Rhonnda, Ronda

Ria Dim. **Victoria** (Lat. "Victor"). Used occasionally as an independent name.
Rea

Riane (Fem. **Ryan**) Ir. last name. Uncommon, but analogous to the more widely used Briana.

Rhiane, Rhianna, Riana, Rianna, Rianne, Ryann, Ryanne

Rica Familiar form of **Erica** (Scan. "Ruler forever") or **Frederica** (OG. "Peaceful ruler") or possibly Sp. "Rich."

Rhica, Ricca, Ricki, Rickie, Ricky, Rieca, Riecka, Rieka, Riki, Rikki, Riqua, Rycca

Ricarda (Fem. **Richard**) OG. "Powerful ruler." One of many feminine forms of a very popular man's name, none of which has been adopted in large numbers.

Richanda, Richarda, Richardella, Richardene, Richardette, Richardina, Richardyne, Richel, Richela, Richele, Richella, Richelle, Richenda, Richenza, Richette, Richia, Richilene, Richina, Richmal, Richmalle

Rickie Dim. **Frederica** (OG. "Peaceful ruler"). Also possibly a feminine version of Richard, and certainly more popular than the longer forms. Occurred most often in the middle of the 20th century. Singer Rickie Lee Jones; actress Ricki Lake.

Rickie, Ricki, Ricky, Ricquie, Rika, Riki, Rikki, Rikky, Ryckie

Rilla Middle German. "Small brook."

Rella, Rilletta, Rillette

Rima Arab. "Antelope."

Risa Lat. "Laughter." A pretty name, but very unusual in English-speaking countries. Opera singer Rise Stevens.

Riesa, Rise, Rysa

Rita Dim. **Margaret** (Gk. "Pearl"). Comes via the Spanish form, **Margarita**. First used on its own some hundred years ago, and quite popular for 50 years. Actresses Rita Hayworth, Rita Moreno; authors Rita Mae Brown, Rita Dove.

Reeta, Reita, Rheeta,Rida, Riet, Rieta, Ritta

Ritsa Gk. Dim. **Alexander** (Gk. "Man's defender").

Riva Var. **Rebecca** (Heb. "Joined"). Also possibly from the French for "shore," but the Jewish families who use it most often probably have the Old Testament associations in mind.

Reba, Ree, Reeva, Reevabel, Reva, Rifka, Rivalee, Rivi, Rivka, Rivke, Rivkah, Rivy

Roanna Var. **Rosanne.**

Ranna, Roanne, Ronni, Ronnie, Ronny

Roberta (Fem. **Robert**) OE. "Bright fame." While **Ricarda,** another simple feminization of an Old German name, never caught on, Roberta was rather widespread between its introduction in the late 19th century and its fall from favor some eighty years later. Singers Roberta Peters, Roberta Flack.

Berta, Bertie, Berty, Bobbe, Bobbee, Bobbette, Bobbie, Bobby, Bobbye, Bobette, Bobi, Bobina, Bobine, Bobinette, Reberta, Roba, Robbee, Robbey, Robbi, Robbie, Robby, Robeena, Robella, Robelle, Robena, Robenia, Robertena, Robertene, Robertha, Robertina, Robetta, Robette, Robettina, Robin, Robina, Robinett, Robinette, Robinia, Robyn, Robyna, Robynna, Ruperta, Rupetta

Robin Dim. **Robert** (OE. "Bright fame"). Originally a boy's nickname (as in Winnie the Pooh's friend Christopher Robin), but appropriated for girls in increasing numbers starting in the middle of the 20th century. Now out of fashion for both sexes. Actresses Robin Givens, Robin Wright Penn.

Robee, Robbey, Robbi, Robbie, Robbin, Robby, Robbyn, Robena, Robene, Robenia, Robi, Robina, Robine, Robinet, Robinett, Robinette, Robinia, Robyn, Robyna, Robynette

Rochelle Fr. Place name: "Little rock." Enthusiastically used as a first name starting in the 1940s, but rare now.

Roch, Rochell, Rochella, Rochette, Roschella, Roschelle, Roshelle, Shell, Shelley, Shelly

Roderica (Fem. **Roderick**) OG. "Renowned ruler."

Rica, Roddie, Roderiga, Roderiqua, Roderique, Rodriga

Rohana Sanskrit. "Sandalwood."

Rohanna

Rolanda (Fem. **Roland**) OG. "Famous land."

Orlanda, Orlande, Rolande, Rollande

Roline Dim. **Caroline** (OG. "Man.") Unusual diminutive that appears from time to time in the South.
Roelene, Roeline, Rolene, Rollene, Rolleen, Rollina, Rolline, Rolyne

Roma It. Place name: the capital city, Rome. Rather widely used since it first appeared in the late 19th century, though of course, it never approached the popularity of **Florence**. Actress Roma Downey.
Romelle, Romilda, Romina, Romma

Romaine (Fem. **Romain**) Fr. "From Rome." A pretty name that might be associated with a common variety of lettuce.
Romane, Romayne, Romeine, Romene

Romola Lat. "Roman woman." Actress Romola Garai.
Romala, Romella, Romelle, Rommola, Romolla, Romula

Rona ONorse. "Rough island." In Britain, used interchangeably with **Rhona**. Both versions cropped up at the turn of the century and have occurred steadily without ever being fashionable. Gossip columnist Rona Barrett.
Rhona, Ronella, Ronelle, Ronna

Ronni (Fem. **Ronald**) OE. "Strong counsel" or Dim. **Veronica** (Lat. "Image").
Ronalda, Ronee, Ronette, Roni, Ronna, Ronnee, Ronnelle, Ronnella, Ronney, Ronnie, Ronny

Rosabel Com. form **Rose** and **Belle**. A combination that appeared in the mid-19th century. Its meaning ("beautiful rose") probably appealed as much to parents of the era as the name itself, which lost favor in the unsentimental 20th century.
Rosabella, Rosabelle

Rosalba Lat. "White rose." Artist Rosalba Carriera.

Rosalie Fr. Var. It. **Rosalia**. Possibly "rose garden." Mostly 19th century use.
Rosalee, Rosaleen, Rosaley, Rosalia, Rosalina, Rosaline, Rosalyne, Roselia, Rosella, Roselle, Rozalia, Rozalie, Rozele, Rozelie, Rozely, Rozella, Rozelle, Rozellia

Rosalind Sp. "Pretty rose" is the most common interpretation, though the name was actually coined in 16th-century Britain. A German form also existed, formed of words that meant "horse" or "renown" and "shield" or "snake." It has been used since the mid-19th century, with a surge in the middle of the 20th century. Actress Rosalind Russell.

Ros, Rosalen, Rosalin, Rosalina, Rosalinda, Rosalinde, Rosaline, Rosalinn, Rosalyn, Rosalynd, Rosalynda, Rosanie, Roselin, Roselina, Roselind, Roselinda, Roselinde, Roseline, Roselinn, Roselyn, Roselynda, Roselynde, Rosina, Roslyn, Roslynn, Roslynne, Roz, Rozali, Rozalia, Rozalin, Rozalind, Rozalinda, Rozalynn, Rozalynne, Rozelin, Rozelind, Rozelinda, Rozelyn, Rozelynda

Rosalyn Com. form. **Rose** and **Lynn** (Sp. "Pretty"). The most common of the modern variants of **Rosalind**. First Lady Rosalynn Carter.

Rosalin, Rosalynn, Roselynn, Roslyn, Rozlynn

Rosamond OG. "Renowned protector." Also translatable (from the Latin) as "rose of the world." More popular in the 19th century than it is today. Author Rosamond Bernier; actress Rosamund Pike.

Ros, Rosamonde, Rosamund, Rosamunda, Rosemond, Rosemonda, Rosmund, Rosmunda, Roz, Rozamond

Rose Lat. Flower name. Scholars actually trace the name (which the Normans imported to Britain in the 11th century) to an Old German name meaning something like "renown," but the flower meaning has had much more currency, particularly given the Christian symbolic meaning of the rose. (The "rosa mystica" is the Virgin Mary.) It reached its peak use at the turn of the 20th century, along with other flower names. An elaboration, **Rosario,** is currently popular in Spain. Actress Rosario Dawson; talk-show host Rosie O'Donnell.

Rasia, Rasine, Rasja, Rasya, Rhoda, Rhodea, Rhodia, Rhody, Rosa, Rosaleen, Rosalia, Rosalie, Rosalin, Rosalina, Rosalind, Rosaline, Rosalinn, Rosalynn, Rosanie, Rosario, Roselia, Roselina, Roseline, Rosella, Roselle, Rosena, Rosenah, Rosene, Rosetta,

Rosette, Rosey, Rosheen, Rosie, Rosina, Rosita,
Roslyn, Rosy, Roza, Rozalie, Rozaline, Rozalyne,
Roze, Rozele, Rozella, Rozene, Rozina, Rozsa, Rozsi,
Rozsika, Rozy, Ruza, Ruzena, Ruzenka, Ruzha, Ruzsa,
Zita

Roseanne Com. form. **Rose** and **Anne**. The pairing of the
two names appeared in the 18th century, and various
forms have drifted in and out of popularity. Actresses
Rosanna Arquette, Roseanne Barr.

Ranna, Roanna, Roanne, Rosanagh, Rosanna,
Rosannah, Rosanne, Roseann, Roseanna,
Rosehannah, Rozanna, Rozanne, Rozeanna

Rosemary Lat. "Dew of the sea" is the correct meaning,
though the name gained great currency with the flower
name fad of the late 19th century. The fact that most parents read it as a combination of **Rose** and **Mary** (both already popular, and with strong religious resonance for
Catholics) can't have hurt. Singer Rosemary Clooney.

Rosemaree, Rosemarey, Rosemaria, Rosemarie,
Rosmarie, Rozmary, Romy

Rowena Welsh. "Slender and fair." This meaning is an ap-
proximation. The name was actually brought to public notice by novelist Sir Walter Scott with his immensely
popular *Ivanhoe,* in the early 19th century.

Roweena, Roweina, Rowina

Roxanne Per. "Dawn." In history, the wife of Alexander the
Great was named Roxane, but 20th century parents may
be more familiar with the Roxane who is the heroine of
Rostand's play *Cyrano de Bergerac,* or the character
played by Daryl Hannah in Ron Howard's film adaptation.

Oksana, Oksanna, Roksanne, Roxana, Roxane,
Roxann, Roxanna, Roxene, Roxey, Roxiane, Roxianne,
Roxie, Roxine, Roxy, Roxyanna, Ruksana, Ruksane,
Ruksanna

Royale OF. "Regal one." Something of a curiosity in the
democratic United States.

Royalla, Royalene, Royalina, Royall, Royalle, Royalyn,
Royalynne

Ruby Jewel name. Launched in the 1870s with other jewel names, but passé by the mid-20th century. Dancer Ruby Keeler.

Rubee, Rubetta, Rubey, Rubi, Rubia, Rubie, Rubina, Rubinia, Rubyna

Rudelle OG. "Renowned." From the same root that produces the male name **Rudolph**.

Rudella

Rufina Lat. "Red haired." Can be considered a feminine version of **Rufus,** which is given to boys regardless of their hair color.

Rufeena, Rufeine, Ruffina, Ruphyna

Ruth Heb. "Friend, companion." The Old Testament Book of Ruth is about the widowed Moabite woman who refuses to leave her Hebrew mother in-law, Naomi, and says, "Whither thou goest, I will go." Her sentiments appealed greatly to Victorian poets. The name has been consistently used ever since the 17th century, peaking at the turn of the century. Actresses Ruth Gordon, Ruth Buzzi; author Ruth Rendell.

Ruthe, Ruthelle, Ruthetta, Ruthi, Ruthie, Ruthina, Ruthine

Ruthann Com. form. **Ruth** and **Ann**.

Ruthanna, Ruthanne

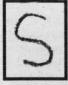

Saba Gk. "From Sheba"; Arab. "Morning." The queen of Sheba is mentioned in the Old Testament as having been hugely rich and very ostentatious.

Sabah, Sheba, Shebah

Sabina Lat. "Sabine." The Sabines were a tribe living in central Italy around the time Romulus and Remus estab-

lished the city of Rome. In an effort to provide wives for
the citizens of Rome, Romulus arranged the mass kidnapping of the Sabine women, which came to be known (and
frequently portrayed in art and literature) as the "Rape of
the Sabines." The name was used among the ancient Romans and in English-speaking countries after the 17th
century, but has been very rare lately.

**Bina, Byna, Sabine, Sabinna, Sabiny, Sabyna,
Sahbina, Savina, Savine, Sebina, Sebinah**

Sabra Origin disputed: may be Heb. "To rest," or possibly
"Cactus." Is now used as a term for a native-born Israeli.

Sabrah, Sebra, Sabrette

Sabrina Lat. Place name: the Latin term for the Severn
River in England. Though Milton (among others) writes
about a Sabrina, she appeared most vividly in modern culture as *Sabrina Fair* in the play and movie. The name was
used in the 19th century and cropped up again in the last
part of the 20th century. Though it resembles many currently popular names it may not be familiar enough to
most parents to seem an appealing choice.

**Brina, Sabreena, Sabrinna, Sabryna, Sebreena,
Sebrina, Zabrina**

Sachi Jap. "Child of joy."

Sachiko

Sadie Dim. **Sarah** (Heb. "Princess"). Use as an independent name occurred mostly at the turn of the 20th century.
Actress Sada Thompson.

**Sada, Sadah, Sadelle, Saida, Saidee, Saidey, Saidie,
Saydie, Sydell, Sydella, Sydelle**

Sadira Pers. "Lotus tree." The lotus has great significance
in several of the Eastern religions.

Saffron Flower name: Saffron refers to a substance (the
dried stamens of saffron crocuses) used as a spice in
Mediterranean and other Southern cuisines. It produces
a bright orange-yellow color, and is sometimes used as
a dye. Monks of some Eastern religions wear saffron
robes, which may explain why the name was used occasionally in the 1960s, an era when saffron robes and

Eastern religions went mainstream. Actress Saffron Aldridge.

Saffran, Saffren, Saffronia, Saphron

Sage Lat. "Wise, healthy." More likely to be a boy's name, perhaps via associations with sagebrush, cowboys, and the Wild West.

Saige, Sayge

Salena Var. **Selina** (Gk. "Moon goddess").

Salina

Salimah Arab. "Healthy, sound." Currently popular in Arabic countries.

Salima, Selima

Sally Dim. **Sarah** (Heb. "Princess"). A popular independent name in the 18th century and again in the 20th. Talkshow host Sally Jessy Raphael; actress Sally Field; astronaut Sally K. Ride.

Sal, Salcia, Saletta, Sallee, Salletta, Sallette, Salley, Sallianne, Sallie, Sallyann

Salome Heb. "Peace." Possibly from the same root that gives us the greeting "Shalom." The most famous biblical Salome is the woman who danced for King Herod and demanded, as her reward, the head of John the Baptist on a platter. In spite of this unsavory antecedent, the name was used somewhat in the 19th century, but its connotations make it an unlikely choice.

Sahlma, Salima, Salma, Salmah, Saloma, Salomea, Salomey, Salomi, Selima, Selma, Selmah, Solome, Solomea

Salvadora Sp. "Savior." Referring, of course, to Jesus Christ.

Salvia Lat. "Whole, healthy." The Latin name for the herb known as sage, which has mild healing powers as well as being an aromatic used in cooking.

Sallvia, Salvina

Samala Heb. "Requested of God."

Samale, Sammala

Samantha (Fem. **Samuel**) Heb. "Told by God." Occasionally used in the 17th-19th centuries, but truly popular in the 1960s and 1970s, possibly triggered by the TV series "Bewitched." Also popular now, having been a top-ten choice for the last decade. Actress Samantha Eggar.

Sam, Samey, Sami, Samentha, Sammantha, Sammee, Sammey, Sammie, Semantha, Semanntha, Simantha, Symantha

Samara Heb. "Under God's rule."

Samaria, Samarie, Sammara, Semara

Samuela (Fem. **Samuel**) Heb. "Told by God." Very scarce, particularly compared with **Samantha**.

Samella, Samelle, Samuella, Samuelle

Sancia Lat. "Sacred."

Sancha, Sanchia, Santsia, Sanzia

Sandra Dim. **Alexandra** (Gk. "Defender of mankind") via It. **Alessandra**. Popular in the middle of the 20th century, but today's parents are more inclined to prefer the full four syllables of the original name. Comedienne Sandra Bernhard; actresses Sandrine Bonnaire, Sondra Locke, Sandra Dee, Sandra Bullock; Supreme Court Justice Sandra Day O'Connor.

Sahndra, Sanda, Sandee, Sandie, Sandreea, Sandrella, Sandrelle, Sandretta, Sandrette, Sandria, Sandrina, Sandrine, Sandy, Sanndra, Sanndria, Sauhndra, Saundra, Sohndra, Sondra, Sonndra, Wysandria, Zandra

Sandy Dim. **Sandra**. Mostly used post-1950.

Sandee, Sandi, Sandie, Sanndi

Sapphire Heb. Jewel name. Unusual biblical name, and the birthstone for September. One of the least used of the jewel names.

Safira, Saphira, Sapphira, Sephira

Sarah Heb. "Princess." In the Old Testament, the wife of the patriarch Abraham. Came into vogue with other biblical names in the 16th century and was enough of a staple for 400 years to have spawned a variety of nicknames (though not as many as the multisyllabic **Elizabeth,** for instance). Sarah was the fourth most popular girls' name in the 1990s and is still in the top ten. It is also very well used in Ireland and Scotland, though not as popular in

England. As **Sara,** it's fashionable in Germany. Actresses Sarah Bernhardt, Sarah Siddons, Sarah Jessica Parker, Sarah Michelle Gellar; singer Sarah Vaughan; poet Sara Teasdale; Sarah Ferguson, Duchess of York; figure skater Sarah Hughes.

Sadee, Sadella, Sadelle, Sadellia, Sadie, Sadye, Saidee, Sal, Sallee, Salley, Sallie, Sally, Sara, Sarai, Saraia, Sareen, Sarely, Sarena, Sarette, Sari, Sarika, Sarina, Sarine, Sarita, Saritia, Sarka, Sarolta, Sarotta, Sarotte, Saroya, Sarra, Sarrah, Sasa, Sera, Serach, Serah, Serita, Shara, Sorcha, Sydel, Sydelle, Zahra, Zara, Zarah, Zaria, Zarita

Sasha Rus. Fem. and Dim. **Alexander** (Gk. "Man's defender"). The "-sha" ending is not necessarily feminine in Russia, and Sasha is more commonly a male nickname there.

Sacha, Sasa, Sascha, Saschenka, Zsazsa

Saskia Dutch name of unknown meaning. It would probably have been forgotten, but it was the name of Rembrandt's wife, who is depicted in some of his finest canvases. Actress Saskia Reeves.

Savannah Sp. "Treeless." Originally familiar as a place name, as in the city in Georgia, or name of a geographical feature: a wide, treeless plain.

Savana, Savanna, Sevanna

Scarlett ME. "Scarlet." Given its fame by the inimitable Scarlett O'Hara, heroine of *Gone With the Wind.* Not hugely popular, possibly because the young lady in the novel is so headstrong. It is nevertheless the middle name of one of Mick Jagger's children with Jerry Hall.

Scarlet, Scarletta, Scarlette

Season Lat. "Time of sowing." The word used as a name. Cropped up in the 1970s (along with **Spring** and **Summer**), when children were given counterculture names, but seems unlikely to endure. Actress Season Hubley.

Sebastiane (Fem. **Sebastian**) Lat. "From Sebastia." Unusual feminization of a name that is very infrequent in America.

Bastia, Bastiana, Sebastiana, Sebastienne

Secunda Lat. "Second."

Seema Heb. "Precious thing, treasure."
   Cima, Cyma, Seemah, Sima, Simah, Sina

Selena Gk. "Moon goddess." Most popular in the 19th century, though the immense fame of the late Tejana pop star of this name may promote its use.
   Celene, Celie, Celina, Celinda, Celine, Cellina, Celyna, Saleena, Salena, Salina, Sela, Selene, Selia, Selie, Selina, Selinda, Seline, Sena

Selima Heb. "Tranquil."
   Saleema, Saleemah, Selimah

Selma (Fem. **Anselm** by way of **Anselma**) OG. "Godly helmet." Selma is the more common form, though it is far from an everyday choice. Actress Selma Blair.
   Anselma, Sellma, Selmah, Zelma

Semiramis Heb. "Highest heaven." Semiramis was an Assyrian queen who, myth has it, built Babylon and turned into a dove after death. Her legend inspired both Voltaire and Rossini.
   Semira

Senalda Sp. "A sign."

Senga Var. **Agnes** (Gk. "Pure"). A rare Scottish name; it is **Agnes** spelled backward.

September Month name. Much less common than **April, May,** or **June**.

Septima Lat. "Seventh." If one has a seventh child, why not celebrate with her name?

Seraphina Heb. "Ardent." The seraphim are the highest-ranking angels in Heaven (above angels, archangels, cherubim, etc.). They have six wings and are noted for their zealous love.
   Sarafina, Serafina, Serafine, Seraphe, Seraphine, Serofina, Serophine

Serena Lat. "Tranquil, serene." Used by Roman Christians, and periodically popular since, though never in a big way. Tennis player Serena Williams.
   Cerena, Reena, Sarina, Saryna, Serene, Serenna, Serina, Serenity, Seryna

Serilda OG. "Armed warrior woman."

Sarilda, Serhilda, Serhilde, Serrilda

Shaina Heb. "Beautiful."

Shaine, Shana, Shanee, Shani, Shanle, Shayna, Shayne

Shaka Modern name: "Sha-," like "La-," is a very fashionable prefix, attached to any number of other particles to form names that have no specific meaning but sound attractive.

Shakeela, Shakelta, Shakeera, Shakette, Shakila, Shakina, Shakira, Shakitra, Shaquina, Shaquita

Shalom Heb. "Peace." Not a name but a greeting to speakers of Hebrew. Nevertheless adapted by some parents for its meaning. Model Shalom Harlow.

Shalome, Shalva, Shalvah, Shelom, Shilom, Sholome

Shana Dim. **Shannon,** or anglicization of **Shaina,** or diminutive of **Shoshana.** Uncommon, but kept in the public eye by journalist and biographer Shana Alexander. Singer Shania Twain.

Shanah, Shania, Shanna, Shannah

Shaneika Modern U.S. Another elaboration of the popular "Sha-" prefix. Some of the more common of these names are the ones that sound like **Ashanti,** the name of an area in Western Africa that was the original home of many American slaves. Other "Sha-" names, like the "La-" names, are limited in form only by parental imagination.

Shandee, Shandeigh, Shandey, Shandeya, Shanecka, Shaneese, Shaneikah, Shanequa, Shaneyka, Shaniece, Shanika, Shanique, Shanisse, Shanneice, Shanta, Shantee, Shanteigh, Shantella, Shantelle, Shantey, Sheniece, Shenika, Sheniqua, Shonyce

Shanelle Modern U.S. name which is a phonetic spelling of "Chanel," the name of the great French couturier. It has double-barreled appeal, since it combines the "Sha-" prefix with an evocation of great feminine elegance.

Shanel, Shanella, Shanelly, Shannel, Shaney, Shanilly, Shanisse, Shanita, Shenell, Shenelle, Shinella, Shonelle, Shynelle

Shannon Ir. Gael. "Old, ancient." The name of an important river, county, and airport in Ireland, used as a first name in this century. Most popular among families with Irish roots, but little found in Ireland. Actresses Shannen Doherty, Shannyn Sossamon; gymnast Shannon Miller.

Channa, Shana, Shandy, Shane, Shani, Shanna, Shannae, Shannen, Shannin, Shanon

Shantal Var. **Chantal** (Fr. place name). Its popularity may be associated with both Shanelle and the other "Sha-" names, rather than with the rather obscure French first name.

Shanta, Shantahl, Shantay, Shantalle, Shante, Shantella, Shantelle, Shontal, Shontalle, Shontelle

Sharlene (Fem and Dim. **Charles**) OG. "Man." Var. **Caroline**. One of the numerous variations that were popular in the 1950s and 1960s.

Sharleen, Sharleyne, Sharlina, Sharline, Sharlyne

Sharon Heb. Place name: "A plain." In the Old Testament, refers to flat land at the foot of Mount Carmel. Not picked up by the 16th-century Puritans, probably since it wasn't a personal name, but by mid-20th century it was quite popular in America. Now much less common. Actresses Sharon Gless, Sharon Stone.

Charin, Cheron, Shara, Sharan, Sharen, Sharene, Shari, Sharie, Sharla, Sharolyn, Sharona, Sharonda, Sharren, Sharrin, Sharronne, Sheran, Sheron, Sherri, Sherry, Sheryn, Sherynn

Shavonne Phonetic var. **Siobhan** (Ir. Gael. var. **Joan**, fem. **John**). Heb. "The Lord is gracious."

Shevon, Shevonne, Shivonne, Shyvon, Shyvonne

Shawn (fem. var. **Sean**, Ir. var. **John**) Heb. "The Lord is gracious." Use of Sean and its variants peaked in the 1970s, but they are still used quite substantially for boys. Girls with this name are a rarity. Actress Sean Young.

Sean, Seana, Seanna, Shana, Shanna, Shaun, Shauna, Shaunee, Shaunie, Shawna, Shawnee, Shawneen, Shawnette, Sianna

Shea Ir. Gael. "From the fairy fort." More commonly an Irish last name. Basketball player Shea Ralph.

Shae, Shay, Shaye, Shayla, Shaylyn

Sheba Heb. "From Sheba." Also a short version of **Bathsheba** (Heb. "Daughter of the oath"). The queen of Sheba is mentioned in the Old Testament as having been hugely rich and very ostentatious.

Saba, Sabah, Scheba, Shebah, Sheeba, Shieba

Sheena Ir. Var. **Jane** (Heb. "The Lord is gracious"). Many of the "Sh" names are Gaelic versions of **Jane, Jean,** and **Joan,** which are in turn variations on that old staple, **John.** Rock star Sheena Easton.

Sheenagh, Sheenah, Sheina, Shena, Shiona, Shionagh, Sina, Sine

Sheila Ir. Var. **Cecilia** (Lat. "Blind"). Popular mid-20th century in Britain and the Commonwealth; in Australian slang, a "sheila" is a woman.

Seila, Selia, Shayla, Shaylah, Sheela, Sheelagh, Sheelah, Sheilagh, Sheilah, Shela, Shelagh, Shelia, Shiela

Shelby OE. Place name: "Estate on the ledge." Used to occur infrequently as a man's name, but it has recently been taken up by parents, reaching into the top 40 U.S. girls' names by 1991. Use since then has tapered off.

Shelbea, Shelbee, Shelbeigh, Shelbey, Shelbie, Shellby

Shelley OE. Place name: "Meadow on the ledge." Last name made famous by the poet Percy Bysshe Shelley. Use as a feminine first name seems to have been related to **Shirley**. Actresses Shelley Winters, Shelley Duvall, Shelley Long.

Schelley, Shellee, Shellie, Shelly

Sherry Var. **Cher** (Fr. "Dear"), **Sharon** (Heb. "The plain"), or **Cheryl** (Var. **Charlotte,** OG. "Man"). In the 1950s and 1960s these three names and their variants were all popular, giving rise to a parade of further forms, spellings, and elaborations. Tracing the exact origin of any of them is difficult. Puppeteer Shari Lewis.

Cheray, Sharee, Shari, Sharie, Sharrie, Sherae, Sheraie, Sheray, Sheree, Sherey, Sheri, Sherice,

Shericia, Sherie, Sherina, Sherissa, Sherita, Sherree, Sherrey, Sherri, Sherryn, Sherye, Sh'rae

Sheryl Var. **Cheryl** (Var. **Charlotte**, OG. "Man"). Actress Sherilyn Fenn; singer Sheryl Crow; basketball player Sheryl Swoopes.

Cheralin, Cheralyn, Cheralynne, Cherilynn, Sheralyn, Sheralin, Sherileen, Sherill, Sherilyn, Sherilynne, Sherrell, Sherrill, Sherryl, Sheryll

Shifra Heb. "Lovely."

Schifra, Shifrah

Shiri Heb. "My song."

Shira, Shirah, Shirit

Shirley OE. Place name: "Bright meadow." Originally a last name, brought to immense fame and popularity as a girl's name with the career of child star Shirley Temple. Now widely neglected. Actress Shirley MacLaine; politician Shirley Chisholm; novelist Shirley Hazzard.

Sherlee, Sherli, Sherlie, Sherrlie, Sheryl, Shirely, Shirl, Shirlea, Shirlee, Shirleen, Shirleigh, Shirlene, Shirlinda, Shirline, Shirlley, Shirly, Shirlyn, Shurlee

Shona Ir. Gael. Var. **John**. While **Sinead** is a Gaelic form of **Janet**, Shona is the equivalent form of **Joan**.

Shonagh, Shonah, Shone, Shuna, Shunagh

Shoshana Heb. "Lily." The more common form is the anglicized **Susan** or **Susanna**. Fashion designer Shoshana Lonstein.

Shosha, Shoshanah, Sosanna, Sosannah

Shulamith Heb. "Peace." Composer Shulamit Ran; writer Shulamith Firestone.

Shula, Shulamit, Sula, Sulamith

Sibyl Gk. "Seer, oracle." In ancient myth, sibyls interpreted the messages from oracles devoted to particular Gods, but their legend was also taken up and Christianized, and the name was common in the Middle Ages. Use dropped off and was revived at the turn of the 20th century, but the name now has a slightly dated aura. Actress Cybill Shepherd.

Cybele, Cybil, Cybill, Cybilla, Sabilla, Sabylla, Sib, Sibbell, Sibel, Sibell, Sibella, Sibelle, Sibilla, Sibyll, Sibylla, Sybel, Sybella, Sybelle, Sybill, Sybilla, Sybille

Sidonie Lat. "From Sidonia." Sidon was an area in the Middle East. Not uncommon in France, but easily confused with **Sidney** in the U.S.
Sidaine, Sidonia, Sidony, Sydona, Sydonah, Sydonia, Syndonia

Sidra Lat. "Of the stars."

Sierra Place name. Sierra is Spanish for "saw," and was the name Spanish settlers gave to the sharp, irregular peaks of some of the Western mountains like the Sierra Nevada (literally, "snowy saw"). Now used from time to time as a proper name, along with other geographical features like **Savannah** and **Mesa**.
Ciera, Cierra, Siera

Sigfreda OG. "Peaceful victory."
Sigfreida, Sigfrida, Sigfrieda, Sigfryda

Sigismonda It. from OG. "Victorious shield."
Sigismunda, Sigmonda, Sigmunda

Signa Unknown Scandinavian meaning: "Victory" is a possibility. The name is very unusual.
Signe, Signild, Signilda, Signilde, Signy

Sigourney Origin unclear, and made familiar almost single-handedly by actress Sigourney Weaver, who was christened **Susan**.
Sigornee, Sigournie

Silvia Var. Sylvia (Lat. "From the woods"). This was the original form of the name, eclipsed by the "-y-" spelling in the 19th century.
Silva, Silvana, Silvanna, Silvie, Silvija, Sirvana, Sirvanna, Silvy, Silvya, Sylvia, Sylvie

Simcha Heb. "Joy."

Simone (Fem. **Simon**) Heb. "listening intently." Used outside of France from the middle of the 20th century. Actress Simone Signoret; writer Simone de Beauvoir; gymnast Simona Amanar.
Shimona, Shimonah, Simeona, Simmina, Simona, Simonetta, Simonette, Simonia, Simonina, Simonna, Simonne, Symona, Symone

Sinead Ir. Var. **Janet** (Fem. **John**, Heb. "The Lord is gracious"). This name and **Siobhan** are a little more common than most Gaelic names, possibly influenced by actresses Sinead Cusack and Siobhan McKenna. **Sheena** is a short version of Sinead. Singer Sinead O'Connor.

Shinead, Seonaid, Sina, Sine

Siobhan Ir. Var. **Joan** (Fem. **John,** Heb. "The Lord is gracious"). Many of the phonetic forms of this name are probably intended as a combination of the "Sha-" prefix and **Yvonne**. Actress Siobhan McKenna.

Chavonne, Chevonne, Chivon, Chyvonne, Shavaun, Shavon, Shervan, Shevon, Shevonne, Shirvaun, Shivahn, Shivaun, Shovonne, Shyvonne, Sh'vonne, Sioban, Siobahn, Siobhian, Syvonne

Sirena Gk. "Entangler." In Greek myth, sirens were creatures that were half-woman, half-bird. They sang so sweetly that men dropped everything to listen, and starved to death. Odysseus outwitted them in his travels.

Sireena, Sirene, Syrena

Sissy Dim. **Cecilia** (Lat. "Blind"). Also a common nickname for a sister, since this is the way a younger sibling may say that word. Actress Sissy Spacek.

Cissee, Cissey, Cissi, Cissie, Cissy, Sissee, Sissey, Sissie

Skye Scot. Place name: the name of a spectacular island off the west coast of Scotland.

Skie, Sky

Skyler Dutch. "Giving shelter." Most probably an adaptation of the Dutch last name of **Schuyler,** which was brought to New York by 17th-century settlers.

Schyler, Schuyler, Skyla, Skylar, Skyllar

Socorro Sp. "Aid, help." Currently well used in Spain. Most likely refers to the aid or help provided by the Almighty.

Secorra, Socaria, Socorra, Sucorra

Solange Fr. "With dignity."

Souline, Zeline

Soledad Sp. "Solitude."

Solveig Scan. "Woman of the house."

Solvag, Solvej

Sondra Var. **Sandra** (Dim. **Alexandra**, Gk. "Defender of mankind"). Actress Sondra Locke.

Saundra, Sohndra, Sonndra, Zohndra, Zondra

Sonia Var. **Sophia** (Gk. "Wisdom"). Used since early in the 20th century. The current Queen of Norway is named Sonja. Skater/actress Sonja Henie; painter Sonia Delaunay.

Sohnia, Sohnnja, Sondja, Sondya, Sonja, Sonje, Sonnja, Sonya

Sophia Gk. "Wisdom." Used in English-speaking countries since the 17th century, though the French form, **Sophie**, has given it much competition in Britain. The famous Istanbul mosque Hagia Sofia was once a Christian church, but it was dedicated, not to Saint Sophia (an obscure and possibly nonexistent martyr), but to the Holy Wisdom, i.e., the Word of God. Sophia is in the top ten names in England and Scotland, in Germany (as Sophia), and in the top twenty in Ireland (Sophie). Actresses Sophia Loren, Sophie Dahl.

Saffi, Sofia, Sofie, Soficita, Sofka, Sofy, Sofya, Sonia, Sonja, Sonnie, Sonya, Sophey, Sophie, Sophy, Zofia, Zofi, Zofya, Zosia

Sophronia Gk. "Sensible, prudent."

Soffrona, Sofronia

Sorcha Ir. Gael. "Bright, shining." Used almost exclusively in Ireland. Actress Sorcha Cusack.

Sorrel Botanical name. Sorrel is a wild herb. Much less common than **Laurel** or **Rosemary.**

Sorel, Sorelle, Sorrell, Sorrelle

Speranza It. "Hope."

Esperance, Esperanza, Speranca

Spring OE. "Springtime." Use as a given name dates from (and is almost exclusive to) the 1970s.

Stacy Gk. "Resurrection." Dim. **Anastasia**. Most popular since the 1970s, and has long since outstripped its source.

Stace, Stacee, Stacey, Staci, Stacia, Stacie, Stasa, Stasee, Stasey, Stasia, Stasie, Stasey, Stasha, Staska, Stasy, Staycee, Staycey, Staysie, Staysy, Tacy, Taisie

Star Word as name. Translations, such as **Stella** (Greek) and **Esther** (Persian), are far more common.
Starla, Starlene, Starletta, Starlette, Starr

Stella Lat. "Star." Use was mostly literary until the 19th century, when the name became fashionable. For a generation of parents brought up on classic movies, it is hard to dissociate from Marlon Brando bellowing "Stella!" in *A Streetcar Named Desire.*
Estelle, Estella, Estrella, Stela, Stelle

Stephanie (Fem. **Stephen**) Gk. "Crowned." Cropped up in the 1920s and current since then. Use peaked in the top ten in the 1990s, and has since dwindled. Tennis star Steffi Graff; actresses Stefanie Powers, Stephanie Zimbalist; poet Stevie Smith.
Fania, Fanya, Phanie, Phanya, Stefa, Stefania, Stefanie, Stefenney, Stefcia, Steffa, Steffaney, Steffanie, Steffenie, Steffie, Stefinney, Stefka, Stefya, Stepa, Stepania, Stepanida, Stepanyda, Stepahnie, Stepfanie, Stepha, Stephana, Stephania, Stephanina, Stephanine, Stephannie, Stephene, Stepheney, Stephine, Stephney, Stephoney, Stesha, Steshka, Stevana, Stevena, Stevie, Stevey, Stevonna, Stevonne

Stina Dim. **Christina** (Gk. "Anointed, Christian").
Stine

Sukey Dim. **Susan** (Heb. "Lily"). Appeared in the 18th century and revived in the 20th, following the popularity of Susan itself.
Soki, Sokie, Sukee, Sukie, Suky

Summer OE. Name of the season. Like Spring and Season, a phenomenon of the 1970s. Swimmer Summer Sanders.
Somer, Sommers, Summers

Sunny Eng. Word as name: most likely to be a nickname characterizing a child's temperament.
Sunnee, Sunnie, Sunshine

Susan Heb. "Lily." After 18th-century use, neglected until a huge surge of popularity made it a top choice in the middle years of the 20th century, thus a name to overlook in the 21st. Suffragette Susan B. Anthony; authors Susan

Cheever, Susan Isaacs; actresses Susan Hampshire, Susan Dey, Susan Sarandon; basketball player Sue Bird.

Sanna, Shoshana, Shoshanah, Shoshanna, Shushana, Shu Shu, Sioux, Siouxsie, Siusan, Soosan, Soosanna, Sosanna, Suanny, Sue, Suesann, Suesonne, Suezanne, Sukee, Sukey, Sukie, Sonel, Sunel, Susana, Susanetta, Susanka, Susann, Susanna, Susannagh, Susannah, Susanne, Suse, Susee, Susette, Susi, Susie, Susy, Suzan, Suzana, Suzane, Suzanna, Suzanne, Suze, Suzee, Suzetta, Suzette, Suzie, Suzon, Suzy, Suzzanne, Zanna, Zanne, Zannie

Susannah Heb. "Lily." The original version of the name, and ripe for revival, combining as it does the nostalgic and the unusual (like **Molly** and **Emma**). Actress Susannah York.

Sanna, Sannah, Shoshanna, Shanna, Shu Shu, Suesanna, Susana, Susanna, Susannagh, Suzanna, Zanna, Zannie

Suzanne Fr. Var. **Susan**. It has more or less followed Susan into and out of fashion. Ballerina Suzanne Farrell; actresses Suzanne Pleshette, Suzanne Sommers.

Suesana, Susanna, Susanne, Suzane, Suzannah, Suzette, Suzzanne, Zanne, Zannie

Sybil Var. **Sibyl**. The most common spelling of the name, though it only became prevalent in the last century. Actress Cybill Shepherd.

Cybele, Cybill, Sibell, Sibilla, Sibyl, Sibylla, Sybel, Sybella, Sybelle, Sybill, Sybilla

Sydney OF. Place name: "Saint Denis." Originally Saint Denis would have been the name of a village, and the name Sydney would have indicated a resident there. The name used to be almost exclusively male, but was given prominence as a woman's name in the 1980s by madam/celebrity Sydney Biddle Barrows. Though many of today's parents like flowery old-fashioned names there is also a strong trend toward formerly male names like this one, which is steadily climbing popularity charts.

Cydney, Cydnie, Sidnee, Sidney, Sidnie, Sydel, Sydelle, Sydnie

Sylvia Lat. "From the forest." The Latin form, **Silvia,** predominated for centuries, but when the name was at its most popular (from the 19th century into the 1940s), Sylvia was the spelling of choice. Poet Sylvia Plath; actress Silvana Mangano.

Silva, Silvaine, Silvana, Silvania, Silvanna, Silvia, Silviana, Silvianne, Silvie, Sylva, Sylvana, Sylvanna, Sylvee, Sylvette, Sylviana, Sylvianne, Sylvie, Sylvine, Sylwia, Zilvia, Zylvia

Tabina Arab. "Muhammad's follower."

Tabitha Aramaic. "Gazelle." New Testament name reintroduced in the 17th century passion for biblical names. Neglected in this century until a minor revival in the 1960s. Journalist Tabitha Soren.

Tabatha, Tabbee, Tabbey, Tabbi, Tabbie, Tabbitha, Tabby, Tabatha, Tabetha, Tabita, Tabotha, Tabytha

Tacita Lat. "Silence." Never a standard, but somewhat more common in eras when a woman's role was to be quiet.

Tace, Tacey, Tacia, Tacie, Tacye

Taffy Welsh. "Loved one."

Tahira Arab. "Virginal, pure."

Talia Heb. "Heaven's dew." May also be a variant of **Thalia,** or a derivative of **Natalie.** A pretty name, but infrequently used. Actress Talia Shire.

Talitha Aramaic. "Young girl." Actress Talitha Soto.

Taleetha, Taletha, Talicia, Talisha, Talita

Tallulah Choctaw Indian. "Leaping water." Not, as one might expect, an invented name, nor even one assumed by its most famous bearer, actress Tallulah Bankhead. It was

a Bankhead family name, and is also a place name in
Georgia. Could not now be used without reference to the
actress, however.
Talley, Tallie, Tallula, Tally, Talula

Tamara Heb. "Palm tree." Old Testament name with a hint
of the picturesque. **Tamar** was the more common version
until this century, when Tamara, the Russian form, over-
took it. Quite fashionable in the 1970s. Skiing champion
Tamara McKinney; author Tama Janowitz.
**Tama, Tamar, Tamarah, Tamarra, Tamary, Tamera,
Tamma, Tammara, Tammi, Tammy, Tamora, Tamra,
Tamrah, Thamar, Thamara, Thamarra, Thamera**

Tamika Modern U.S. name of unknown origin. Some
sources suggest a Japanese root meaning "people," but
this seems farfetched since the name is not used in the
Japanese community. More likely to be a variant of the
popular **Tanisha.** Basketball player Tamika Catchings.
**Tameka, Tameeka, Tameika, Tamiecka, Tamieka,
Tamike, Tamiko, Taminique, Tamiqua, Temeequa,
Temika, Timeeka, Tomika, Tonica, Tonique,
Tymmeeka, Tymmiecka**

Tammy Dim. **Tamara** (or other "Tam-" names). A nickname that took on a life of its own in the 1950s and 1960s,
and was probably used without much interest in its source
or meaning. Now out of fashion. Actress Tammy Grimes;
singer Tammy Wynette; evangelist Tammy Faye Bakker.
Tami, Tamie, Tammee, Tammey, Tammie

Tamsin Var. **Thomasina** (Heb. "Twin"). Very old name that
was revived by British parents in the middle of the 20th
century.
**Tamasin, Tamasine, Tamsine, Tamsinne, Tamsyn,
Tamzen, Tamzin**

Tanisha Modern name of unclear meaning, though several
sources propose an African origin. Its popularity may
stem from a contemporary fondness for 3-syllable names
ending in "-a." And while the "Ta-" prefix doesn't ap-
proach the popularity of "La-" or "Sha-," the similarity of
sound probably contributes to Tanisha's widespread use.

This is probably a combination of "Ta-" and the much-favored **Aisha**.

Taneesha, Taniesha, Tanitia, Tannicia, Tanniece, Tannisha, Teinicia, Teneesha, Tinecia, Tiniesha, Tynisha

Tansy Gk. "Everlasting life." Also the name of a fairly unusual herb. Used mostly since the 1960s.

Tanazia, Tandie, Tandy, Tansee, Tansey, Tansia, Tanzey, Tanzia

Tanya Dim. **Tatiana,** an ancient Italian name. This diminutive has been more popular than the full name, especially in the 1970s. Photographer Tana Hoban; country singer Tanya Tucker.

Tana, Tanazia, Tahnee, Tahnya, Taneea, Tania, Tanita, Tanja, Tarnya, Tawnya, Tonnya, Tonya, Tonyah

Tara Ir. Gael. "Rocky hill." Though Irish legends mention a place called Tara, its real prominence came in the 1940s when most Americans knew that Scarlett O'Hara's plantation home was called Tara. This seems to have launched the use of the name. Actress Tara Reid.

Tarah, Tarra, Tarrah

Taryn Var. **Tara,** or re-spellling of a group of names that was popular in the 1950's and '60s, **Karen, Sharon,** and **Darren**.

Taran, Tarin, Tarina, Tarnia, Tarren, Tarryn, Taryna, Teryn

Tasha Dim. **Natasha** (Rus. "Christmas"). Author Tasha Tudor.

Tahsha, Tashey, Tashina, Tasia, Tasenka, Taska, Tasya

Tatiana Rus. Var. of an ancient Italian name. Has penetrated the U.S. somewhat in recent years. Opera star Tatiana Troyannos.

Tania, Tanya, Tati, Tatianna, Tatie, Tatijana, Tatiyana, Tatjana, Tatyana, Tatyanna, Tonya

Taylor ME. Occupational name: "Tailor." The "last name as first name" trend brought Taylor streaking into the nation's top ten names for girls during the mid-nineties, but it has since begun to fade almost as fast as it became popular.

Tahlor, Tailor, Tayler

Tecla Gk. "Fame of God." Traditionally Saint Thecla, converted by Saint Paul, was the first female Christian martyr, but her legend seems to be largely fantastic. The name has been most popular in Greece.

Teccla, Tekla, Tekli, Telca, Telka, Thecla, Thekla

Temira Heb. "Tall."

Temora, Timora

Temperance Puritan virtue name.

Tempest OF. "Storm." Rare usage is probably a matter of a family name transposed, since few parents wish for a child with a stormy temperament. Actress Tempestt Bledsoe.

Tempesta, Tempeste, Tempestt

Terena (Fem. **Terence**) Roman clan name. Used mostly in the middle of the 20th century.

Tareena, Tarena, Tarina, Tereena, Terenia, Terenne, Terriell, Terriella, Terina, Terrena, Terrene, Terrin, Terrina, Teryl, Teryll, Teryna, Therena

Teresa Popular alternate spelling of **Theresa**. Actress Teresa Wright; basketball player Teresa Weatherspoon.

Techa, Terasa, Terasina, Terasita, Terecena, Teresia, Teresina, Teresita, Tereska, Teresse, Tereza, Terezilya, Terezita, Terosina, Terrie, Terrosina, Terry, Tersa, Tersia, Terushka, Teruska, Tesa, Tesia, Teskia, Tess, Tessa, Tessie, Tessy

Terry Terry Dim. **Theresa**. This and other nicknames for Theresa were at their most popular in the middle of the 20th century. Actresses Theresa Russell, Teri Garr.

Terall, Terea, Teree, Tereigh, Terell, Terella, Terelynn, Terelynn, Teri, Terie, Terree, Terreigh, Terrey, Terri, Terrye

Tertia Lat. "Third." Unusual, as most of these number names (**Prima, Secunda**) are. Curiously, **Octavia** (which means "eighth") is the only one that has taken on a life of its own.

Tercia, Tersia, Tersha

Tessa Dim. **Theresa**. Some sources also suggest Gk. "Fourth child." Pretty, simple, and uncommon.

Tess, Tessie, Tessy, Teza

Thaddea (Fem. **Thaddeus**) Gk., meaning unsure: "Brave" is one possibility.

Tada, Tadda, Taddie, Thada, Thadda, Thadée, Thaddie

Thalassa Gk. "Sea, ocean."

Talassa

Thalia Gk. "Blooming, in flower." In Greek legend Thalia is one of the Three Graces (along with Aglaia and Euphosyne); she is also one of the nine Muses, daughters of Zeus and Mnemosyne, each of whom represents an art or a science. Thalia represents Comedy.

Talia, Talie, Talley, Tally, Thaleia, Thalie, Thalya

Thana Arab. "Thanksgiving."

Thea Gk. "Goddess." Also dim. **Dorothea** (Gk. "gift of God"). Actress Téa Leoni.

Tea, Theia, Thia

Thelma Gk. "Will." Literary name coined in the late 19th century, at its peak in the first third of this century. It has the aura of a bygone era, but not so bygone that it is attractive to modern parents.

Telma, Thellma

Theodora Gk. "Gift of God." Much less common than its synonym, **Dorothy.** At its peak in the middle third of the 20th century, but never a standard. Actress/vamp Theda Bara.

Dora, Fedora, Feodora, Fyodora, Teddey, Teddie, Tedra, Teodora, Teodory, Theadora, Theda, Theo, Theodosia, Todora

Theodosia Gk. "Gift of God." Little-used variant given some prominence by Anya Seton's 1941 historical novel *My Theodosia,* about Aaron Burr's daughter.

Docia, Dosia, Feodosia, Theda, Teodosia, Tossa, Tossia

Theone Gk. "Name of God." Costume designer Theoni V. Aldredge.

Teone, Teoni, Theoni

Theophania Gk. "God's appearance." Immensely popular in its contracted modern form, **Tiffany,** but almost unheard of in this full version.

Theofania, Theophanie, Teofanie, Teophania, Teophanie

Theophila Gk. "God-loving."
Teofila, Teophile, Teophila, Theofila

Theresa Gk. "Harvest." May also stem from a Greek place name. The name owes its popularity to two important Catholic saints, the astringent, intellectual mystic St. Teresa of Avila, and the humble young nun, St. Thérèse of Lisieux. It seems to have spread from Catholic families to wider acceptance, and was especially common in the 1960s. Actresses Theresa Russell, Teresa Wright, Teri Garr; humanitarian Mother Teresa; basketball player Theresa Edwards.
Resi, Rezi, Rezka, Taresa, Tera, Terasa, Teresa, Terese, Teresia, Teresina, Teresita, Teressa, Tereza, Terezinha, Terezsa, Teri, Terrasa, Terresa, Terresia, Terri, Terrosina, Terry, Terrya, Tersa, Tersina, Tersita, Terza, Tess, Tessa, Tessey, Tessi, Tessie, Tessy, Thérèse, Theresina, Theresita, Theressa, Tracey, Tracie, Tracy, Treesa, Tresa, Tressa, Trescha, Treza, Zita

Thomasina (Fem. **Thomas**) Heb. "Twin." **Thomasin** was the earliest form, replaced by Thomasina in the Victorian era, and **Tamsin** a hundred years later. Now quite scarce.
Tammi, Tammie, Thomasa, Thomasin, Thomasine, Thomazine, Toma, Tomasina, Tomasine, Tomina, Tommie, Tommy

Thora Scan. "Thor's struggle." Thor is the Norse god of thunder. Actress Thora Birch.
Thordia, Thordis, Thyra, Tyra

Thurayya Arab. "Star."
Soraya, Surayya, Surayyah, Thuraia

Tia Sp. "Aunt." Probably used as a first name with little reference to its actual meaning, but fondness for its sound. Actress Tia Carrere.
Thia, Tiana, Tiara

Tiberia Lat. Place name: The river Tiber flows through Rome, and Tiberius was a Roman clan name.
Tibbie, Tibby, Tyberia

Tiffany Gk. "God's appearance." Literally, **Theophania**. Traditionally used for babies born on Epiphany, the day when the Three Kings first saw the Christ Child. Now associated with Tiffany & Co., the New York City jeweler. The name has become shorthand for upper-class luxury, and was hugely popular in the 1980s. By 1990 it was sliding down the list of popularity. Actress Tiffani Thiessen.

Theophanie, Tifara, Tifennie, Tiffaney, Tiffani, Tiffanie, Tiffeny, Tiffenie, Tiffie, Tiffney, Tiffy, Tiphanie, Tiphara, Tiphenie, Tipheny, Tyffany, Tyffenie

Tilda Dim. **Matilda** (OG. "Battle-mighty"). Actress Tilda Swinton.

Thilda, Thilde, Tildie, Tildy, Tilley, Tillie, Tilly

Timothea (Fem. **Timothy**) Gk. "Honoring God." Uncommon feminization of a well-established boy's name.

Thea, Timaula, Timmey, Timmi, Timmie, Timotheya

Tina Dim. **Christina**, etc. Used in the 20th century, but especially popular in the 1960s. Rock star Tina Turner; actress Tina Louise; playwright Tina Howe; basketball player Tina Thompson.

Teena, Teenie, Teina, Tena, Tine, Tiny

Tirza Heb. "Pleasantness." Although many versions of the name exist, it is rarely used in modern times. It is one of the few Old Testament female names that was not used widely in the Puritan era.

Thersa, Thirsa, Thirza, Thirzah, Thursa, Thurza, Tierza, Tirzah, Tyrzah

Tita Probably derived from Spanish diminutives like **Martita**; may be considered a feminization of **Titus** (or **Tito**).

Teeta, Tyta

Titania Gk. "Giant." The Titans in Greek myth were a race of giants. A more familiar use of the name, though, is the Queen of the Fairies in Shakespeare's *A Midsummer Night's Dream*. Easily confused with the more familiar **Tatiana**.

Tania, Tita, Titaniya, Titanya, Tiziana

Toby Heb. "God is good." More commonly a boy's name, used from time to time for girls.

Taube, Taubey, Taubie, Thobey, Thobie, Thoby, Tobe, Tobee, Tobey, Tobi, Tobiah, Tova, Tovah, Tove

Toni Dim. **Antoinette** (Lat. "Beyond price, invaluable"). Author Toni Morrison; actress Toni Colette.

Toinette, Toinon, Tola, Tona, Tonee, Toney, Tonia, Tonie, Tonina, Tony, Tonya, Twanette

Topaz Lat. Jewel name. Less common than **Ruby** or **Pearl**, but a good candidate for a November baby (it is that month's birthstone) or for a baby with topaz (golden) coloring.

Tori Dim. **Victoria** (Lat. "Victory"). Actresses Tori Spelling, Tori Amos.

Torey, Toria, Torie, Torrey, Torrye, Tory

Toya Modern U.S. name, perhaps a diminutive of **Latoya,** one of the most popular "La-" names. It has no particular meaning.

Toia

Tracy Dim. **Theresa** (Gk. "Harvest"). First used in numbers in the 1940s, probably in response to the film *The Philadelphia Story* whose main character is named Tracy Lord. This touched off a long period of popularity that is now distinctly fading. Actress Tracey Ullman; tennis player Tracy Austin; singer Tracy Chapman; swimmer Tracy Caulkins.

Trace, Tracee, Tracey, Traci, Tracie, Trasey, Treacy, Treasa, Treasey, Treasa

Traviata It. "One who goes astray." As in the great Verdi opera, *La Traviata.*

Tricia Dim. **Patricia** (Lat. "Aristocratic"). Choreographer Trisha Brown.

Treasha, Trichia, Tris, Trisa, Trish, Trisha, Trisia, Trissina

Trilby Literary name coined at the turn of the 20th century. Trilby, the central character of the eponymous novel and play, became a great singer. (The name may refer to vocal trills.) A trilby hat, worn by the character in the 1895 stage production, is a soft felt hat with a dented crown.

Trilbea, Trilbee, Trilbeigh, Trilbey, Trilbie, Trillby

Trina Dim. **Katrina** (Gk. "Pure").

Treena, Treina, Trine, Trinette, Trinnette

Trinity Lat. "Triad." Refers to the Holy Trinity, the three forms of God in the Christian faith. Used mostly among Spanish-speaking families. Actress Trini Alvarado.
Trini, Trinidad, Trinidade, Trinita, Trinitee, Trinitey

Trista Lat. "Sad." An inauspicious name for a baby, however pretty it sounds. A short-lived 2002 reality show called "The Bachelorette" featured a woman named Trista Rehn.

Trixie Dim. **Beatrice** (Lat. "Bringer of gladness").
Trix, Trixee, Trixy

Trudy Dim. **Gertrude** (OG. "Strength of a spear"). Cropped up in the middle of the 20th century, but little heard now.
Truda, Trude, Trudey, Trudi, Trudie, Trudye

Tsifira Heb. "Crown, diadem."

Tuesday OE. Day of the week. Given exposure by actress Tuesday Weld, but not in general use.
Tuesdee

Twyla Modern name of uncertain meaning and derivation. Choreographer Twyla Tharp.
Tuwyla, Twila, Twilla

Tyler Occupational name: "Maker of tiles." The name of one of the country's less memorable presidents (John Tyler, 1841–1845). Very unusual as a girl's name, but one of the country's top ten for boys in the mid-1990s.
Tyller

Tzipporah Var. **Zippora** (Heb. "Bird.") Zipporah was the wife of Moses. Despite its Biblical prominence, the name is not popular.
Tzipora, Tzippora, Zipporah

Tzigane Hung. "Gypsy."
Tsigana, Tsigane

Udele OE. "Wealthy."
> **Uda, Udella, Udelle, Yewdelle, Yudella, Yudelle**

Ula Celt. "Gem of the sea."
> **Eula, Ulla, Ulli, Yulla**

Ulima Arab. "Astute, wise."
> **Uleema, Ulima, Ullima**

Ulrica (fem. **Ulric**) OG. "Power of the wolf" or "Power of the home." Very unusual outside of Germany.
> **Rieka, Rica, Ricka, Uhlrike, Ulka, Ullrica, Ullricka, Ulrika, Ulrike, Uulrica**

Ultima Lat. "End, farthest point." In English, hard to dissociate from "ultimate."
> **Ulltima, Ultimata**

Ulva OG. "Wolf."

Uma Sanskrit. "Flax or turmeric." Uma is also the name of the Indian goddess Sakti, in her guise as light, and is a Hebrew name meaning "nation." For all the fame of actress Uma Thurman, the name may be too exotic for widespread use.
> **Ooma**

Una Lat. "One." The origin of the name may be Irish, though its Celtic meaning is lost. Very unusual.
> **Euna, Oona, Oonagh, Unah**

Undine Lat. "Little wave." In myth, Undine is the spirit of the waters. Edith Wharton created a character in *The Custom of the Country* who was named Undine for the hair-curling (or "waving") tonic that had made her father rich.
> **Ondina, Ondine, Undeen, Undene, Undina**

Unity ME. "Oneness." Used by the Puritans and extremely uncommon. Most people have heard of it only in connection with Unity Mitford, one of the famous English Mitford sisters.
> **Unita, Unite, Unitey**

Urania Gk. "Heavenly." Urania was one of the Greek Muses, the nine daughters of Zeus and Mnemosyne identified with particular arts and sciences. Urania was in charge of astronomy.
Ourania, Ouranie, Urainia, Uraniya, Uranya

Urbana Lat. "Of the city." The male form, **Urban**, is a bit more familiar, having been used by eight popes.
Urbanna

Urit Heb. "Brightness."
Urena, Urina, Uriya, Urith

Ursula Lat. "Little female bear." Saint Ursula was a much-venerated virgin martyr, allegedly executed by Attila the Hun, though her story has little basis in fact. The name was most popular in the 17th century. Fans of Disney cartoons will be bound to associate it with the overweight octopus sea-witch in *The Little Mermaid*. Author Ursula K. Le Guin; actress Ursula Andress.
Orsa, Orsala, Orsola, Orsolla, Seula, Sula, Ulla, Ursa, Ursala, Urselina, Ursella, Ursie, Ursley, Ursola, Ursule, Ursulette, Ursulina, Ursuline, Ursy, Urszula, Urszuli

Uta Origin unclear: possibly dim. **Otthild** (OG. "Prospers in battle"). Actress Uta Hagen.
Ute, Utte, Yuta

 Val Dim.**Valentina, Valerie**. Occasionally an independent name.
Vala OG. "Singled out."
Valla

Valda (Fem. **Waldemar**) OG. "Renowned ruler." Occurs in some Northern European countries, and from time to time in Britain, but very scarce in the U.S.

Vallda, Velda

Valentina Lat. "Strong." This name and **Valerie** come from the same Latin root. **Valentia** was the earliest form, but it entered the modern age as Valentina. **Valentine** is used for both boys and girls, and the early Christian martyr for whom the holiday is named was male. Cosmonaut Valentina Tereshkova.

Teena, Teina, Tena, Tina, Val, Vale, Valeda, Valena, Valencia, Valenteen, Valenteena, Valentia, Valentijn, Valentine, Valenzia, Valera, Valida, Valina, Valja, Vallatina, Valli, Vallie, Vally, Velora

Valerie Lat. "Strong." The French form of an early Christian name (**Valeria**) that was revived at the turn of the 20th century. It was very popular in the middle of the 20th century, less so now. Actresses Valerie Harper, Valerie Bertinelli, Valerie Perrine.

Val, Valaree, Valarey, Valaria, Valarie, Vale, Valeree, Valeria, Valeriana, Valery, Valerye, Valka, Vallarie, Valleree, Vallerie, Vallery, Vallie, Vallorey, Vallorie, Vallory, Valorie, Vallrie, Valry, Valka

Valeska (Fem. **Vladislav**) Old Slavic. "Splendid leader."

Valonia Lat. Place name: "Shallow valley."

Vallonia, Valonya

Valora Lat. "Courageous."

Vallora, Valoria, Valorie, Valory, Valorya, Valoura, Valouria

Vanda Var. **Wanda**. OG. tribal name. Mostly used at the turn of the century.

Vahnda, Vannda, Vohnda, Vonda

Vanessa Literary name, invented by *Gulliver's Travels* author Jonathan Swift. Suddenly leapt into everyday use in the middle years of the 20th century, achieving some popularity in the 1970s, and quite considerable use recently. Actresses Vanessa Redgrave, Vanessa Williams; celebrity Vanna White.

Nessa, Nessie, Nessy, Van, Vanesa, Vanesse, Vanetta, Vannessa, Vannetta, Vania, Vanija, Vanna, Vannie, Vanya, Venesa, Venessa, Venetta, Vinessa, Vonessa, Vonesse, Vonnessa

Vanora Old Welsh. "White wave."
  Vannora
Varda Heb. "Rose."
  Vardia, Vardice, Vardina, Vardis, Vardit, Vardith
Varvara Var. **Barbara** (Gk. "Stranger"). In Greek pronunciation the "V" and "B" sounds are quite close, hence the ties between these names.
  Varenka, Varina, Varinka, Varka, Varya, Vava, Vavka
Vashti Per. "Lovely." In the Old Testament, the wife of the proud King Ahasuerus of Persia. Passed over by the Puritans (perhaps because she became a divorcée), but revived very slightly in the 19th century.
  Vashtee
Veda Sanskrit. "Knowledge, wisdom." The Vedas are the four sacred books of the Hindus.
  Vedis, Veeda, Veida, Veta, Vida
Vedette It. "Sentry, scout." By extension, because a sentry or a scout is often singled out or separated from the group, the French term *vedette* means something (like a headline) that is singled out graphically. And by further extension, in everyday usage, *vedette* is the French word for a movie star.
  Vedetta
Vega Arab. "Falling," Swedish from Latin, "Star." Vega is the name of one of the largest and brightest stars.
  Vaga, Vaiga, Vayga
Velda Var. **Valda**.
  Vellda
Velika Old Slavic. "Great, wondrous."
Velma Origin disputed. Possibly dim. **Wilhelmina** (OG. "Will-helmet"), possibly a late-19th-century invention. In general use since the 1920s, but not fashionable.
  Vehlma, Vellma
Venetia Place name. Never reached the stature of that other great Italian tourist mecca, **Florence**. Cropped up from the 17th century onward; use increased in the 19th century, but the name would still be considered a bit fanciful. The English form, **Venice,** is also used occasionally.
  Vanecia, Vanetia, Venecia, Venetta, Venezia, Venice,

Venise, Venita, Venize, Venitia, Vennice, Vinetia, Vonitia, Vonizia

Venus Name of the Roman goddess of love and beauty. Used in Britain in the 16th century through the 19th, but very scarce now. It creates a lot of expectations for a female baby. Tennis star Venus Williams has endowed the name with some of her own powerful glamor, however.

Venusa, Venusette, Venusina, Venusita

Vera Slavic. "Faith"; Lat. "Truth." Use by two popular novelists in the late 19th century promoted the name to high fashion, but it is hardly found now. Actress Vera Miles; fashion designer Vera Wang.

Veradis, Verasha, Veera, Veira, Vere, Verena, Verene, Verina, Verine, Verinka, Verka, Verla, Verochka, Veroshka, Veruschka, Verushka

Verbena Lat. "Holy plants." Originally referred to olive, laurel, and myrtle, plants with spiritual significance to the Romans. In modern times, a class of plants with medicinal properties and, frequently, pleasant scents.

Verbeena, Verbeina, Verbina, Verbyna

Verdad Sp. "Truth."

Verena Lat. "True." Derives from the same root as **Vera**. Primarily English use.

Varena, Varina, Vereena, Verina, Veruchka, Veruschka, Veryna

Verity Lat. "Truth." Puritan virtue name, much less common than **Constance, Prudence, Hope,** etc.

Veretie, Verety, Verita, Veritie

Verna Lat. "Springtime." Use spans the late years of the 19th century to the middle of the 20th, but the name has a dated air and is rare today. Actress Virna Lisi.

Verda, Verne, Verneta, Vernetta, Vernette, Vernice, Vernie, Vernis, Vernise, Vernisse, Vernita, Virna

Verona Dim. **Veronica.** Also the name of a northern Italian city well-known to tourists, so it may be used by reminiscent parents.

Varona, Veron, Verone, Verowna

Veronica Lat. "True image." Or Var. **Bernice** (Gk. "She who brings victory"). According to a legend that sprang up in the Middle Ages, a young girl wiped Jesus' sweating brow on his way to Calvary. The handkerchief she used later showed a perfect image of his face. (Three separate Italian churches now claim to own this holy relic.) The name first appeared in Britain in the 17th century, spread beyond Catholic families in the 19th century, and became popular in the 1950s. Possibly reminiscent of the Archie and Veronica comic books. Actress Veronica Lake.

Rana, Ranna, Roni, Ronica, Ronika, Ronna, Ronnee, Ronni, Ronnica, Ronnie, Ronny, Veera, Veira, Vera, Veranica, Veranique, Verinique, Vernice, Vernicka, Vernika, Verohnica, Verohnicca, Veronice, Veronicka, Veronika, Veronike, Veroniqua, Véronique, Veronka, Veronqua, Vonnie

Vespera Lat. "Evening star."

Vesperina, Vespers

Vesta Lat. The Roman household goddess. Her altar was tended by six virgins (the "vestal virgins"), who were kept under severe discipline. They were buried alive if they lost their virginity. Most common late 19th to early 20th century.

Vicky Dim. **Victoria**. Author Vicki Baum; actress Vicki Lawrence.

Vicci, Vickee, Vickey, Vicki, Vicky, Vicqui, Vikkey, Vikki, Vikky, Viqui

Victoria (Fem. **Victor**) Lat. "Victory." Extremely common in Christian Rome, but curiously not fashionable during the reign (1837-1901) of the woman who gave her name to the Victorian age. Most recently popular in the 1950s and 1960s, but daughters in those days were probably called "Vicky." Parents who use it now are more likely to insist on the whole mouthful, or **Tori** in a pinch. For the past dozen years, Victoria has hovered in the top 20% of American girls' names. Actress Victoria Principal.

Tori, Toria, Torie, Tory, Toya, Vic, Vicci, Vickee, Vickey, Vicki, Vickie, Vicky, Victoriana, Victorie, Victorina, Victorine, Victory, Vika, Vikkey, Vikki,

Vikky, Viktoria, Viktorija, Viktorina, Viktorine, Viktorka, Viqui, Vitoria, Vittoria

Vida Dim. **Davita** (Heb. "Loved one") or Sp. "Life."
Veda, Veeda, Vidette, Vieda, Vita, Vitia

Vidonia Port. "Branch of a vine."
Veedonia, Vidonya

Vigilia Lat. "Wakefulness."

Vigdis Nor. "War goddess."
Vigdess

Vilhelmina Var. **Wilhelmina** (OG. "Will-helmet").
Vilhelmine, Villhelmina, Wilhelmina

Villette Fr. "Small town." The name of one of Charlotte Brontë's lesser-known novels.

Vilma Rus. Dim. **Vilhelmina**.
Wilma

Vina Dim. **Davina, Lavinia,** etc or. Sp. "Vineyard." In either case, probably a name whose use was promoted by the feminine ending "-a."
Veena, Vena, Veina, Vinetta, Vinette, Vinia, Vinica, Vinita, Vinya, Vyna, Vynetta, Vynette

Vincentia (Fem. **Vincent**) Lat. "Conquering." An unusual feminization of a name that has not been very common in America.
Vicenta, Vicentia, Vincenta, Vincentena, Vincentina, Vincentine, Vincenza, Vincenzia, Vincetta, Vinetta

Violet Lat. "Purple." A flower name in longer use than most. Occurred first in the 1830s and lasted nearly a hundred years, but always more popular in Britain (whose cool, damp climate is more hospitable to the spring flowers). **Viola** has been a less-used choice. Ballerina Violette Verdy.
Eolande, Iolande, Iolanthe, Jolanda, Jolande, Jolanta, Jolantha, Jolanthe, Vi, Viola, Violaine, Violanta, Violante, Violanthe, Viole, Violeine, Violetta, Violette, Viollet, Violletta, Viollette, Vyolet, Vyoletta, Vyolette, Yolanda, Yolande, Yolane, Yolantha, Yolanthe

Virginia Lat. "Virgin." The name probably derives from a Roman clan name, but the current meaning has been assumed for hundreds of years. A great favorite in the U.S. from the mid-19th century to the mid-20th; the first child born in the U.S. was Virginia Dare, in 1597. The state of Virginia was named in compliment to the Virgin Queen, Elizabeth I. A good candidate for 21st century revival. Author Virginia Woolf; tennis player Virginia Wade.

Geena, Geenia, Geenya, Genia, Genya, Gigi, Gina, Ginella, Ginelle, Ginger, Gingia, Ginia, Ginnee, Ginni, Ginnie, Ginny, Ginya, Jenell, Jenella, Jenelle, Jinia, Jinjer, Jinnie, Jinny, Verginia, Verginya, Virge, Virgenya, Virgie, Virgine, Virginie, Virginnia, Virgy

Viridis Lat. "Green."

Virdis, Viridia, Viridian, Viridiana, Viridianna, Viridianne

Vita Lat. "Life." Also occasionally a nickname for **Victoria**, as in the case of English writer Vita Sackville-West.

Veeta, Vitel, Vitella, Vitka

Viveca Scan. "Alive." Var. **Viva**. Actresses Viveca Lindfors, Vivica Fox.

Vivecka, Viveka, Vivica, Vivika

Viva Lat. "Alive." Most familiar from the expression meaning "Long live . . ." as in *"Viva l'Espana"* or *"Vive la France."* Actress Viva.

Veeva, Viveca, Vivva

Vivian Lat. "Full of life." Used for boys in Britain (although infrequently), generally for girls in the U.S. In spite of the early martyr Saint Vivian, the name has been current only since the 19th century, and has never been a real favorite. Actresses Vivien Leigh, Vivian Vance.

Bibi, Bibiana, Bibiane, Bibianna, Bibianne, Bibyana, Vevay, Vi, Vibiana, Viv, Vivee, Vivi, Vivia, Viviana, Viviane, Vivianna, Vivianne, Vivie, Vivien, Vivienne, Vivyan, Vivyana, Vivyanne, Vyvyan, Vyvyana, Vyvyanne

W **Walburga** OG. "Strong protection." Saint's name very rarely trotted out in modern times. Saint Walburga was an 8th-century missionary in Germany whose feast day was May 1, the traditional pagan festival day. Walpurgisnacht has come down in legend as the night of the witches' sabbath.

Walberga, Wallburga, Walpurgis

Walda (Fem. **Waldo**) OG. "Ruler." Extremely unusual feminization of a name that is also unusual for boys.

Waldena, Waldette, Waldina, Wallda, Welda, Wellda

Walker OE. Occupational name: "Cloth-walker." The era that saw the rise of last names was also the great English era of the wool trade, giving us such cloth-manufacturing names as **Fuller, Tailor,** and **Weaver**. In that medieval era, workers trod on the wool to clean it. This name is very unusual for girls.

Wallker

Wallis Var. **Wallace** (OE. "From Wales"). Famous as a feminine name because of Wallis Simpson, the woman who very badly wanted to be queen of England, but became Duchess of Windsor instead.

Walless, Wallie, Walliss, Wally, Wallys

Wanda Probably a Slavic tribal name, though some sources suggest OG. "Wanderer." Use has been pretty well confined to the middle of the 20th century. Harpsichordist Wanda Landowska.

Vanda, Wahnda, Wandah, Wandie, Wandis, Wandy, Wannda, Wenda, Wendaline, Wendall, Wendeline, Wendy, Wohnda, Wonda, Wonnda

Wanetta OE. "Pale-skinned." From the same root that gives us "wan," which is not exactly a complimentary term. In the U.S. this name is more likely a phonetic spelling or variant of **Juanita**.

Waneta, Wanette, Wanita

Warda (Fem. **Ward**) OG. "Guardian."

Wardia, Wardine

Wendy Literary name: coined by James Barrie for the human heroine of *Peter Pan*. The parents who used it in great numbers in the middle of the 20th century may have been inspired by either the musical play or the animated movie. Some, wishing to call a daughter Wendy, no doubt named her **Gwendolyn,** but the names aren't actually related. Ballerina Wendy Whelan; playwright Wendy Wasserstein; actress Dame Wendy Hiller.

Wenda, Wendaline, Wendee, Wendeline, Wendey, Wendi, Wendie, Wendye, Windy

Whitney OE. Place name: "White island." Boy's name that became hugely popular for girls in the early 1980s, possibly because of its connotations of old wealth. It was sliding out of the top 100 names by the early 1990s and is now almost an oddity. Singer Whitney Houston.

Whitnea, Whitneigh, Whiteney, Whitnee, Whitni, Whitnie, Whitny, Whittaney, Whittany, Whittney, Whittnie

Wilda OE. "Willow" or OG. "Untamed."

Willda, Wylda

Wilhelmina OG. "Will-helmet." Despite the number of variants spawned by the name, it hasn't been very popular in any form. Probably used more often to honor a beloved relative named **William** rather than on its own merits. Actress Billie Burke; author Willa Cather.

Billa, Billee, Billey, Billie, Billy, Ellma, Elma, Guglielma, Guillelmina, Guillelmine, Guillema, Guillemette, Guillemine, Helma, Helmina, Helmine, Helminette, Min, Mina, Minna, Minnie, Minny, Valma, Velma, Vilhelmina, Villhelmina, Villhelmine, Vilma, Wileen, Wilene, Wilhelmine, Willa, Willabella, Willabelle, Willamina, Willamine, Willeen, Willene, Willemina, Willetta, Willette, Williamina, Willie, Williebelle, Wilmette, Willmina, Willmine, Willy, Willybella, Wilma, Wilmette, Wilmina, Wilna, Wylma

Willow Tree name. A phenomenon of the 1970s. TV reporter Willow Bay.

Wilma Dim. **Wilhelmina**. Less of a mouthful than its source, but reminiscent of the dizzy Stone Age housewife Wilma Flintstone in the TV cartoon show "The Flintstones." Track star Wilma Rudolph.

Valma, Vilma, Willma, Wilmina, Wylma

Wilona OE. "Longed-for."

Wilone

Winifred Welsh. "Holy peacemaking." Also often explained as Old German "Friend of peace." Popular in Britain for fifty years around the turn of the 20th century, but little used otherwise.

Fred, Freddie, Freddy, Fredi, Fredy, Wina, Winafred, Winefred, Winefride, Winefried, Winfreda, Winfrieda, Winifryd, Winne, Winnie, Winnifred, Wynafred, Wynifred, Wynn, Wynne, Wynnifred

Winola OG. "Charming friend."

Winona Sioux Indian. "Firstborn daughter." Actress Winona Ryder; country singer Wynonna Judd.

Wenona, Wenonah, Winnie, Winnona, Winoena, Winonah, Wynnona, Wynona, Wynnona

Winter OE. Season name. Like **Summer,** used mostly in the 1970s.

Wintar

Wren OE. Bird name: A wren is a small brown songbird.

Wynne Welsh. "Fair, pure." Uncommon, simple, but distinctive in a way that may appeal to today's parents.

Win, Winne, Winnie, Winny, Wyn, Wynn

Xanthe Gk. "Yellow." A description of someone's coloring. Almost unknown.
    Xantha, Xanthia, Zanthe

Xaviera (Fem. **Xavier**). Basque. "New house." Given some exposure by Xaviera Hollander, the author of a book that caused some stir in the early 1970s. It was called *The Happy Hooker*.
Exaviera, Exavyera, Xavienna, Xavyera, Zaveeyera, Zaviera

Xenia Gk. "Welcoming." Occasionally spelled with the "X"; occurs once in a while with a "Z."
Xeenia, Xena, Xiomara, Zeena, Zena, Zenia, Zina, Zyna

Xylia Gk. "Wood-dweller." Related to the far more common Sylvia.
Xylina, Xylona, Zylina

Yaffa Heb. "Lovely."
    Jaffa, Yaffah

Yalena Rus. Var. **Helen** (Gk. "Light").
    Yelena, Lenuschka, Lenushka, Lenya, Lenyushka

Yaminah Arab. "Suitable, proper."
Yamina, Yemina

Yancey Name of unclear origin: possibly a Native American word that, misunderstood by its hearers, resulted in the term "Yankee." Carries a whiff of the West about it courtesy of Edna Ferber's novel *Cimarron,* whose hero was named Yancey. Rare for boys or girls. Actress Yancey Butler.

Yancee, Yancie, Yancy

Yasmin Arab. "Jasmine." A variation of a flower name that was quite popular in the late eighties and early nineties. Princess Yasmin Aga Khan; model Yasmin Le Bon.

Yasamin, Yasiman, Yasmeen, Yasmeena, Yasmena, Yasmene, Yasmina, Yasminda, Yasmine

Yetta OE. Dim. **Henrietta** (OG. "Ruler of the house"). Used at the turn of the 20th century, but virtually unheard-of now.

Yette

Ynez Sp.Var. **Agnes** (Gk. "Pure").

Ines, Inez, Ynes, Ynesita

Yoko Jap. "Good, positive." Would probably be unknown outside Japanese families without the fame of Beatle wife Yoko Ono.

Yolanda Gk. "Violet flower." The Spanish version of **Violet**. Used in English-speaking countries in the 20th century, particularly during the 1960s.

Eolande, Eolantha, Iola, Iolanda, Iolande, Iolantha, Iolanthe, Jolan, Jolanna, Jolanne, Jolanta, Jolantha, Jolanthe, Yalinda, Yalonda, Yola, Yolaiza, Yoland, Yolande, Yollande, Yolantha, Yolanthe, Yolette, Yolie, Yulanda

Yonina Heb. "Dove."

Jona, Jonati, Jonina, Yona, Yonah, Yonina, Yoninah, Yonit, Yonita

Yosepha (fem. **Joseph**) Heb. "Jehovah increases." A possibility for parents who don't like **Josephine**.

Josefa, Josepha, Yosefa, Yuseffa

Ysabel Var. **Elizabeth** (Heb. "Pledged to God") via **Isabel**.

Yabell, Yabella, Yabelle, Ysabell, Ysabella, Ysabelle, Ysbel, Ysbella, Ysobel

Ysanne Modern name, combination of **Ysabel** and **Anne**. Found in Britain.

Ysande, Ysanna

Yudit Heb. "Praise."
   Yehudit, Yudelka, Yudif, Judit, Judith, Yudita, Yuta
Yuliya Rus. Var. **Julia** (Lat. "Youthful").
   Youliya, Yula, Yulenka, Yulinka, Yulka
Yvette Dim. **Yvonne**. Actress Yvette Mimieux.
   Ivett, Ivetta, Ivette, Yevette, Yvedt, Yvetta
Yvonne (Fem. **Ivo**) Fr. from OG. "Yew wood." Since yew
wood was used for bows, Ivo may have been an occupa-
tional name meaning "archer." The most common male
form is probably **Yves,** but Yvonne is more widespread in
English-speaking countries. It was particularly popular in
Britain in the 1970s. Tennis star Evonne Goolagong; ac-
tress Yvonne DeCarlo.
   Eevonne, Evonne, Ivonne, Yevette, Yvetta, Yvette

Zada Arab. "Fortunate, prosperous." Author
Zadie Smith.
   Zadie, Zaida, Zayeeda, Zayda
Zahavah Heb. "Gilded."
   Zachava, Zachavah, Zahava, Zechava, Zehavah,
   Zehavit
Zahira Arab. "Brilliant, shining."
   Zaheera, Zahirah
Zahra Arab. "White," or "Flower." Currently popular in
Arabic-speaking countries.
   Zahrah
Zandra Var. **Sandra,** dim. **Alexandra** (Gk. "Defender of
mankind"). Fashion designer Zandra Rhodes.
   Zahndra, Zandie, Zandy, Zanndra, Zohndra, Zondra
Zanna Dim. **Susanna** (Heb. "Lily").
   Zana, Zanne, Zannie
Zara Heb. "Eastern brightness, dawn." May also be a form

of **Sarah** (Heb. "Princess"). Literary name used often over the centuries for exotic characters. Taken up in the 1960s in Britain (Princess Anne's daughter is named Zara), but unusual in the U.S.

Zaira, Zarah, Zaria, Zarina, Zarinda, Zayeera

Zelda Dim. **Griselda** (OG. "Gray fighting maid"). The original name has long been eclipsed by this nickname, which was made famous by F. Scott Fitzgerald's glamorous but unstable wife.

Selda, Zelde, Zellda

Zelia Origin unclear; perhaps Gk. "Zeal" or Fr. "Solemn," from a saint's name. Rare.

Zalia, Zailie, Zaylia, Zele, Zelene, Zelie, Zelina, Zeline

Zelma Dim. **Anselma** (OG. "God-helmet"). A less common form than **Selma**.

Zellma

Zena Var. **Xenia** (Gk. "Welcoming"). This is the slightly more common form of the name. Tennis player Zina Garrison.

Zeena, Zeenia, Zeenya, Zenia, Zenya, Zina

Zénaïde Var. **Zenobia**.

Zenaida

Zenobia Gk. "Power of Zeus." A 3rd-century empress of Palmyra, whose name was revived in the 19th century but has a rather quaint sound today.

Cenobia, Cenobie, Zeba, Zeena, Zena, Zenaida, Zénaide, Zenayda, Zenda, Zenina, Zenobie, Zenna

Zephyr Gk. "West wind."

Cefirina, Sefira, Sefarina, Sephira, Tzefira, Tzephira, Tzephyra, Tzifira, Zefeera, Zefir, Zefiryn, Zephira, Zephirine, Zephyra, Zephyrine

Zerlinda Heb./Sp. "Beautiful dawn."

Zerlina

Zetta Heb. "Olive."

Zeta, Zetana

Zia Lat. "Grain."

Zea

Zigana Hung. "Gypsy."

Tsigana, Tsigane, Tzigana, Tzigane, Ziganna

Zilla Heb. "Shadow." Old Testament name revived by the Puritans and again in the 19th century, when it was more popular than one might suppose, given its current obscurity.
Zila, Zillah, Zylla

Zinnia Lat. Flower name. In this case the flower itself was named for its classifier, 18th-century German botanist Johann Zinn.
Zinia, Zinnya, Zinya

Zippora Heb. "Bird." Another Old Testament name; Zipporah was the wife of Moses. This biblical prominence has not translated into great popularity for the name, which sounds to some people like a way to do up a skirt.
Zipora, Ziporah, Zipporah

Zita Gk. "Seeker." Also dim. **Teresita, Rosita,** etc. The name of the last Hapsburg empress, who was given the name when it was at its most popular, at the turn of the century.
Zeeta, Zyta

Ziva Heb. "Brilliance, brightness."
Zeeva, Ziv

Zizi Hung. Dim. **Elizabeth** (Heb. "Pledged to God"). Analogous to the Hungarian diminutive for **Susan, Zsa Zsa.** French singer Zizi Jeanmaire.
ZsiZsi

Zoe Gk. "Life." Currently popular in Greece, and catching on strongly in English-speaking countries, especially in Britain. A variant, **Zooey,** comes from J.D. Salinger's novel entitled *Frannie and Zooey*—although the character Zooey is actually a young man named Zachery. Actresses Zoe Caldwell, Zooey Deschanel.
Zoee, Zoelie, Zoeline, Zoelle, Zoey, Zoie, Zoya

Zola It. "Lump of earth." Like **Zona,** probably used more for its sound than for its meaning. Runner Zola Budd.
Zoela

Zona Lat. "Belt, girdle." The name given to the constellation in Orion's belt. Generally U.S. use.
Zonia

Zora Slavic. "Dawn's light." Author Zora Neale Hurston.
Zorah, Zorana, Zorina, Zorine, Zorra, Zorrah, Zorya

Zoya Rus. Var. **Zoe.**
  Zoia, Zoyenka, Zoyya
ZsaZsa Hung. Dim. **Susan** (Heb. "Lily"). Made famous by
  actress and celebrity Zsa Zsa Gabor.
  Zsuzsa, Zsuzsanna
Zsofia Hung. Var. **Sofia** (Gk. "Wisdom").
Zuleika Arab. "Brilliant and lovely." Inseparable from Max
  Beerbohm's comic heroine in the eponymous novel
  Zuleika Dobson, for the sake of whose love all the under-
  graduates of Oxford University drown themselves. Not,
  perhaps, an inspiring example for parents.
  Zulaica, Zuleica

If it's a
BOY

A

Aaron Heb. "Exalted, on high." In the Old Testament, Aaron was the brother of Moses. The name was unusual until the 17th century, when so many Old Testament names first came into prominence. It has been widely used, especially in the U.S., since the 1970s, and is currently quite a favorite in Scotland. U.S. Vice President Aaron Burr; baseball star Hank Aaron; composer Aaron Copeland; actor Aaron Eckhart.

Aaran, Aaren, Aarron, Aaronas, Aeron, Aharon, Arand, Arend, Ari, Arin, Arnie, Arny, Aron, Aronne, Arran, Arron, Arun, Erin, Haroun, Ron, Ronnie, Ronny

Abbey Dim. **Abbot, Abelard, Abner**. Political activist Abbie Hoffman.

Abbie, Abby

Abbott Heb. "Father." An abbot is the head of a monastic community, so the original bearers of this name (as a surname) may have worked for an abbot. Its use as a first name occurred mostly in the 19th century. In the 1940s and early 1950s Bud Abbott served as straight man to short chubby comedian Lou Costello.

Ab, Abad, Abba, Abbe, Abe, Abbey, Abbie, Abbot, Abby, Abot, Abott

Abda Arab. "Servant."

Abdul Arab. "Servant of." Often used in combination with another name, as in "Abdullah," or "servant of Allah." Basketball star Kareem Abdul-Jabar.

Ab, Abdal, Abdall, Abdalla, Abdallah, Abdel, Abdell, Abdella, Abdellah, Abdoul, Abdoull, Abdoulla, Abdoullah, Abdull, Abdullah, Del

Abe Dim. **Abraham**. Heb. "Father of many."

Abey, Abie

Abel Heb. "Breath." Abel was the younger son of Adam and Eve, who was slain by his older brother, Cain. Abel has survived with steady use ever since the 6th century, and surprisingly enough, **Cain** also occurs from time to time. Abel is currently a top-ten name in Spain.

Abe, Abell, Abey, Abie, Able

Abelard OG. "Highborn and steadfast." Made famous by the 12th-century French philosopher Pierre Abelard, who fell in love with and seduced his student Heloise. Her uncle and guardian had him emasculated, even though he married Heloise. She became a nun, he became a monk.

Ab, Abbey, Abby, Abe, Abel

Abiah Heb. "My father is the Lord." Another Old Testament name, used for women as well as men in the Bible. Unusual in real life.

Abia, Abija, Abijah

Abida Heb. "God knows."

Abidan

Abiel Heb. "My father is God." Old Testament name that the Puritans used in the U.S., but rare since.

Abiell, Abyel, Abyell, Ahbiel

Abimelech Heb. "My father is king." Occurred occasionally in the 19th century.

Abir Heb. "Strong."

Abeer, Abeeri, Abiri

Abisha Heb. "Gift of God."

Abidja, Abidjah, Abijah, Abishai

Abner Heb. "My father is light." Old Testament name that came to some prominence in the late 16th century. Use fell off in this century, and the name is now mostly associated with Al Capp's comic strip *Li'l Abner.* Inventor of baseball Abner Doubleday.

Ab, Abbey, Abbie, Abby, Abna, Abnar, Abnor, Avner, Eb, Ebbie, Ebby, Ebner

Abraham Heb. "Father of many." First of the Hebrew patriarchs. In the Bible, Abraham has a son named Isaac when he is 100 and his wife Sarah is 90. The name was popular while Abraham Lincoln was president (even more so after his assassination), but has faded from use since 1900.

Abarran, Abe, Abey, Abie, Abrahamo, Abrahan, Abram, Abrami, Abramo, Abran, Avram, Avrom, Bram, Ibrahim

Abram Heb. "He who is high is father." Var. **Abraham**.

Abe, Abey, Abie, Abramo, Avram, Avrom, Bram

Absalom Heb. "Father is peace." The handsome son of King David who connived to steal his father's throne. He died in battle, and his father lamented, "Would God I had died for thee, O Absalom, my son, my son!" Also the title of a tragic novel by William Faulkner. Little used today.

Absalon, Abshalom, Absolom, Absolon, Avshalom, Avsholom

Ace Lat. "Unity." Connotations of superiority come from the fact that the ace is the playing card with highest face value.

Acer, Acey, Acie

Achilles Gk. Place name; also hero of the *Iliad,* as the greatest of the Greek heroes fighting the Trojans. He was all but invulnerable, having been dipped in the River Styx by his mother. She held him, however, by the heel, which was thus his one weak point: hence "Achilles' heel."

Achill, Achille, Achillea, Achilleus, Achillios, Achillius, Akil, Akilles, Akillios, Akillius, Aquil, Aquiles, Aquilles, Quilo

Achim Heb. "God will judge."

Acim, Ahim

Ackerley OE. Place name: "Oak meadow." Surname transferred to first name.

Accerly, Acklea, Ackleigh, Ackley, Acklie, Ackerlea, Ackerleigh, Ackerly

Acton OE. Place name: "Oak tree settlement." Another surname transferred to a first name: also the pseudonym used by Charlotte Brontë's sister Anne, who wrote as "Acton Bell." (The three sisters purposely chose masculine-sounding pseudonyms.)

Adair Scot. Gael. Place name: "Oak tree ford." Recently becoming more popular.

Adaire, Adare, Adayre

Adalard OG. "Noble and courageous."

Adelard, Adellard

Adalfieri It. from Ger. "Noble oath."

Adelfieri, Edelfieri

Adam Heb. "Son of the red earth." In the Bible, God created Adam—the first man—out of the "red earth" and breathed life into him. An appropriate name for the first boy in a family that has produced many girls. Currently very popular in Ireland. Congressman Adam Clayton Powell, Jr.; actor Adam Sandler.

Ad, Adamo, Adams, Adan, Adao, Addam, Addams, Addem, Addie, Addis, Addison, Addy, Ade, Adem, Adhamh, Adnet, Adnon, Adnot

Adamson OE. "Son of Adam."

Adamsson, Addamson

Adar Heb. "Noble."

Addison OE. "Son of Adam." Transferred surname. The English poet and essayist Joseph Addison was popular and influential through the 18th century.

Ad, Addeson, Addie, Addy, Adison, Adisson

Addy Teut. "Awe-inspiring; highborn." Also short for Adam, etc.

Addie, Ade, Adi, Ado

Adel OG. "Noble, highborn." More familiar as a particle of other names.

Adal, Edel

Adelar OG. "Noble eagle." Var. **Abelard.**

Adal, Adalar, Adalard, Adelard

Adelphe Fr. from Gk. "Brother."

Adelfo, Adelfus, Adelpho, Adelphus

Aden Possibly place name (for a region of South Yemen, formerly a British colony) or a variation on Aidan.

Aiden

Adham Arab. "Black."

Adlai Heb. "My ornament." Used in the Old Testament, and very rare, though brought to public notice by statesman Adlai Stevenson.

Ad, Addie, Addy, Adley

Adler OG. "Eagle." More common as a surname, especially in the U.S.

Ad, Addler, Adlar

Adnah Heb. "Ornamented."

Adin

Adney OE. Place name: "The noble's island."

Adolph OG. "Noble wolf." The Latinized form Adolphus arrived in Britain in mid-19th century, having been a German and Swedish royal name and also a saint's name. Almost unheard of since the rise of Adolf Hitler and World War II. Filmmaker Adolph Zukor; Actor Adolphe Menjou; fashion designer Adolfo; beer magnate Adolph Coors.

Ad, Addolf, Addolph, Adolf, Adolfo, Adolfus, Adollf, Adolphe, Adolpho, Adolphus, Dolf, Dolph, Dolphus

Adonis Gk. In Greek myth, Adonis was a young man so beautiful that Aphrodite, goddess of love, became enamored of him. The name has come to epitomize male beauty.

Addonis, Adohnes, Adones

Adrian Lat. "From Adria"—a north Italian city. First popular in the 1950s in Britain, and used also as a woman's name, though it seems to be holding steady as a choice for male children. Hollywood costume designer Adrian; 12th-century pope Adrian IV (the only English pope in history); actor Adrien Brody.

Ade, Adiran, Adrain, Adrean, Adreean, Adreyan, Adreeyan, Adriano, Adrien, Adrin, Adrino, Adryan, Aydrean, Aydreean, Aydrian, Aydrien, Hadrian, Hadriano, Hadrien, Haydrian, Haydrien

Aeneas Gk. "He who is praised." The Trojan hero of Virgil's *Aeneid*. Legend has it that he founded the Italian colony that was the origin of Rome. Football player Aeneas Williams.

Aenneas, Aineas, Aincias, Aineis, Ainneas, Eneas, Enné, Enneas, Enneis, Enneiss

Afif Arab. "Chaste."

Afton OE. Place name. A surname that has come into use as a first name.

Affton

Agnolo It. "Angel."

Ahab Heb. "Father's brother." Pleasant way to honor an uncle, though literary types may be reminded of the mad sea captain in Herman Melville's novel *Moby Dick.*

Ahearn Celt. "Horse-lord."
  Ahearne, Aherin, Ahern, Aherne, Hearn, Hearne, Herin, Hern

Ahmed Arab. "Greatly praised." Name often used for the prophet Muhammad, and favored by Muslims in the U.S. The name is in fact commonly used throughout the Islamic world. Football player Ahmad Plummer.
  Achmad, Achmed, Ahmaad, Ahmad, Ahmod, Amahd, Amed

Ahsan Arab. "Compassion."
  Ehsan, Ihsan

Aidan Gaelic. "Fire." Saint Aidan was a 7th-century Irish monk. The name is also used for women. Actor Aidan Quinn.
  Aidano, Aiden, Edan, Eden, Eidan, Eiden

Aiken OE. "Made of oak." English writer Conrad Aiken.
  Aicken, Aikin, Ayken, Aykin

Aimé Fr. "Much loved." More common as **Aimée,** a girl's name, or even as **Esmé,** a variant once well used in Scotland.

Aimery Teut. "Hardworking ruler."
  Almerey, Aimeric, Amerey, Aymeric, Aymery, Imre

Aimon Fr. from Teut. "House." Also possibly phonetic variant of the Irish **Eamon,** in turn a version of **Edmund.**
  Aimond, Aymon, Haimon, Heman

Ainsley Scot. Gael. Place name: "His very own meadow." A last name converted to a first name, used by both sexes.
  Ainsley, Ainsleigh, Ainslie, Ansley, Aynslee, Aynsley, Aynslie

Akbar Arab. "Great."

Akim Rus. Dim. **Joachim.** Heb. "God will judge."

Akmal Arab. "Perfect."
  Aqmal

Alaire Fr. from Lat. "Joyful." Var. Hilary. The root is the same as "hilarious," though the meaning has shifted a bit.
  Alair, Helier, Hilaire, Hilary, Larie, Lary

Alan Ir. Gael. Possible meanings are "rock" or "comely." Widely used in the Middle Ages, then again from the 19th century to the late 20th, with a boom around the 1950s influenced by the popularity of actor Alan Ladd. Now waning, like most fifties names. South African author Alan Paton; lyricist Alan Jay Lerner; playwright Alan Bennett; astronaut Alan Shepard; actors Alan Alda, Alan Cumming; poet Allen Ginsberg; basketball player Allen Iverson.

Ailean, Ailin, Al, Alain, Alair, Aland, Alann, Alano, Alanson, Alen, Alin, Allan, Allayne, Allen, Alley, Alleyn, Alleyne, Allie, Allin, Allon, Allyn, Alon, Alun

Alard OG. "Noble and steadfast."

Adlar, Adlard, Al, Allard

Alaric OG. "Ruler of all" or "Highborn ruler." Alaric I was the 5th-century king of the Visigoths who sacked Rome.

Al, Alarick, Alarico, Aleric, Alerick, Allaric, Allarick, Alleric, Allerick, Alric, Alrick, Ullrich, Ulrich, Ulrick

Alastair Gael. var. **Alexander** (Gk. "man's defender"). Generally a Scottish name, though it appears occasionally throughout the English-speaking world. Most of the variants are different phonetic spellings of the name. TV commentator Alistair Cooke; actor Alistair Sim.

Al, Alasdair, Alasteir, Alaster, Alastor, Alaisdair, Alaistair, Alaister, Aleister, Alester, Alistair, Alistar, Alister, Allaistar, Allaster, Allastir, Allistair, Allister, Allistir, Allysdair, Allysdare, Allystair, Allyster, Alysdair, Alysdare, Alystair, Alyster

Alban Lat. "From Alba," a city on a "white" hill, the oldest city in the ancient kingdom of Latium. The first Christian martyr on British soil was Saint Alban. Not to be confused with **Albin**, which has a different root.

Al, Albain, Alban, Albany, Albie, Albin, Albinet, Albion, Albis, Alby, Albys, Alvan, Alvin, Alvy, Auban, Auben, Aubin

Albern OG. "Noble courage."

Albert OE. "Highborn, brilliant." Most widely used during the lifetime of Queen Victoria's German prince consort, Albert. Her many children and grandchildren carried the name to most of the royal families in Europe, but her eldest son's first move as king was to drop it. Out of style since the 1920s. Scientist Albert Einstein; Prince Albert of Monaco; actor Albert Finney; philosopher Albert Camus; artist Albrecht Durer; baseball star Albert Belle; politician Al Gore.

Adalbert, Adalbrecht, Adelbert, Adelbrecht, Ailbert, Al, Alberto, Albie, Albrecht, Albrekt, Alvert, Alvertos, Aubert, Bert, Bertie, Berty, Dalbert, Delbert, Elbert, Elbrecht, Ulbricht

Albin Lat. "White, pale-skinned." From the root that gives us the word "albino." Common in Roman and medieval times, but not in the modern era.

Al, Alben, Albinson, Alpin, Aubin

Albion Celtic. "Mountain." Used in England until the 1930s; "Albion" is a poetic name for Britain.

Alcander Gk. "Strong."

Alcinder, Alcindor, Alkander, Alkender

Alcott OE. Place name: "The old cottage."

Alcot, Allcot, Allcott, Alkott

Alden OE. "Old friend." Surname transferred to first name, but unusual.

Al, Aldin, Aldwin, Aldwyn, Aldwynn, Elden, Eldin, Eldwin, Eldwyn, Eldwynn

Aldo OG. "Old." An Italian name that is occasionally used in the U.S.

Aldus, Alldo

Aldous OG. "Old." Medieval name that was brought back in the 19th century to slight popularity. Made famous by writer Aldous Huxley.

Al, Aldis, Aldivin, Aldo, Aldon, Aldus, Alldo, Eldin, Eldis, Eldon, Eldous

Aldred OE. "Old counsel."

Alldred, Eldred, Eldrid, Elldred

Aldrich OE. "Old leader."

Al, Aldric, Aldridge, Aldrige, Aldritch, Alldrich, Alldridge, Allric, Alrick, Audric, Eldrich, Eldridge, Eldritch, Elldrich, Rich, Richie, Richy, Ritch, Ritchey, Ritchie, Ritchy

Aldwin OE. "Old friend." See **Alden.**
 Aldwinn, Aldwinne, Aldwyn, Aldwynne, Alswynn,
 Elden, Eldin, Eldwin, Eldwyn, Eldwynn
Alejandro Sp. Var. **Alexander.**
 Alejo
Alem Arab. "Wise man."
 Alerio
Alex Dim. **Alexander.** Baseball players Alex Ochoa, Alex
 Rodriguez.
 Alec, Aleco, Aleck, Alecko, Aleko, Aleks, Alick, Alik, Elex
Alexander Gk. "Man's defender." Given great prominence
 by Alexander the Great, and steadily used worldwide, as
 the numerous variants show. It was a royal name in Scot-
 land, where it is still highly popular, and it is widely used
 in the U.S. without having attained trendy status. Variant
 Alek is very fashionable in Russia. English poet Alexan-
 der Pope; U.S. statesman Alexander Hamilton; actors Sir
 Alec Guinness, Alec Baldwin; U.S. Secretary of State
 Alexander Haig; Soviet writer and dissident Aleksandr
 Solzhenitsyn; writer Alexandre Dumas; hockey player
 Aleksei Kovalev.
 Al, Alasdair, Alastair, Alaster, Alcander, Alcinder,
 Alcindor, Alec, Aleco, Alejandro, Alejo, Alek,
 Aleksander, Aleksandr, Alessandre, Alessandri,
 Alessandro, Alex, Alexandre, Alexandro, Alexandros,
 Alexei, Alexi, Alexio, Alexis, Alic, Alicio, Alick, Alik,
 Alisander, Alissander, Alissandre, Alistair, Alister,
 Alistir, Alix, Allistair, Allister, Allistir, Alsandair,
 Alsandare, Iskander, Sacha, Sander, Sandero,
 Sandor, Sandro, Sandros, Sandie, Sandy, Sascha,
 Sasha, Saunder, Saunders, Sikander, Xander, Zander,
 Zandro, Zandros
Alexis Gk. "Helper." Usually thought of as a diminutive of
 Alexander, though it has a different etymological root.
 More commonly a girl's name.
 Alejo, Aleksei, Aleksi, Aleksio, Aleksios, Aleksius,
 Alexei, Alexey, Alexi, Alexios, Alexius, Alexy
Alford OE. Place name: "The old river-ford."
 Aldford, Allford

Alfred OE. "Counsel from the elves." After wide medieval use, the name fell out of sight until a 19th-century revival; Queen Victoria even named her second son Alfred. Out of fashion since the 1920s. English King Alfred the Great; poet Alfred Tennyson; film director Alfred Hitchcock.

Ahlfred, Ailfred, Ailfrid, Ailfryd, Al, Alf, Alfeo, Alfey, Alfie, Alfre, Alfredas, Alfrey, Alfredo, Alfredos, Alfy, Avery, Elfred, Fred, Freddie, Freddy, Fredo

Alger OE. "Spear from the elves." Possibly a diminutive of **Algernon**. Medieval name revived with the 19th-century hunger for a picturesque past, but never common. State Department Official Alger Hiss.

Al, Algar, Allgar, Allger, Elgar, Elger, Ellgar, Ellger

Algernon OF. "Wearing a mustache." A first name in several hugely powerful English aristocratic families, and given wider use in the latter half of the 19th century in Britain. Oscar Wilde used it for a brainless fop in *The Importance of Being Earnest.* All but unknown now. English poet Algernon Swinburne.

Al, Alger, Algernone, Algey, Algie, Algy, Aljernon, Allgernon

Algis OG. "Spear."

Ali Arab. "The high, exalted one."

Aly

Alison OE. "Son of the highborn." More common as a girl's name.

Alisson, Allcen, Allison, Allisoun, Allson, Allyson

Allard OE. "Highborn and courageous."

Adelard, Adelhard, Alhard, Alhart, Allart

Alonzo Var. **Alphonse** (OG. "Ready for battle").

Alanso, Alanzo, Allonso, Allonzo, Allohnso, Allohnzo, Alohnso, Alohnzo, Alonso, Lonnie, Lonny

Aloysius OG. "Famous fighter." Latinized version of **Luigi** or **Louis,** also related to **Clovis** and **Ludwig.** The 16th-century Italian Saint Aloysius is patron saint of students.

Ahlois, Aloess, Alois, Aloisius, Aloisio, Aloys, Lewis, Louis, Ludwick, Ludwig, Lutwick

Alpheus Heb. "He who follows after." Biblical, used in the 19th century, now very unusual.

Alfaeus, Alfeos, Alfeus, Alpheaus, Alphoeus

Alphonse OG. "Ready for battle." Alfonso is a royal name in Spain, thus very popular there. French writer Alphonse Daudet.

Affonso, Al, Alfie, Alfo, Alfons, Alfonso, Alfonsus, Alfonzo, Alfonzus, Alford, Alfy, Alonso, Alonzo, Alphonso, Alphonsus, Alphonzo, Alphonzus, Fons, Fonz, Fonzie, Phauns, Phons, Phonz

Alpin Gael. "Fair one."

Alpine, Macalpin, McAlpin, McAlpine

Alston OE. Place name: "Noble one's settlement."

Alsdon, Alsten, Alstin, Allston, Allstonn

Altman OG. "Old man." Last name occasionally used as a first name. Film director Robert Altman; department store magnate Bernard Altman.

Alterman, Altermann, Altmann, Eltman, Elterman, Eltermann

Alton OE. Place name: "Old town." Activist Alton Maddox.

Aldon, Allton, Alten

Alured Lat. Var. Alfred.

Ailured

Alva Heb. Possibly "Brilliance"; also related to Latin **Albin**. Old Testament name rarely used for men or women, in spite of Thomas Alva Edison's fame.

Alba, Alvah

Alvar OE. "Army of elves." Very rare. Architect Alvar Aalto.

Albaro, Alvaro, Alvarso, Alverio

Alvin OE. Several possible sources: the second element, "vin," means "Friend," but Al could indicate "Elf," "Noble," or "Old." Choreographer Alvin Ailey.

Ailwyn, Al, Aloin, Aluin, Aluino, Alva, Alvan, Alven, Alvie, Alvy, Alvyn, Alwin, Alwyn, Alwynn, Aylwin, Elvin, Elwin, Elwyn, Elwynn

Alvis Origin unclear. Possibly from an Old Norse legend involving the dwarf Alviss; possibly a modern blend reminiscent of **Elvis**. First appeared in the mid-20th century, but never widespread.

Alviss, Alwis, Alwyss

Amadeo Sp. from Lat. "Loved by God." The Latin version is Amadeus, given great prominence by the 1984 film about Mozart.

Amadee, Amadei, Amadeus, Amadi, Amadieu, Amadis, Amado, Amando, Amati, Amato, Amatus, Amedeo, Amyas, Amyot

Amadour Fr. from Lat. "Lovable." A Saint Amadour, purportedly founder of a French shrine (Rocamadour), has been venerated by the Catholic church, but recent research indicates he probably never lived.

Amador, Amadore

Amasa Heb. "Bearing a burden." Occasionally used in the 19th century, but little-known today.

Ambrose Gk. "Ever-living." Saint Ambrose was the 4th-century Bishop of Milan who baptized Saint Augustine. The name is more widely found on the Continent than in English-speaking countries. Writer Ambrose Bierce; Civil War General Ambrose E. Burnside.

Ambie, Ambroeus, Ambrogio, Ambroise, Ambros, Ambrosi, Ambrosio, Ambrosios, Ambrosius, Amby, Brose

Amerigo It. Var. **Emery** (OG. "Home ruler"). Italian explorer Amerigo Vespucci.

America, Americo, Americus, Amerika, Ameriko, Amerikus

Amiel Heb. "God of my people."

Amyel

Amory OG. "Home ruler." Var. **Emery**. Scott Fitzgerald used this name for Amory Blaine, the hero of his first best-selling novel, *This Side of Paradise*. Writer Cleveland Amory.

Aimory, Amery, Amorey

Amos Heb. "Borne, carried." A prophet of the Old Testament. The name has been little used in this century. Novelist Amos Oz.

Amoss

Amyas Lat. "Loved one." Possibly an anglicized version of

Amadeus, though sometimes considered a masculine variant of **Amy**. Unusual.

Amias, Amyes, Amyess

Anastasius Gk. "Resurrection." Much more common in the feminine version, **Anastasia**.

Anastas, Anastase, Anastagio, Anastasio, Anastatius, Anastice, Anastius, Anasto, Anastos, Anstas, Anstasios, Anstasius, Anstice, Stasio, Stasius

Anatole Gk. "From the east." Anatolia is a region of Turkey, which, of course, is east of Greece. French novelist Anatole France.

Anatol, Anatolio, Anatoly, Antal, Antol, Antole, Antolle, Antoly

Anders Scan. Var. **Andrew**.

Ander, Anderson, Andersson

André Fr. Var. **Andrew**. Traditionally parents have chosen English-style names for boys in the U.S., but this preference seems to be changing, and names with a foreign flair are inching into acceptability, if not into trendiness. In Russia, **Andrey** is currently very well used. Pianist André Watts; actor André Gregory; composer/conductor André Previn; tennis player Andre Agassi.

Andrae, Andras, Andrei, Andrej, Andrey, Andres, Andris, Ohndrae, Ohndre, Ondre, Ondrei, Ohnrey, Ondrey

Andrew Gk. "Masculine." In the Bible, Andrew was the first of the twelve apostles. Legend has it that after his crucifixion on an X-shaped cross, his bones were transported to Scotland, where he is patron saint. The "Saint Andrew's Cross," representing Scotland, appears on the flag of the United Kingdom. U.S. Presidents Andrew Jackson, Andrew Johnson; industrialist Andrew Carnegie; Prince Andrew, Duke of York; actors Andy Devine, Andy Griffith, Andy Garcia; artists Andrew Wyeth, Andy Warhol; baseball player Andruw Jones.

Aindrea, Aindreas, Anders, Andie, Andonis, Andor, André, Andrea, Andreas, Andrei, Andrej, Andres, Andresj, Andrewes, Andrews, Andrezj, Andrey,

Andrius, Andro, Andros, Andru, Andruw, Andy, Dandie, Dandy, Drew, Dru, Drud, Drugi, Ohndrae, Ohndre, Ondre, Ondrei, Ohnrey, Ondrey

Aneurin Welsh. "Honor." Mostly limited to Wales.
Aneirin, Nye

Angel Gk. "Messenger." **Angelo** is most often used now, even in English-speaking countries, as Angel is usually considered a girl's name (although in Thomas Hardy's 1891 novel *Tess of the D'Urbervilles,* a major character is named Angel Clare). Both forms are popular in Spanish-speaking countries. Jockey Angel Cordero.
Ange, Angell, Angie, Angelmo, Angelo, Angy, Anjel, Anjelo, Anyoli, Ohngel, Ohnjel, Onjel, Onjello, Onnjel, Onnjelo

Angus Scot. Gael. "Sole or only choice." In Celtic myth Angus Og is a god of such attractive traits as humor and wisdom.
Anngus, Ennis, Gus

Annan Celt. "From the brook."

Anscom OE. Place name: "Valley of the awesome one." "Combe" is an Old English term for a deep, narrow valley.
Anscomb, Anscombe, Anscoombe

Ansel OF. "Follower of a nobleman" or variant of **Anselm**. Photographer Ansel Adams. Ancell, Ansell

Anselm OG. "God-helmet." Saint Anselm was Archbishop of Canterbury in the 12th century, and one of the formative influences on medieval Christian thought. Painter Anselm Kiefer.
Anse, Ansel, Anselme, Anselmi, Anselmo, Anshelm, Anso, Elmo, Selmo

Ansley OE. Place name: "The awesome one's meadow."
Ainslea, Ainslee, Ainsleigh, Ainsley, Ainslie, Ainsly, Annslea, Annsleigh, Annsley, Anslea, Ansleigh, Anslie, Ansly

Anson Unclear origin and meaning, perhaps OG. Possibly "son of Ann," though "Son of the divine" seems more likely. Baseball great Cap Anson.
Annson, Ansson, Hanson

Anstice Var. Anastasius.
  Anstiss
Anthony Lat. Clan name of the Romans, possibly meaning "Beyond price, invaluable." The 3rd-century hermit Saint Anthony, who, according to legend, lived alone in the wilderness for over 80 of his hundred-some years, is patron saint of the poor. In England the name is usually spelled—and pronounced—without the *h*. German variant Anton is currently very popular in that country. Actors Anthony Quinn, Anthony Hopkins, Anthony Perkins, Tony Curtis, Antonio Banderas; photographer Antony Armstrong-Jones, Earl of Snowdon; composer Anton Bruckner; playwright Anton Chekhov; basketball player Anthony Mason; singer Marc Antony.
  Anntoin, Antin, Antoine, Anton, Antone, Antonello, Antoney, Antoni, Antonin, Antonino, Antonio, Antonius, Antons, Antony, Antuwan, Antwahn, Antwohn, Antwon, Antwuan, Toney, Toni, Tony
Antoine Fr. Var. Anthony. Popular in the U.S. in recent years. Football player Antone Davis.
  Antione, Antjuan, Antuan, Antuwain, Antuwaine, Antuwayne, Antuwon, Antwahn, Antwain, Antwaine, Antwan, Antwaun, Antwohn, Antwoin, Antwoine, Antwon, Antwone
Anwar Arab. "Shafts of light." Made famous by Egyptian President Anwar Sadat.
Anwell Welsh-Celt. "Loved one."
  Anwel, Anwil, Anwill, Anwyl, Anwyll
Apollo Gk. "Manly." In classical myth, Apollo is the god who drives the sun across the sky in a carriage, and also rules over healing and prophecy, speaking through the famous oracle at Delphi.
  Apollon, Apollos, Apolo
Aquila Lat. "Eagle." Despite the feminine "-a" ending, used in the 19th century as a revival of an ancient Roman name.
  Acquila, Acquilino, Acquilla, Akila, Akilino, Akilla, Aquilina, Aquilino, Aquilla
Archard Anglo-Ger. "Holy, powerful."
  Archerd

Archelaus Gk. "Ruler of the people." Not uncommon in the ancient world; Herod the Great had a son of that name who is mentioned in the Bible. Rare today.
Archelaios, Arkelaos, Arkelaus

Archer OF. "Bowman." Originally surname indicating occupation (like **Miller, Smith,** or **Baker**), mildly popular in the 19th century. Philanthropist Archer Huntington.

Archibald OG. "Noteworthy and valorous." Brought to Britain with the Norman Conquest, and popular largely in Scotland, where it was in the top 20 until the 1930s. Virtually invisible in the U.S. Poet Archibald MacLeish.
Arch, Archaimbaud, Archambault, Archer, Archibaldo, Archibold, Archie, Archimbald, Archimbaldo, Archy, Arquibaldo, Arquimbaldo

Arden Lat. "Burning with enthusiasm." The Forest of Arden in Shakespeare's *As You Like It* is a magically beautiful place.
Ard, Arda, Ardie, Ardin, Ardon, Ardy, Arrden

Ardley OE. Place name: "Home-lover's meadow."
Ardly, Ardsley, Ardsly

Ardmore Lat. "More zealous."
Ardmorr

Argus Gk. "Vigilant guardian." In Greek myth, a creature with 100 eyes, who was later changed into a peacock with eyes on his tail-feathers.
Argos

Argyle Scot. Place-name. Also given to the indigenous knitting pattern of interlocking diamonds.
Argyll

Aric OG. "Ruler." Also an element of many other names like **Alaric** and **Frederick**.
Arick, Arric, Arrick, Eric, Erick, Errick, Erik, Rick, Rickie, Ricky

Ariel Heb. "Lion of God." In Shakespeare's *The Tempest,* Ariel is a sprite who can disappear at will. The name has the connotation of something otherworldly, and though Shakespeare's Ariel is male, the name is used mostly for girls. Israeli statesman Ariel Sharon.

Aeriell, Airel, Airyel, Airyell, Arel, Arie, Ariell, Arik, Aryel, Aryell

Aries Lat. "A ram." The name of the astrological sign for those born from March 21 to April 19.

Ares, Arese, Ariese

Aristotle Gk. "Superior." Indelibly associated with the Greek philosopher Aristotle, though given prominence in recent years by the fame of Jacqueline Kennedy's second husband, shipping magnate Aristotle Onassis.

Ari, Arle, Aristotelis, Aristotellis, Arri, Ary

Arledge OE. Place name: "Lake with the hares." TV magnate Roone Arledge.

Arlidge, Arlledge, Arrledge

Arlen Ir. Gael. "Pledge, oath."

Arlan, Arlenn, Arles, Arlin, Arlyn, Arllen, Arrlen

Arley OE. Place name: "Hare-meadow."

Arlea, Arleigh, Arlie, Arly

Arlo Sp. "Barberry tree." Enjoyed a spurt of popularity in the early 1970s, possibly attendant on the fame of singer Arlo Guthrie.

Arlow, Arlowe, Arrlo

Armand Fr. Var. **Herman** (OG. "Army man"). Actor Armand Assante.

Almando, Arman, Armande, Armando, Armani, Armin, Armon, Armond, Armonde, Armondo, Ormond, Ormonde, Ormondo

Armstrong OE. "Strong arm."

Arnaud Fr. Var. Arnold.

Arnald, Arnaldo, Arnauld, Arnault

Arne OG. "Eagle." Var. Arnold.

Arney, Arni, Arnie

Arnett OF./Eng. "Little eagle." Broadcaster Peter Arnett.

Arnat, Arnet, Arnot, Arnott, Ornet, Ornette

Arno OG. "Eagle-wolf."

Arnoe, Arnou, Arnoux, Arnow, Arnowe

Arnold OG. "Strength of an eagle." Brought to Britain with the Norman invasion, faded out after the 13th century, and briefly revived in the late 19th century. Unusual today.

English novelist Arnold Bennett; golfer Arnold Palmer; actor and governor Arnold Schwarzenegger.

Arnaldo, Arnaud, Arnauld, Arnault, Arndt, Arne, Arney, Arni, Arnie, Arnoldo, Arnot, Arny

Arran Scot. Place name. The Isle of Arran is off the Atlantic coast. Also possibly a phonetic variant of **Aaron,** even though the sources are unrelated.

Arren, Arrin, Arron

Arrio Sp. "Belligerent."

Ario, Arryo, Aryo

Artemus Gk. Probably "follower of the goddess Artemis." New Testament name occasionally used in the 19th century. Author Artemas Ward.

Art, Artemas, Artemis, Artie, Artimas, Artimis, Artimus, Arty

Arthur Celt. Possibly "bear" or "rock." Linked with King Arthur, the legendary British hero of the Round Table, and often used in the Middle Ages, but unfashionable until the early 19th century, when Arthur Wellesley, the Duke of Wellington, vanquished Napoleon. The Victorian enthusiasm for the romance of the past probably promoted its use, and the name's popularity only began to wane in the 1920s. In Spain, **Arturo** is currently fashionable. Columnist Art Buchwald; actor Art Carney; tennis star Arthur Ashe; writer Arthur C. Clarke; playwright Arthur Miller.

Arrt, Art, Artair, Arte, Arther, Arthor, Arthuro, Artie, Artor, Artro, Artur, Arturo, Artus, Arty

Arundel OE. Place name: "Eagle valley."

Arondel, Arondell, Arundale, Arundell

Arvad Heb. "Exile, voyager."

Arpad, Arv, Arvid, Arvie

Arvin OGer. "People's friend."

Arv, Arvid, Arvie, Arvy, Arwin, Arwyn

Asa Heb. "Doctor." Another Old Testament name made popular by the Puritans in the 17th century. Now unusual.

Ase

Ascot OE. Place name: "Eastern cottage." More specifically the name of England's famous racetrack near Windsor Castle, and also a style of tying a cravat.

Ascott, Escot, Escott

Ashby OE. Place name: "Ash tree farm."

Ash, Ashbie, Ashbey, Ashburn, Ashton

Asher Heb. "Felicitous." Old Testament name brought into English use by the Puritans.

Ash, Asser

Ashford OE. Place name: "Ford near ash trees." Musician Nick Ashford.

Ash, Ashenford

Ashley OE. Place name: "Ash tree meadow." Originally a surname that migrated to first-name status, possibly helped along by Ashley Wilkes in Margaret Mitchell's *Gone With the Wind*. Though originally used for boys, it is now so hugely popular for girls that an infant named Ashley will be presumed to be feminine.

Ash, Ashely, Asheley, Ashelie, Ashlan, Ashleigh,
Ashlen, Ashli, Ashlie, Ashlin, Ashling, Ashlinn, Ashly,
Ashlyn, Ashlynn

Ashton OE. Place name: "Ash tree settlement." More popular in the 19th century than now, though this is the kind of name Anglophile parents of the 21st century may make more popular. Choreographer Sir Frederick Ashton; museum executive Ashton Hawkins; actor Ashton Kutcher.

Assheton, Ashtun

Ashur Semitic. "Warlike one." A name used by various Assyrian kings, who lived up to its meaning.

Asher

Aston OE. Place name: "Eastern town." Famous for an English sports car, the Aston Martin.

Aswin OE. "Spear-friend."

Aswinn, Aswyn, Aswynn

Atherton OE. Place name: "Town by the spring."

Athelstan OE. "Highborn rock." Used by Anglo-Saxon royalty and revived slightly by Sir Walter Scott's use of it in *Ivanhoe*. Now extremely rare.

Athol Scot. Place name, meaning unclear.

Atholl

Atley OE. Place name: "The meadow." Indicates an ances-

tor who, once upon a time, lived in a house near (or "at")
a meadow. English politician Clement Attlee.

Atlea, Atlee, Atleigh, Attlee, Attleigh, Attley

Atwater OE. Place name: "The water."

Attwater

Atwell OE. Place name: "The well."

Atwood OE. Place name: "The wood."

Atwoode

Atworth OE. Place name: "The farmstead."

Auberon OG. "Highborn and bearlike." Also possibly a
form of **Aubrey.** Better-known, though no more common
for it, as Oberon, King of the Fairies in Shakespeare's *A
Midsummer Night's Dream.* English writer Auberon
Waugh.

Auberron, Oberon, Oberron, Oeberon

Aubrey OF. "Elf ruler." Originally a man's name that arrived in England with the Norman Conquest. Now used by
girls as well, thus no doubt dooming its use as a boy's
name. The 19th-century artist Aubrey Beardsley; biographer John Aubrey.

**Alberic, Alberick, Alberik, Aube, Auberon, Aubry,
Averey, Averie, Avery, Oberon**

Audley OE. Place name of uncertain meaning.

Audric OG. "Noble ruler." Var. **Aldrich.**

August Lat. "Worthy of respect." The feminine version,
Augusta, and the longer Latin version, **Augustus,** are
more widely (though still infrequently) used in English-
speaking countries. Sculptor Auguste Rodin; painter Auguste Renoir.

**Agostino, Agosto, Aguistin, Agustin, Agustino, Augie,
Auguste, Augustin, Augustine, Augustino, Augusto,
Augustus, Augie, Augy, Austen, Austin, Gus, Guss**

Augustine Lat. Dim. **August.** The 5th-century bishop Saint
Augustine is famous for the frank *Confessions,* in which
he says, "Oh God, make me chaste—but not yet."

**Aguistin, Agustin, Augie, Augustin, Augy, Austen,
Austin, Austyn**

Augustus Lat. "Worthy of respect." Given historical
glamor by Roman emperors and German princely fami-

lies, who brought it to Britain in the 18th century, when it became very fashionable. Now little used. Sculptor Augustus Saint-Gaudens; painter Augustus John; beer magnate Augustus Busch.

Augie, Augustin, Augy, Austen, Austin, Austyn, Gus, Guss

Aurelius Lat. "Golden."

Aurelio, Aurelo, Oriel

Austin Oral form of **Augustine,** contracted by everyday speech. Now most often a family name transferred to a first name.

Austen, Austyn, Ostyn, Ostynn

Avenall OF. Place name: "Oat pasture."

Aveneil, Aveneill, Avenel, Avenell, Avenil, Avenill

Averill Most likely derivation is OE. "Boar-warrior," though may also be related to French *avril* or "April." Industrialist and statesman Averell Harriman.

Ave, Averel, Averell, Averil, Averyl, Averyll, Avrel, Avrell, Avrill, Avryll, Haverelll, Haverill

Avery OE. "Elf-ruler." Var. **Alfred, Aubrey.** Philanthropist Avery Fisher.

Averey

Avram Heb. Var. **Abraham.**

Aviram

Axel OGer. "Father of peace" and Scan. Var. **Absalom.** Rock star Axl Rose.

Aksel, Ax, Axe, Axell, Axil, Axill, Axl

Aylmer OE. "Highborn and renowned." The homonym **Elmer** is the more common form of this very old English name.

Aillmer, Ailmer, Allmer, Ayllmer, Elmer, Eylmer

Aylward OE. "Awesome guardian" or "Highborn guardian."

Azuriah Heb. "Aided by Jehovah." Although 28 different biblical characters are known by this name, it is all but obsolete today. Actor Hank Azaria.

Azaria, Azariah, Azria, Azriah, Azuria

Bailey OF. "Bailiff." Occupational name: in the Middle Ages a bailiff was a minor officer of the law.

Bail, Bailee, Bailie, Baillee, Baillie, Baily, Baley, Baylee, Bayley, Bayly

Bainbridge Ir. Gael. "Pale bridge."

Bain, Banebridge, Baynbridge, Bayne, Baynebridge

Baird Gael. "One who sings ballads."

Bar, Bard, Barde, Barr, Bayerd, Bayrd

Baker OE. Occupational name transferred to surname and, in the 19th century, to a first name. Politician James Baker.

Balbo Lat. "Mutterer."

Bailby, Balbi, Balbino, Ballbo

Baldemar OG. "Bold and renowned."

Baldomar, Baldomero, Baumar, Baumer

Balder OE. "Courageous army." In Norse myth the god Balder is called "the good," and reigns over summer, light, and innocence

Baldor, Baldur, Baudier

Baldric OG. "Brave ruler."

Balderic, Balderik, Baldrick, Baudric

Baldwin OG. "Brave friend." Unusual in English-speaking countries, though **Baudoin** is a royal name in Belgium. Author James Baldwin.

Bald, Baldewin, Baldovino, Balduin, Balduino, Baldwinn, Baldwyn, Baldwynn, Balldwin, Baudoin

Balfour Gael. "Grazing land." Also the name of a town in northern Scotland.

Balfer, Balfor, Balfore, Ballfour

Ballard OG. "Brave and strong."

Balthasar Gk. "God save the king." Along with Caspar and Melchior, one of the Three Kings who brought gifts to the baby Jesus, though they are not named in the Bible. Actor Balthazar Getty.

Baldassare, Baltasar, Baltazar, Balthasaar, Balthazaar, Balthazar, Balto, Belshazzar

Bancroft OE. Place name: "Field of beans." Many of the most common Anglo-Saxon place names that have become first names refer to simple, homely agricultural landmarks.

Ban, Bancrofft, Banfield, Bank, Binky

Banning Ir. Gael. "Small fair one" or "Son of the fair one."

Barclay OE. Place name: "Where birches grow." This is the form most favored in Scotland; **Berkeley** is more common elsewhere. Basketball player Charles Barkley.

Bar, Barcley, Barklay, Barkley, Barklie, Barrclay, Berk, Berkeley, Berkie, Berkley, Berklie, Berky

Bard Ir. Var. Baird.

Bar, Barde, Bardo, Barr

Bardolf OE. "Axe-wolf." A drunken fool named Bardolph figures in four of Shakespeare's plays.

Bardolph, Bardou, Bardoul, Bardulf, Bardulph

Bardrick Teut. "Axe-ruler." Just as many of the Anglo-Saxon names relate to farming, numerous Teutonic names relate to fighting.

Bardric, Bardrich

Barker OE. Possibly "shepherd." Used more often in the 19th century. In the U.S. a barker is also someone who delivers a glib sales talk to attract customers.

Birk

Barlow OE. Place name: "The bare hillside."

Barlowe, Barrlow

Barnabas Heb. "Son of comfort." In the New Testament, Barnabas is a companion of Paul's and uncle of the gospeler Mark. **Barnaby** is used more often now in Britain. One of Charles Dickens's lesser-known novels is entitled *Barnaby Rudge*.

Barna, Barnaba, Barnabé, Barnabee, Barnabey, Barnabie, Barnabus, Barnaby, Barnebas, Barnebus, Barney, Barni, Barnie, Barny, Bernabé, Burnaby

Barnes OE. Place name: "Near the barns."

Barnett OE. Place name: "From the land that was burned." Or possibly a contraction of the English aristocratic title "baronet." **Duke, Earl,** and **Baron,** other ranks of English nobility, are used as first names from time to time.

Barnet, Barney, Barnie, Baronet, Baronett, Barrie, Barron, Barry

Barney Var. Barnabas.

Barny

Barnum OE. Possibly a contraction of "baron's home." In the U.S. inseparable from Phineas T. Barnum, founder of Barnum & Bailey's circus and one of America's great showmen.

Barnham

Baron OE. The title of nobility used as a first name.

Baronicio, Barren, Barron

Barret OG. "Bear-strength." Used as a first name mostly in the 19th century, possibly because of the fame of English poet Elizabeth Barrett Browning.

Baret, Barrat, Barratt, Barrett, Barrey, Barrie, Barry

Barrington Eng. Place name now fairly common as a first name in Britain. Perhaps a bit of a mouthful for the more democratic U.S.

Barry Gael. "Sharp, pointed." Also a place name turned into a first name used by both sexes. Possibly influenced by the fame of Sir James Barrie, author of *Peter Pan,* since it cropped up as a first name during the height of his renown. Barry (with the "-y") was quite popular in the 1950s. Senator Barry M. Goldwater; singer Barry Manilow; baseball player Barry Bonds.

Barree, Barrey, Bari, Barrie, Baris

Bart Dim. Bartholomew. Football player Bart Starr.

Barrt

Bartholomew Heb. "Farmer's son." One of the twelve apostles. The name was common in the Middle Ages but was not revived in the 19th century, as so many medieval names were.

Bart, Bartel, Barth, Barthelemy, Bartho, Barthold, Bartholoma, Bartholomaus, Bartholomé, Barthlomeo, Barthol, Barthold, Bartholomeus, Bartlet, Bartlett,

Bartolome, Bartolomeo, Bartolommeo, Bartome, Bartow, Bartt, Bat, Bertel

Bartlet Dim. Bartholomew.
Bartlett, Bartlitt

Barton OE. Place name: "Barley settlement," or possibly "Bart's town."
Bart, Barten, Barrton

Bartram OE. "Bright raven." See **Bertram**.
Barthram

Baruch Heb. "Blessed." American philanthropist Bernard Baruch.
Baruchi, Boruch

Basil Gk. "Royal, kingly." Brought to England by the Crusaders, having been common in the eastern Mediterranean. Unusual in the U.S., but more often used in Britain. Also the name of a common herb. British actor Basil Rathbone; film director Baz Luhrmann.
Basile, Basilic, Basilides, Basileios, Basilie, Basilio, Basilius, Bazeel, Bazeelius, Bazil, Bazyli, Vasilios, Vasilis, Vasilius, Vasilus, Vassilij, Vassily, Wassily

Bassett OE. "Little person." Descriptive surname transferred to first name. Also the name of a very short-legged hunting dog, the basset hound, possibly called that because its torso is so low (*bas* in French) to the ground.
Basset

Baxter OE. Occupational name: "Baker."
Bax, Baxley

Bayard OE. "Russet-haired." A famous French knight of the 15th century, the Seigneur de Bayard, was known as "the irreproachable and fearless."
Baiardo, Bajardo, Bay

Beacher OE. Place name: "Near the beech trees." Generally a last name. The 19th-century preacher Henry Ward Beecher.
Beach, Beachy, Beech, Beecher, Beechy

Beagan Ir. Gael. "Small one."
Beagen, Beagin, Beegan, Beegin

Beal OF. "Handsome." Var. Beau.
Beale, Beall, Bealle, Beals

Beaman OE. Occupational name: "Beekeeper." Athlete Bob Beamon.

Beamann, Beamen, Beeman, Beamon, Beemon

Beamer OE. "Trumpet player."

Beemer

Beattie (masc. **Beatrice**) Ir. Gael. from Lat. "Bringer of gladness."

Beatie, Beatty, Beaty

Beau Fr. "Handsome." Dim. **Beauregard**. Used somewhat in the U.S. in the last 30 years. English dandy Beau Brummel; actor Beau Bridges; sports star Bo Jackson.

Beal, Beale, Bo, Boe

Beaufort OF. Place name: "The beautiful fort."

Beaumont OF. Place name: "The beautiful mountain." More common in the 19th century than it is today. English playwright Francis Beaumont.

Beauregard Fr. "Beautiful gaze." Could also be taken to mean, in modern parlance, "easy on the eye." A lot for a boy to live up to.

Beau

Beck OE. Place name: "Small stream." The term is still in use in rural Scotland. Singer Beck.

Becker

Bede OE. "Prayer." Saint Bede was an influential 7th-century English church historian.

Beda

Belden OE./OF. Place name: "Pretty valley."

Beldene, Beldon, Bellden, Belldene, Belldon

Bellamy OF. "Handsome friend." Actor Ralph Bellamy.

Belamy, Bell, Bellamey, Bellamie, Bellemy

Ben Heb. "Son." Also dim. **Benedict, Benjamin, Benson,** etc. Now given as an independent name, and especially popular in Ireland. Playwright Ben Jonson; actors Ben Gazzara, Ben Stiller, Ben Vereen, Ben Affleck.

Benn, Benny

Benedict Lat. "Blessed." Saint Benedict, founder of a monastic order, brought the name to prominence. **Bennett** is the more common form, especially in the U.S., where every schoolchild learns the tale of Revolutionary War traitor Benedict Arnold. Italian dictator Benito Mussolini; actor Benicio del Toro.

Ben, Bendick, Bendict, Benedetto, Benedick, Benedicto, Benedictos, Benedictus, Benedikt, Benedikte, Bengt, Benicio, Benito, Bennedict, Bennedikt, Bennet, Bennett, Bennie, Bennito, Bennt, Benoit, Bent, Venedictos

Benjamin Heb. "Son of the right hand." In the Old Testament, the younger son of Jacob and Rachel. Brought into use by the Puritan fondness for Old Testament names, and persistent until the end of the 19th century. After several decades of disuse, came back to great popularity by the 1970s, and is now quite standard. Currently popular in Spain. Diplomat and inventor Benjamin Franklin; U.S. President Benjamin Harrison; jazz musician Benny Goodman; pediatrician and oracle Benjamin Spock; British Prime Minister Benjamin Disraeli; actor Benjamin Bratt.

Ben, Benejamen, Beniamino, Benjaman, Benjamen, Benjamino, Benjamon, Benjee, Benjey, Benji, Benjie, Benjiman, Benjimen, Benjy, Benn, Bennie, Benno, Benny, Benyamin, Benyamino, Binyamin, Binyamino, Venyamin, Yamin, Yamino, Yemin

Bennett Fr. Var. **Benedict**. Choreographer Michael Bennett; humorist Bennett Cerf; author William Bennett; aviation pioneer Floyd Bennett.

Benet, Benett, Bennet, Benoit

Benoni Heb. "Son of my sorrow." In the Old Testament, Rachel, mother of Benjamin, knew she was dying after his birth and called him Benoni, but Jacob, his father, changed the name to Benjamin.

Benson "Son of Ben." Originally a surname, transferred to a first name in the 19th century.

Bensen, Benssen, Bensson

Bentley OE. "Meadow with coarse grass." Place name become surname become first name, more common for boys but used occasionally for girls. Irresistibly linked in most minds with the luxurious English cars.

Ben, Bentlea, Bentlee, Bentley, Bentlie, Bently, Lee

Benton OE. Place name. As in Bentley, refers to a kind of "bent" or coarse grass. Artist Thomas Hart Benton; film director Robert Benton.

Beresford OE. Place name: "Ford where barley grows." Used as a first name principally at the turn of the century. Film director Bruce Beresford.

Berg Ger. "Mountain." Often found as a suffix in German surnames.

Berger, Bergh, Burg, Burgh

Bergen Scan. "Lives on the hill." Bergen is a major port city in Norway.

Bergin, Birgin

Berger Fr. Occupational name: "Shepherd." Game show host Tom Bergeron.

Bergeron

Berkeley OE. Place name: "Where birches grow." In the U.S. probably most famous as the San Francisco suburb that is home to a branch of the University of California.

Bar, Barcley, Barklay, Barkley, Barklie, Barrclay, Berk, Berkeley, Berkie, Berklee, Berkley, Berky, Birkeley, Birkley

Bern OG. "Bear." Also possible nickname for **Bernard**.

Berne, Bernie, Berny, Bjorn

Bernal OG. "Strength of a bear." Occasionally used in English-speaking countries, but more common on the Continent.

Bernald, Bernhald, Bernhold, Bernold

Bernard OGer. "Bear/courageous." Brought to England with the Norman Conquest. Two famous medieval saints bore the name; one was a founder of a monastic order. The other, for whom the shaggy brown and white dogs are named, is patron saint of mountain climbers. A fairly common name until the 18th century and revived a bit around 1920, but now unusual. Playwright George Bernard Shaw; statesman Bernard M. Baruch; film director Bernardo Bertolucci; art critic Bernard Berenson; comedian Bernie Mack.

Barnard, Barnardo, Barney, Barnhard, Barnhardo, Barnie, Barny, Bear, Bearnard, Bern, Bernardo,

Bernarr, Bernd, Berndt, Bernhard, Bernhardo, Bernie, Bernis, Bernt, Burnard

Berry Botanical name used for both boys and girls, though the boy's name is more likely a derivative of Bernard or a transferred surname. Pop music impresario Berry Gordy.

Bert OE. "Shining brightly." Dim. **Albert, Egbert, Robert,** etc. Used more often as a nickname. Its popularity among show-business types of a certain age (Miss America emcee Bert Parks; actors Burt Lancaster and Burt Reynolds) suggests a jaunty, masculine connotation.

Bertie, Berty, Burt, Burty, Butch

Berthold OG. "Bright strength." Unusual in English-speaking countries, but not unheard-of. Playwright Bertolt Brecht.

Bert, Bertell, Bertil, Berthoud, Bertol, Bertoll, Bertold, Bertolde, Berton

Berton OE. Place name: "Bright settlement."

Bert, Bertie, Burt, Burton

Bertram OG. "Bright raven." Norman name revived in the Victorian era. Rare since the 1930s. Archictect Bertram Goodhue.

Bart, Bartram, Beltran, Beltrano, Berton, Bertran, Bertrand, Bertrando, Bertranno

Bertrand OG. "Bright shield." Also possibly a variation on **Bertram**. Philosopher Bertrand Russell.

Berwyn OE. "Bear friend" or "Bright friend."

Berwin, Berwynn, Berwynne

Bevan Welsh. "Son of Evan." Mostly 20th-century use. British politician Aneurin Bevan.

Beavan, Beaven, Bev, Beven, Bevin, Bevon, Bevvan, Bevvin, Bevvon, Bivian

Beverly OE. "Of the beaver-stream." Originally an English place name transferred to a surname, then a first name for both sexes. Probably still most famous as a place name, referring to Beverly Hills. The English spelling is usually **Beverley**. In the U.S., this is more likely to be considered a girl's name.

Beverlea, Beverleigh, Beverley, Beverlie

Bevis OF. Place name: Beauvais is a town in France famous

for the manufacture of tapestries. This anglicized version is very unusual, and the popularity of the cartoon "Beavis and Butthead" won't do much for its eligibility as a baby name.
Beauvais, Beavess, Beavis, Beviss

Bickford OE. Place name: "Axe-man's ford."

Bill Dim. **William**. Used occasionally as an independent name. Before mid-19th century, Will was the more common nickname. Actors Bill Cosby, Bill Bixby, Billy Crystal, Billy Crudup, Billy Bob Thornton; designer Bill Blass; singer Billy Joel.
Billie, Billy, Byll

Bing OG. Place name: "The hollow shaped like a pot." Another source claims that modern use of the name is inspired by singer Bing Crosby, who was given the nickname after a comic-strip character.

Birch OE. Place name: "Where birch trees grow." Not uncommon in the 19th century. Senator Birch Bayh.
Birk, Burch

Birkett ME. Place name: "Birch coastland."
Birket, Birkit, Birkitt, Burket, Burkett, Burkitt

Birkey ME. Place name: "Island of birch trees."
Birkee, Birkie, Birky

Birley OE. Place name: "Meadow with the cow byre." Not related to the homonym **Burleigh**.
Birlie, Birly

Birney OE. Place name: "Island with the brook."
Birnie, Birny, Burney, Burnie

Birtle OE. Place name: "Hill of birds."
Bertle

Bishop OE. "Bishop." Probably originally meant "One serving the bishop," or "Bishop's man."
Bishopp

Bjorn Scan. Var. **Bernard**. The fame of tennis player Bjorn Borg is probably responsible for the use of this name in English-speaking countries.
Bjarn, Bjarne, Bjorne

Black OE. "Dark-skinned."

Blackburn OE. Place name: "Black brook." Used as a first

name mostly in the 19th century. In Scotland, burn is still the term for a little brook.
Blackburne, Blagburn

Blagden OE. Place name: "Dark valley."

Blaine Ir. Gael. "Slender." Surname used since the 1930s as a first name, mostly for boys but occasionally for girls. Magician David Blaine.
Blane, Blayne

Blair Scot. Gael. Place name: "Plain" or "Flat area." Surname now used as first name, again more common for boys. Like many similarly transferred names, Blair was used for girls in greater numbers starting in the early 1980s. Actor Blair Underwood.
Blaire, Blayr, Blayre

Blaise Lat./Fr. "One who stutters." Used for both sexes, though more common for men. Extremely popular in France. The alternate spelling of **Blaze** probably refers to fire instead. French philosopher Blaise Pascal.
Biagio, Blaize, Blas, Blase, Blasio, Blasios, Blasius, Blayse, Blayze, Blaze

Blake OE. Paradoxically, could mean either "Pale-skinned" or "Dark." Surname used as a first name for either sex, most often in the U.S. Director Blake Edwards; "Dynasty" character Blake Carrington.

Blakely OE. Place name: "Dark meadow" or "Pale meadow." See **Blake**.
Blakelee, Blakeleigh, Blakeley, Blakelie

Blanco Sp. "Fair, white."
Bianco

Blanford OE. Place name: "Gray man's ford."
Blandford

Blaze Lat. "One who stutters." Anglicized form of **Blaise.**
Biaggio, Biagio, Blaise, Blaize, Blase, Blasien, Blasius, Blayse, Blayze

Bliss OE. "Intense happiness."

Blythe OE. "Happy, carefree." Made famous by the opening lines of Shelley's poem "To a Skylark" ("Hail to thee, blithe spirit!") and Noel Coward's play *Blithe Spirit.*
Bligh, Blithe

Bo Dim. **Robert, Beauregard**. Rare as a given name, more likely to be a nickname. Football coach Bo Schembechler; sports star Bo Jackson.
Boe

Boaz Heb. "Swiftness." Used for several Old Testament characters (including the second husband of Ruth), and revived with the Puritan passion for Old Testament names. Now very rare.
Boas, Boase

Bob Dim. **Robert**. OE. "Bright fame." Used independently from time to time. The usual habit for naming, however, is to give the full form of a name, even if the parents never intend to use anything but the nickname. Comedian Bob Hope; singer Bob Dylan; chess master Bobby Fischer; actor Billy Bob Thornton.
Bobbee, Bobbey, Bobbie, Bobby

Boden OF. "One who brings news."
Bodin, Bowden, Bowdoin

Bogart OF. "Bow strength." In current use probably always refers to actor Humphrey Bogart.
Bogey, Bogie, Bogy

Bonar OF. "Gentle, mannerly." From the French *debonnaire*. The famous line from the Sermon on the Mount, "Blessed are the meek," translates into French as "*Heureux sont les debonnaires.*" In English, "debonair" now means something closer to "nonchalant" or "urbane," as personified by Fred Astaire. British politician Bonar Law.
Bonnar, Bonner

Bond OE. Occupational name: "Man of the soil." Or as any moviegoer can tell you, "Bond. James Bond."

Boniface Lat. "Fortunate, of good fate." Also commonly, though erroneously, taken to mean "doing good." Name of a number of early popes.
Boni, Bonifacio, Bonifacius

Booker Uncertain origin; may allude to "the Book," i.e., the Bible. American reformer Booker T. Washington.

Boone OF. "Good." The French adjective is *bon* or *bonne*.

Backwoods connotations courtesy of 19th-century explorer Daniel Boone.

Booth OG. Place name: "Dwelling place." Surname whose 19th-century use as a first name was probably a tribute to Salvation Army founder William Booth. In the U.S. made famous also by Lincoln's assassin John Wilkes Booth. Author Booth Tarkington.
Boot, Boote, Boothe, Both

Borden OE. Place name: "Vale of the boar."
Bordin

Boris Slavic. "Warrior." Russian playwright Pushkin and composer Mussorgsky both based works on the career of the bloodthirsty 16th-century czar Boris Godunov. Horror-movie actor Boris Karloff; author Boris Pasternak; tennis player Boris Becker.
Boriss, Borris, Borys

Botolf OE. "Messenger wolf." An obscure 7th-century English saint who was very popular in the Middle Ages. He founded a monastery in England, which is thought to have been in the Lincolnshire town of Boston (Botolph's town).
Botoliff, Botolph, Botulf, Botulph

Bourne OE. Place name: "The stream." A little stream is still called a *burn* in Scotland. Or possibly OFr. "Boundary, milestone." Scottish poet Robert Burns.
Born, Borne, Bourn, Burn, Burne, Byrn

Bowen Welsh. "Son of the young one."
Bowin

Bowie Scot. Gael. "Blond." Col. James Bowie, scout and originator of the knife that bears his name. Former baseball commissioner Bowie Kuhn.
Bow, Bowen

Boyce OF. Place name: "Woods."
Boice, Boise

Boyd Scot. Gael. "Blond." Possibly also a place name, for the Scottish Isle of Bute. Actor Boyd Gaines.
Boid

Boyne Ir. Gael. "White cow."
Boine, Boyn

Brad OE. "Broad." Also diminutive for **Bradley** and other "Brad-" names. Quite scarce as a given name. Actors Brad Pitt, Brad Renfro.
Bradd

Bradburn OE. Place name: "Wide stream."

Braden OE. Place name: "Wide valley."
Bradan, Bradin, Bradon, Braiden, Braidin, Brayden, Braydon

Bradford OE. Place name: "Wide river-crossing." Name of the first governor of the Plymouth colony, William Bradford.
Braddford, Bradfurd

Bradley OE. Place name: "Wide meadow." Used since the mid-19th century, more in the U.S. than in other English-speaking countries. Actor Bradley Whitford; Senator Bill Bradley.
Brad, Bradd, Bradlea, Bradleigh, Bradlie, Bradly, Bradney, Lee

Bradshaw OE. Place name: "Broad forest."

Brady OE. Place name: "Wide island." Football player Tom Brady.
Bradey, Bradie, Braedy, Braidie, Braidy, Braydie

Brainard OE. "Courageous raven."
Brainerd, Braynard

Bram Ir. Gael. "Raven." It is curious that so many names refer to the raven, a bird that historically has stood for death and destruction. Bram, of course, can also be a shortened version of **Abraham**. *Dracula* author Bram Stoker.
Bramm, Bran, Brann

Bramwell OE. Place name: "Well where the broom grows" or "Raven well." Author Branwell Brontë.
Brammell, Bramwel, Bramwyll, Branwell, Branwill, Branwyll

Brand OE. "Firebrand." Also, diminutive of **Brandon**.
Brander, Brandt, Brant, Brantley, Brantlie

Brandon OE. Place name: "Broom-covered hill." Also a variant of **Brendan,** which does not quite share its popularity: Brandon was on and off lists of the top ten baby names through the nineties. TV executive Brandon Tartikoff.

Brand, Branden, Brandin, Brandyn, Brannon, Branton

Brant OE. "Proud." Media executive Peter Brant.

Brandt, Brannt, Brantt

Brawley OE. Place name: "Meadow at the slope of the hill."

**Brauleigh, Braulie, Brauly, Brawlea, Brawleigh,
Brawlie, Brawly**

Brendan Ir. Gacl. "Smelly hair." Very few names actually mean anything as negative as this. The Irish Saint Brendan, known as "the Voyager," is supposed to have sailed as far as the Canary Islands in the sixth century. Playwright Brendan Behan; actor Brendan Fraser.

**Brendano, Brendin, Brendon, Brendyn, Brennan,
Brennen, Brennon**

Brent OE. Place name: "Mount, hilltop." Use as a first name dates back only 60 years or so, and has been particularly strong in Canada. Sportscaster Brent Musburger.

**Brennt, Brentan, Brenten, Brentin, Brenton, Brentt,
Brentyn**

Brett Celt. "Man from Britain." Publicized by American writer Bret Harte. Quite popular in Australia and steadily used in the U.S. Baseball players Brett Butler, Brett Saberhagen; football player Brett Favre.

Bret, Brette, Bretton, Brit, Briton, Britt, Britte

Brewster OE. Occupational name: "Brewer." Transferred to a surname, thence to a first name.

Brewer, Bruce

Brian Ir. Gael. Ancient name of obscure meaning, though many sources translate it as "strength." Ireland's most famous King, Brian Boru, liberated the country from the Danes in 1014, and the name has been much favored in Ireland. A spell of popularity lasted from the 1920s to the 1970s, and though Brian is no longer trendy, it is still well used. Actors Brian Dennehy, Bryan Brown; film director Brian De Palma.

**Briano, Briant, Brien, Brion, Bryan, Bryant, Bryen,
Bryent, Bryon**

Brice Var. **Bryce**. The *i* spelling was more common in the 19th century.
Bricio, Brizio

Bridgely OE. Place name: "Bridge meadow."
Bridgeley

Bridger OE. "Lives near the bridge."
Bridge

Brigham OE. Place name: "Little village near the bridge." Most uses of the name probably honor Mormon leader Brigham Young.
Brigg, Briggham, Briggs

Brinley OE. Place name: "Burnt meadow." Used mostly in England and Wales.
Brindley, Brindly, Brinlee, Brinleigh, Brinly, Brynly

Brock OE. "Badger." Unusual transferred surname with mostly American use.
Broc, Brocke, Brok

Brockley OE. Place name: "Meadow of the badger."
Brocklea, Brocklee, Brocklie, Brockly

Broderick ONorse. "Brother." Traveled from Ireland to Scotland as a surname. Actor Broderick Crawford.
Brod, Broddy, Broder, Broderic, Brodric, Brodrick, Ric, Rick, Rickey, Rickie, Ricky

Brody Ir. Gael. "Ditch."
Brodee, Brodey, Brodie, Broedy

Bromley OE. Place name: "Meadow where broom grows." Broom is a shrub related to heather.
Bromlea, Bromlee, Bromleigh, Broomlie

Bronson OE. "Brown one's son." Actors Charles Bronson, Bronson Pinchot.
Bron, Bronnson, Bronsen, Bronsin, Bronsonn, Bronsson

Brook OE. Place name: "Near the stream or brook." Wide fame of actress Brooke Shields will probably go far to terminate use of this name for boys. Critic Brooks Atkinson.
Brooke, Brookes, Brookie, Brooks

Broughton OE. Place name: "Settlement near the fortress."

Brown ME. "Russet-complected."

Bruce OF. "From the brushwood thicket." Norman place

name brought to fame by the Scottish king Robert Bruce, who won Scotland's independence from England in 1327. Naturally popular as a first name in Scotland, and among Americans who cherish Scottish ancestry. Singer Bruce Springsteen; actors Bruce Willis, Bruce Lee.
Brucey, Brucie

Bruno OG. "Brown-skinned." Saint Bruno was the 11th-century founder of the Carthusian order of monks. Orchestral conductor Bruno Walter; actor Bruno Kirby.
Bruin, Bruino

Bryan Var. **Brian**. Actor Bryan Brown; singer Bryan Ferry.
Bryen

Bryant Var. **Brian**. TV commentator Bryant Gumbel.

Bryce Unclear origin; may refer to followers of a 5th-century French bishop, Saint Brice. Bryce Canyon, in Utah, is one of the great natural splendors of the West.
Brice

Buck OE. "Buck deer." "Buck" was also a 19th-century term for a dandy, or a young man who cut a fine figure. It may have been used first as a nickname. Probably not related to the slang word for "dollar." Actor Buck Henry.
Buckey, Buckie, Bucky

Buckley OE. Place name: "Meadow of the deer." Author William F. Buckley.

Bud Modern slang, short for "buddy." Some sources think this is a child's pronunciation of "brother." Rarely given as a first name, but fairly common as a nickname in the middle years of the 20th century. Actor Buddy Ebsen; comedians Bud Abbott, Buddy Hackett.
Budd, Buddey, Buddie, Buddy

Burchard OE. "Castle strong."
Bucardo, Burckhardt, Burgard, Burgaud, Burkhart

Burford OE. Place name: "Ford near the castle."
Bufford, Buford

Burgess OE. "Citizen." Related to the French word *bourgeois,* which has come to mean something like "middle class." Generally a transferred last name. Actor Burgess Meredith; poet Gelett Burgess.
Burges, Burgiss, Burr

Burke OF. "From the fortified settlement."
Berk, Berke, Birk, Bourke, Burk

Burleigh OE. Place name: "Meadow with knotty-trunk trees."
Burley, Burlie, Byrleigh, Byrley

Burnaby ONorse. "Fighter's estate."

Burne OE. Place name: "The brook." Related to **Bourne**.
Beirne, Bourn, Bourne, Burn, Burnis, Byrn, Byrne, Byrnes.

Burnell OF. "Small brown one."
Burnel, Brunel, Brunell

Burnet OE. Transferred surname of unclear origin, mostly used in the 19th century.
Bernet, Bernett, Burnett

Burney OE. Place name: "Island of the brook."
Beirney, Beirnie, Burnie

Burton OE. Place name: "Fortified enclosure." Like many of the older place names, used as a first name in the 19th century. The exploits of African explorer and writer Sir Richard Burton may have influenced its use. Actors Burt Lancaster, Burt Reynolds.
Bert, Burt, Burtt

Busby Scot./ONorse. Place name: "Village in the thicket." A busby is also a tall military hat made of fur, such as those worn by the British soldiers who guard Buckingham Palace. Choreographer Busby Berkeley.
Busbee, Busbey, Busbie, Bussby

Buster Nickname of unknown origin, made famous by silent film star Buster Keaton. A hugely popular comic strip character of the 1930s was called Buster Brown. His pageboy haircut, sailor hat, and round collar were all dubbed "Buster Brown" after him. The name continued into the early 1960s as a brand of shoe with an advertising jingle that ended, ". . . with the boy and the dog and the foot inside." Swimmer/actor Buster Crabbe.

Butcher OE. Occupational name: "Butcher." Nickname Butch is sometimes used to address a stranger in a slightly derogatory way: "Listen, Butch . . ."
Butch

Byford OE. Place name: "By the ford."

Byram OE. Place name. Var. **Byron**.

Byrd OE. "Birdlike."
  Bird, Byrdie

Byron OE. Place name: "Barn for cows." The term "byre" is still used. Use as a first name probably in tribute to the poet Lord Byron, since it dates from the 1850s.
  Beyren, Beyron, Biren, Biron, Buiron, Byram, Byran, Byren, Byrom

Cadby OE. "Fighting man's settlement."
  Cadbee, Cadbey, Cadbie

Caddock Welsh. "Eagerness for war."
  Cadog

Cadell Welsh. "Battle." Political consultant Patrick Cadell.
  Caddell, Cadel

Cadman Anglo-Welsh. "Battle man."

Cadmus Gk. "From the east." In Greek myth, Cadmus is the founder of the city of Thebes, who ultimately turned into a serpent. He is also credited with the invention of writing in letters.
  Cadmar, Cadmo, Cadmos, Cadmuss, Kadmos, Kadmus

Caesar Lat. Clan name of obscure meaning, possibly "hairy, hirsute." The term "caesarean" for a surgical delivery of a baby came about because the famous Roman emperor Julius Caesar was born that way. It has become a generic term for emperor, translated into German (*kaiser*) and Russian (*czar*). Actor César Romero.
  Caezar, Casar, C;aaesar, Cesare, Cesaro, Kaiser, Seasar, Sezar

Cain Heb. "Spear." Adam and Eve's elder son, who slew his brother Abel. Surprisingly enough, used with some frequency, at least in the 19th century. Homonym **Kane** has a different source. Actor Michael Caine.

Caine, Kain, Kaine

Caius Lat. "Rejoice." Var. **Gaius**.

Cai, Caio, Kay, Kaye, Keye, Keyes, Keys

Cal Dim. Calhoun, Calvin, etc. Baseball star Cal Ripken, Jr.

Calder OE. "Stream." Little rivulets are such important features in the English landscape that regional terms for them abound, and several (Brook, Burn) have traced the typical path from geographical feature to place name to surname to given name. Sculptor Alexander Calder.

Caldwell OE. Place name: "Cold well."

Caleb Heb. Either "Dog" or "Courageous." An Old Testament name brought to America with the Puritans, where it was fairly common until around 1920. Author Caleb Carr.

Cal, Cale, Cayleb, Kaleb, Kayleb, Kaylob

Caley Ir. Gael. "Lean, slight."

Cailey, Caily, Kayley

Calhoun Ir. Gael. Place name: "The narrow woods."

Callhoun, Colhoun, Colquhoun

Calum Scot. Var. **Columba** (Lat. "Dove"). Saint Columba was a 6th-century Irish missionary who founded a monastery on the Scottish island of Iona. Calum and its variant **Callum** are both extremely popular in Scotland, where they may be considered variants of **Malcolm**.

Callum, Colm, Colum

Calvert OE. Occupational name: "Calf-herder." English surname. In the U.S. borne by George Calvert, founder of Maryland.

Calbert

Calvin Lat. "Hairless." Roman clan name turned surname. Transferred to first name as a tribute to 16th-century Swiss religious reformer John Calvin, whose thinking deeply influenced the Presbyterian, Methodist, and Huguenot branches of Protestantism. U.S. use may have been influenced by President Calvin Coolidge. Composer Calvin Hampton; Italian author Italo Calvino.

Cal, Calvino, Kalvin, Vinnie

Camden Scot. Gael. Place name: "The twisting valley."
Camdin, Camdon

Cameron Scot. Gael. "Crooked nose." Clan name derived
from the facial feature. In Scotland, the Camerons were a
powerful clan. Little used as a first name until the middle
of this century but currently extremely popular in Scotland.
**Cam, Camaeron, Camedon, Camron, Camry,
Kameron, Kamrey**

Campbell Scot. Gael. "Crooked mouth." Name of a very
famous Scottish clan, again referring to a distinguishing
feature. Use as a first name dates back only to the 1930s.
Actor Campbell Scott.
Campbel

Canning Fr. Occupational name: "Official of the church."
Var. **Cannon**.
Cannan

Canute Scan. "Knot." Brought to Britain by the 11th-
century King Canute of Denmark, who became King of
England in 1016. Very rare, except in those of Scandinavian descent. Football coach Knute Rockne.
Cnut, Knut, Knute

Carey Welsh. Place name: "Near the castle." Distinct from
Cary, which has another source. By the 1950s, this form
was usually a girl's name, often a nickname for **Caroline**.
Actor Jim Carrey.
Carrey

Carl Var. **Charles** (OG. "Man"). Use in America was fairly
steady 1850–1950 (probably as a result of intensive German and Scandinavian immigration), but dropped off in
the 1960s. Poet Carl Sandburg; journalist Carl Bernstein;
astronomer/author Carl Sagan; psychologist Carl Jung.
Carel, Karel, Karl

Carleton OE. Place name: "Farmer's settlement." Only
used as a first name since around 1880. In the U.S., usually spelled without the *e*.
Carl, Carlton, Charlton

Carlin Ir. Gael. "Little champion." Comedian George Carlin.
Carling, Carly

Carlisle OE. Place name: "The fortified tower." Also the name of a very old city in northwest England. Historian Thomas Carlyle.
Carley, Carlile, Carly, Carlyle

Carlos Sp. Var. **Charles** (OG. "Man"). Film directors Carlos Saura, Carlo Ponti.
Carlo, Carrlos

Carmichael Scot. Gael. "Follower of Michael." Possibly referring to partisans of Saint Michael.

Carmine Lat. "Song." Though carmine also means "purplish red" (from an Aramaic word meaning "crimson"), the Latin source is more likely, since the name is almost exclusively used by families of Italian descent.
Carman, Carmen, Carmin, Carmino, Karman, Karmen

Carney Ir. Gael. "The winner."
Carny, Kearney

Carollan Ir. Gael. "Little champion." In the U.S., likely to be confused with a variant of **Caroline.**
Carlin, Carling, Carolan

Carr Scan. "From the swampy place."
Karr, Ker, Kerr

Carroll OG. "Man." An anglicized version of **Charles,** occurring from time to time as a family name, though it is too much like **Carol** (which was very popular in the '60s) to be an appealing boy's name for most parents. Author Lewis Carroll; Signer of the Declaration of Independence Charles Carroll.
Carolus, Carrol, Caroll, Cary, Caryl, Caryll

Carson OE. "Son of the marsh-dwellers." TV hosts Johnny Carson, Carson Daley.

Carswell OE. Place name: "Well where the watercress grows."
Caswell

Carter OE. Occupational name: "One who drives carts." Former President Jimmy Carter; football player Cris Carter.
Cartier

Carvell OF. "Swampy dwelling." Political strategist James Carville.
Carvel, Carvil, Carville

Carver OE. Occupational name: "One who carves wood."

Cary OE. Place name: "Pretty brook." Distinct from **Carey**. Use in the 19th century as a first name was quite rare, but when actor Archibald Leach renamed himself Cary Grant, numerous families suddenly found the name Cary appealing.

Casey Ir. Gael. "Vigilant." Possibly also a short form of **Casimir**. Made famous by the song about the engineer of the Cannonball Express train, Casey Jones. Baseball personality Casey Stengel; radio disc jockey Casey Kasem; actor Casey Affleck.

Cacey, Cayce, Caycey, Kasey

Cash Dim. **Cassius** (Lat. "Vain"). Also a slang word for money, of course. Singer Johnny Cash.

Casshe

Casimir Slavic. "Bringing peace." Associated with Poland for her famous 11th-century king, who brought peace to the nation.

Casimeer, Casimire, Casimiro, Casmir, Kasimiro, Kazimierz, Kazimir

Casper Origin unclear, though many sources suggest Per. "He who guards the treasure." Originally **Jasper,** Germanicized to Caspar. French is **Gaspard**. Traditionally one of the Three Kings (perhaps the one carrying the gold) was named Caspar. A 1960s TV series featured Casper the Friendly Ghost. Defense secretary Caspar Weinberger.

Caspar, Cass, Gaspar, Gaspard, Gasparo, Gasper, Jasper, Kaspar

Cassidy Ir. Gael. "Ingenious, clever."

Cassady, Cassedy, Cassidey

Cassius Lat. "Vain." Historically, Cassius was a Roman politician who was behind the plot to murder Julius Caesar. In Shakespeare's play, Caesar says, "Yon Cassius has a lean and hungry look; He thinks too much: Such men are dangerous." Boxer Cassius Clay (now Muhammad Ali).

Cash, Cass, Cassio

Castor Gk. "Beaver." In classical myth, along with Pollux, one of the heavenly twins immortalized in the constellation Gemini. They were considered the patron gods of seafarers, appearing to them in St. Elmo's fire.

Caster, Castorio, Kastor

Cato Lat. "All-knowing." Cato was a particularly high-minded Roman statesman of the time of Julius Caesar.

Cayto, Kaeto, Kato

Cavan Ir. Gael. "Handsome."

Kavan

Cecil Lat. "Blind one," from a Roman clan name. Used in Roman times, then resurfaced in the Victorian era, possibly given a boost by the fame of industrialist (and founder of Rhodesia) Cecil Rhodes. Little used in this century. Film director Cecil B. De Mille; photographer Cecil Beaton.

Cecil, Cecilio, Cecilius, Celio

Cedric OE. "War leader." Used in two 19th-century literary landmarks (*Ivanhoe* and *Little Lord Fauntleroy*), which probably increased its popularity in Britain. Actors Sir Cedric Hardwicke, Cedric the Comedian.

Caddaric, Ced, Cedrick, Cedro, Rick, Sedric, Sedrick, Sedrik

Cephas Heb. "Rock." New Testament name; what Jesus called his apostle Simon. **Peter** is the Latin translation by which he is more commonly known. Cephas was in steady (if infrequent) use until the 20th century.

Chad Origin cloudy; possibly OE. "Fierce." Saint Chad was a 7th-century English bishop. The name enjoyed a burst of popularity beginning in the late 1960s. Actors Chad Everett, Chad Lowe; football players Chad Morton, Chad Pennington.

Chadd, Chaddie

Chadwick OE. Place name: "The fighter's settlement." Has been used commercially as a generic WASP name.

Chadwyck

Chaim Heb. "Life." Male version of **Eve. Hyman** is more common in English-speaking countries. Author Chaim Potok.

Chayim, Chayyim, Haim, Hayvim, Hayyim, Hy, Hyman, Hymen, Hymie, Manny

Chance ME. "Good fortune." Also var. **Chauncey**.
Chanse, Chantz, Chanze

Chancellor ME. Occupational name: "Chief secretary, record keeper." Broadcaster John Chancellor.
Chance, Chancelor, Chansellor, Chaunce

Chandler OF. Occupational name: "Candle merchant."

Chaney Fr. "Oak tree." Actor Lon Chaney.
Chainey, Chany, Cheney

Channing OF. Occupational name: "Official of the church." Related to **Cannon**.
Canning, Cannon, Canon

Chapman OE. "Peddler."
Chap, Chappy, Manny

Charles OG. "Man." The English term "churl," meaning "serf," comes from the same root. Has been a staple ever since the era of the Emperor Charlemagne, and a royal name in many European countries, including England, where the next king will probably be Charles III. In America, it was one of the top 5 names for the first three-quarters of this century, but has since been displaced by other classics like **Nicholas, Christopher,** and **Andrew**. Naturalist Charles Darwin; French president Charles de Gaulle; author Charles Dickens; actor Charlie Chaplin; basketball player Charles Barkely.
Carel, Carl, Carlo, Carlos, Carrol, Carroll, Cary, Caryl, Chad, Charley, Charlie, Charlot, Charls, Charlton, Charly, Chas, Chay, Chaz, Chazz, Chick, Chip, Chuck, Karel, Karl, Karol, Karolek, Karolik, Karoly

Charlton OE. Place name: "Charles's dwelling." Also possibly a variation on **Carlton**. Used as a given name for the last hundred years. Actor Charlton Heston.
Carleton, Carlton, Charleston, Charleton

Chase OF. "Hunter." Quite steadily used. Painter William Merritt Chase.
Chace, Chayce, Chayse

Chauncey ME. Contraction of **Chancellor**.
Chance, Chancey, Chaunsey, Chaunsy, Chawncey

Chester Lat. "Soldier's camp." Place name from Roman

Britain, gradually evolved into a first name most common in the U.S. Virtually unused now, however. President Chester Arthur; newscaster Chet Huntley.
Cheston, Chet

Chetwin OE. Place name: "Little house on the twisted path."
Chetwen, Chetwyn, Chetwynd, Chetwynn

Chevalier Fr. "Knight." Comedian Chevy Chase.
Chevy

Chick Dim. **Charles** (OG. "Man"). Musician Chick Corea.
Chic, Chik

Chico Sp. Dim. **Francis** (Lat. "Frenchman") via **Francisco**.

Chilton OE. Place name: "Farm near the well."
Chelton, Chill

Chris Dim. **Christian, Christopher**. Actors Chris Cooper, Chris O'Donnell, Chris Sarandon; comedians Chris Rock, Chris Tucker; basketball player Chris Webber.
Chriss, Kris

Christian Gk. "Anointed, Christian." A girl's name that (contrary to the usual movement) became a male name, possibly after the huge success of John Bunyan's *Pilgrim's Progress* (1684), whose hero is called Christian. In Britain and Australia, especially popular in the 1970s. French fashion designers Christian Dior, Christian Lacroix; Dr. Christiaan Barnard; actor Christian Slater.
Chrestien, Chretien, Chris, Christer, Christiano, Christie, Christo, Christy, Cristian, Cristiano, Cristino, Cristy, Kit, Kris, Krister, Kristian, Kristo, Krystian, Krystiano

Christmas Name of the holiday, used occasionally through the 19th century for Dec. 25 babies, but now usually replaced by the French, and somewhat subtler, form, **Noel**.

Christopher Gk. "Carrier of Christ." The much-loved story of Saint Christopher is that he lived alone by a river, carrying travelers across the ford on his back. A child whom he was carrying became almost too heavy to bear, and proved afterward to be the Christ child. Actually the tale has little basis in fact, and probably springs from the literal translation of the name, which originally meant carrying Christ in one's heart. Nevertheless, Christopher is still venerated as patron saint of travelers and drivers. In the modern era the name was little used until a revival in the 1940s, possibly influenced by the popularity of A. A. Milne's *Winnie the Pooh,* whose human hero is called Christopher Robin. Hugely popular right through the 1980s and 1990s, the name is still among the top ten boys' names nationwide. As **Christophe** it is equally popular in France. Explorer Christopher Columbus; actors Christopher Plummer, Christopher Reeve; architect Christopher Wren.

Chris, Christie, Christof, Christoffer, Christoforo, Christoforus, Christoph, Christophe, Christophoros, Christos, Cris, Cristobal, Cristoforo, Cristovano, Kester, Kit, Kitt, Kris, Kriss, Kristo, Kristofel, Kristofer, Kristoffer, Kristofor, Kristoforos, Kristos, Krzysztof, Stoffel, Tobal, Topher

Chuck Dim. **Charles** (OG. "Man"). Cartoon director Chuck Jones; musician Chuck Mangione; aviation pioneer Colonel Chuck Yaeger.

Churchill OE. Place name: "Hill of the church." Use as a first name is probably homage to English statesman Sir Winston Churchill.

Churchil

Cicero Lat. "Chickpea." Most famous for the Roman orator and statesman who lived in the 1st century B.C. Like Cato and Cassius, probably came to the U.S. as a slave name.

Clancy Ir. Gael. "Red-haired fighter's child." An almost stereotypically Irish name.

Clancey, Claney

Clare Dim. **Clarence**. Very unusual for boys.

Clair, Claire, Clarey, Clayre

Clarence Lat. "Bright." An alternate source is the title Duke of Clarence, created for a 14th-century royal prince who married a girl from the Clare family. The bearers of the title have been ill-fated: The third, for example, was said to have drowned in a barrel of wine. In the late 19th century, prompted by the Victorian interest in the picturesque and medieval, Clarence was immensely popular, but gradually acquired the connotations of effete aristocracy and has been neglected recently. Lawyer Clarence Darrow.

Clair, Claran, Clarance, Clare, Clarens, Claron, Clarons, Claronz, Clarrance, Clarrence, Klarance, Klarenz

Clark OF. Occupational name: "Cleric, scholar." Surname transferred to first name, heavily influenced by the fame of actor Clark Gable. Also made famous by "mild-mannered" Clark Kent, alter ego of Superman in the popular comic strip.

Clarke, Clerc, Clerk

Claude Lat. "Lame." Name of a Roman clan that produced the emperor immortalized in Robert Graves's novel (and subsequent TV dramatization) *I, Claudius.* **Claud** was used in the 19th century, but not in great numbers. Painter Claude Monet; composer Claude Debussy; Congressman Claude Pepper; actor Claude Rains.

Claudan, Claudell, Claudianus, Claudicio, Claudien, Claudino, Claudio, Claudius, Claudon, Clodito, Clodo, Clodomiro, Klaudio

Claus Dim. **Nicholas** (Gk. "People of victory"). Very popular in Germany. Actor Klaus Kinski.

Claes, Clause, Klaus

Clay OE. Occupational or place name involving clay. Most famous modern bearer was probably Cassius Clay, later Muhammad Ali, the boxing champion; he, in turn, had originally been named for a 19th-century abolitionist, American statesman Henry Clay.

Klay

Clayborne OE. Place name: "Brook near a clay-bed" or "Border near a clay-bed."

Claiborn, Claiborne, Clay, Claybourne, Clayburn, Klaiborn, Klaibourne

Clayton OE. Place name: "Settlement near the clay-bed." Given as a first name since the early 19th century.

Klayton

Cleary Ir. Gael. "Learned one."

Clement Lat. "Mild, giving mercy." A name borne by fourteen popes as well as the author (Clement Clark Moore) of "A Visit from St. Nicholas." Nevertheless, little used in English-speaking countries. Artist Francesco Clemente, baseball player Roberto Clemente.

Clem, Clemencio, Clemens, Clemente, Clementino, Clementius, Clemmie, Clemmons, Clemmy, Klemens, Klement, Klementos, Kliment

Cleon Gk. "Renowned."
Kleon

Cleveland OE. Place name: "Hilly area." During the fame of U.S. President Grover Cleveland, several towns were named after him, and the surname became a first name, though only in the U.S. Writer Cleveland Amory.

Cleavon, Cleaveland, Cleavland, Cleon, Cleve, Clevon

Cliff OE. "Steep slope." Or dim. **Clifford, Clifton.** Actor Cliff Robertson; singer Cliff Richard.

Cliffe, Clyff, Clyffe

Clifford OE. Place name: "Ford near the cliff." Surname transferred to first name, most popular in the late 19th century. Playwright Clifford Odets.

Cliff, Clyff, Clyfford

Clifton OE. Place name: "Town near the cliff." Another transferred surname, more common in the U.S. than in Britain.

Cliff, Cliffeton, Clift, Clyffeton, Clyfton, Clyffton

Clinton OE. Place name: "Settlement near the headland." An illustrious 18th-century governor of New York, De Witt Clinton, left his name on many New York City locations. Cannot be used now without reference to former President Bill Clinton. Actor Clint Eastwood; singer Clint Black.

Clint, Clintt, Klint

Clive OE. Place name: "Cliff." Given some publicity by a famous English soldier, Robert Clive, for his exploits in India. Thackeray used it as a first name in an 1855 novel, but its real popularity in England didn't come for another hundred years. Never widely used in the U.S. Critic Clive Barnes; author Clive Staples (C.S.) Lewis.

Cleve, Clyve

Clovis OG. "Renowned fighter." Early form of the name that would eventually become **Ludwig** or **Louis**. King Clovis I was the first Christian king of the Franks, and later kings' use of the name Louis probably harks back to the dynasty he founded in the 5th century. The name is rare, however, in the 20th century. Fashion designer Clovis Ruffin.
Clodoveo, Clovisito, Clovio, Clovito

Cluny Ir. Gael. "From the meadow."

Clyde Scot. place name: The River Clyde penetrates western Scotland as far as Glasgow.
Clydell

Cody OE. "Pillow." Some sources suggest "son of Odo." Use as a first name was probably influenced by the fame of Buffalo Bill Cody, frontier scout and entrepreneur, who took his "Wild West Show" around the U.S. and Europe at the turn of the century.
Codey, Codie, Kody

Colbert OE. "Renowned mariner."
Cole, Colt, Colvert, Culbert

Colby OE. Place name: "The dark farmstead."
Colbee, Colbey, Colbie, Collby

Cole Dim. **Nicholas** (Gk. "people of victory") and names beginning with Cole, such as **Coleman**. Composer Cole Porter; outlaw Cole Younger.

Coleman OE. "Follower of Nicholas." Also contraction of the Latin word for "dove"; probably influenced by the Irish Saint Columba.
Colman

Colin Gael. "Young creature." Also dim. **Nicholas** (Gk. "People of victory"). Well-known in the Middle Ages, and popular in Britain in the middle of this century, but didn't spread in any numbers to the U.S. until quite recently. Secretary of State Colin Powell; actors Colin Firth, Colin Farrell.
Colan, Cole, Collin, Colyn

Colley OE. "Dark-haired." Use as a first name is rare. Philanthropist Collis Huntington.
Collie, Collis

Collier OE. Occupation name: "Coal miner."
   Colier, Colis, Collayer, Collis, Collyer
Collins Ir. Gael. "Holly." Author Wilkie Collins.
Colter OE. Occupational name: "Colt-herd."
Colton OE. Place name: "Dark settlement" or possibly "colt-settlement" or "Cole's settlement."
   Coleton, Coilton, Colston
Colville OF. Place name of Norman origin and obscure meaning.
   Colvile, Colvill
Colwyn Welsh. Place name, for a river in Wales.
   Colwin, Colwynn
Conan Ir. Gael. "High, lifted up." Taken to Ireland some time after the Norman Conquest, but almost unknown until the fame of Sherlock Holmes's creator, Sir Arthur Conan Doyle. A more modern example is the movie character Conan the Barbarian, whose creators were probably unaware of the name's previous use or origin. Talk show host Conan O'Brien.
   Con, Conant, Conn, Connie
Conlan Ir. Gael. "Hero."
   Conlen, Conley, Conlin, Conlon, Connlyn
Connor Ir. Gael. "High longing" or possibly "lover of wolves." Currently very popular in Ireland. Irish author Conor Cruise O'Brien.
   Conor
Conrad OG. "Courageous advice." Despite occasional increases in its numbers, a name that has never been widely popular in English-speaking countries. Anthropologist Konrad Lorenz; hotelier Conrad Hilton; author Joseph Conrad.
   Con, Connie, Conrade, Conrado, Corrado, Cort, Curt, Konrad, Kort, Kurt
Conroy Ir. Gael. "Wise man."
Constantine Lat. "Steadfast." The form **Constant** was popular among the Puritans (as a virtue name) and was revived in the 19th century to occasional modern use. Constantine, the Latin form, was the name of the first Roman

emperor, eleven Byzantine emperors, and a royal name in Greece. Steady 19th-century use has now dwindled to neglect.

Constans, Constanz, Constant, Constantin, Constantino, Constantius, Costa, Konstantin, Konstantio, Konstanz

Conway Welsh. "Holy river" or Ir. Gael. "Hound of the plain." Rare. Musician Conway Twitty.

Conwy

Cook Lat. "Cook." Occupational name, one of the 50 most common surnames in England, but an unusual first name in the 20th century.

Cooke, Cookie

Cooper OE. Occupational name: "Barrel maker." Novelist James Fenimore Cooper; actor Gary Cooper.

Coop

Corbin Lat. "Dark as a raven." Most common in the 19th century. Actors Corbin Bernsen, John Corbett.

Corbet, Corbett, Corbie, Corbit, Corbitt, Corby, Corbyn, Cory, Korbyn

Corcoran Ir. Gael. "Ruddy."

Cochran, Cork, Korcoran

Cordell OF. Occupational name: "Rope maker." Football player Kordell Stewart.

Cord, Cordas, Cordelle, Kordell, Kordelle

Corey Ir. Gael. Place name: "The hollow." Transferred to a surname and used as a first name for either sex. Also diminutive for "Cor-" names.

Correy, Corrie, Corry, Cory, Currie, Curry

Cormick Gael. "Chariot driver."

Cormac, Cormack, Cormic

Corliss OE. "Benevolent, cheery."

Corless, Corley

Cornelius Lat. "Like a horn." Comes from a famous Latin clan name, and was often used under the Roman Empire. Railroad millionaire Cornelius Vanderbilt.

Con, Connie, Cornall, Corneille, Cornelious, Cornell, Cornelus, Corney, Cornilius, Kornelious, Kornelis, Kornelius, Neal, Neel, Neil, Neely

Cornell Fr. Var. **Cornelius**.
  Cornall, Cornel, Corney
Cornwallis OE. "Man from Cornwall." Surname transferred to a first name in the 19th century. Famous English general in the Revolutionary War, George Cornwallis.
Cort OG. "Brave." Actor Bud Cort.
  Corty, Court, Kort
Corwin OE. "Heart's friend or companion."
  Corwan, Corwinn, Corwyn, Corwynn
Corydon Gk. "Battle-ready."
  Coridon, Coryden, Coryell
Cosgrove Ir. Gael. "Victorious champion."
  Cosgrave
Cosmo Gk. "Orderliness, organization." Saint Cosmas, a martyr, was patron saint of the Italian city of Milan, and the name was further spread there by the fame of Cosimo de' Medici, Grand Duke of Tuscany. His friend the Duke of Gordon took the name to Britain in the 17th century, but it was never widely used.
  Cosimo, Cosme, Kosmo
Coulson Surname derived from **Nicholas** (Gk. "People of victory"), mostly 19th-century use.
  Colson
Courtland OE. Place name: "Land of the court."
  Cortland, Cortlandt, Court, Courtlandt
Courtney OE. "Court-dweller." Surname transferred to first name; usually feminine in U.S., though still given to boys. Immensely popular for girls in the late eighties, which will probably limit its use as a boys' name for some time. Actor Tom Courtenay.
  Cortney, Courtenay, Courtnay, Curt
Covell OE. Place name: "Slope with the cave."
Cowan Ir. Gael. Place name: "Hollow in the hill."
  Coe
Coyle Ir. Gael. "Follows the battle."
Craddock Welsh. "Love." Anglicization of a Welsh name, more common as a surname.
  Caradoc, Caradog, Cradock
Craig Gael. "Rock." (Think "crag.") Surname that has be-

come a standard first name since its introduction as a first
name only 50 years ago.

Graig, Craigie, Craik, Kraig

Crandall OE. Place name: "Valley of cranes."

Crandal, Crandell

Cranley OE. Place name: "Meadow with the cranes."

Cranlee, Cranleigh, Cranly

Cranston OE. Place name: "Settlement of cranes." U.S.
Senator Alan Cranston.

Craven OE. Last name, formerly place name, of unclear
meaning. As an adjective, however, the usual definition is
"cowardly." Mostly 19th-century use.

Crawford OE. Place name: "Ford of the crows." Particularly well used in Scotland, as both a surname and a given
name.

Crawfurd

Creighton OE. Place name: "Rocky spot."

Crayton, Crichton

Cresswell OE. Place name: "Well where watercress
grows."

Carswell, Creswell, Creswill

Crispin Lat. "Curly-haired." Saint Crispin, supposedly a
3rd-century martyr (though there is some doubt about his
legend), is patron of shoemakers, and Henry V fought the
battle of Agincourt on his feast day, October 25. The name
was somewhat popular in Britain in the 17th and 18th centuries, and was revived in the 1960s, but has not spread to
the U.S. in significant numbers. Actor Crispin Glover.

Crepin, Crispian, Crispino, Crispo, Crispus, Crisspin

Crofton OE. "Settlement of the cottages."

Croft, Crofft, Croffton

Cromwell OE. Place name: "Winding stream." Limited use
as a first name, probably out of admiration for 17th-
century English reformer Oliver Cromwell. Actor James
Cromwell.

Crosby Scan. Place name: "At the cross." Singer Bing
Crosby.

Crosbey, Crosbie

Crosley OE. Place name: "Meadow of the cross."

Croslea, Crosleigh, Crosly, Crosslee, Crossley,
Crosslie

Crowther OE. Occupational name: "Fiddler."
Crothers

Cullen Ir. Gael. "Handsome." Poet William Cullen Bryant.
Cullan, Cullin, Cullinan

Culley Ir. Gael. Place name: "The woods."
Cully

Culver OE. "Dove."
Colver, Cully

Cunningham Ir. Gael. "Village of the milk pail." Football
player Randall Cunningham.
. Conyngham, Cunninghame

Curran Ir. Gael. "Hero."
Currey, Currie, Curry

Curt Dim. **Courtney, Curtis, Conrad**. Most common in
the U.S. Musician Kurt Cobain; actor Kurt Russell; football player Kurt Warner.
Kurt

Curtis OF. "Polite, courteous." Surname used as first name,
notably in the U.S. since the 1950s. Used quite steadily.
General Curtis Le May; golfer Curtis Strange; football
player Curtis Martin.
Curcio, Curt, Curtell, Curtice, Curtiss, Kurtis

Cuthbert OE. "Famous, brilliant." Saint Cuthbert was a
much-loved 7th-century English bishop. He was most famous in northern England and Scotland, and his name was
most common there, though it fell out of favor after the
1930s. Never popular in America.

Cutler OE. Occupational name: "Knife maker."

Cyprian Gk. "From Cyprus." Steadily used in Britain until
the 17th century, but never transferred to the U.S.
Cipriano, Ciprien, Cyprien

Cyrano Gk. "From Cyrene." Use is bound to recall Edmond
Rostand's popular play *Cyrano de Bergerac* (1897), based
on the life of the 17th-century author and swashbuckler of
that name.

Cyril Gk. "The lord." Popularity confined to Britain, from
the turn of the century to the 1930s. Actor Cyril Ritchard.

Ciril, Cirilio, Cyrill, Cyrille, Cirillo, Cyrillus, Cirilo, Kiril, Kyril

Cyrus Per. "Sun or throne." Famous Persian emperor who appears in the Old Testament; he allowed exiled Jews to rebuild Jerusalem. Puritan use brought it to the U.S., where it was somewhat popular, but faded in modern times. Inventor Cyrus McCormick; former Secretary of State Cyrus Vance.

Ciro, Cy

Dacey Ir. Gael. "From the south" or Lat. "From Dacia," an area that is now Romania. The form **Dacian** enjoyed a burst of popularity in the 1970s along with other "-ian" names like **Damian** and **Dorian**.

Dace, Dacian, Dacius, Dacy, Daicey, Daicy

Dag Scan. "Daylight." In Norse mythology the god Dag is the son of light. Diplomat and author Dag Hammarskjold.

Dagget, Daggett, Dagny

Dagan Heb. "Grain, the earth."

Dagon

Dagwood OE. Place name: "Shining forest." Virtually pre-empted by a character from the popular comic strip *Blondie.* Dagwood was the harassed husband of a dizzy blonde.

Dalbert OE. "Bright-shining one."

Del, Delbert

Dale OE. Place name: "Valley." Originally a surname meaning "one who lives in the valley." The term "dale" is still used in parts of England. Most famous as a first name in the 1930s. Success guru Dale Carnegie.

Daile, Daley, Dallan, Dalle, Dallin, Dayle

Dallas Scot. Gael. Place name of a village in northeastern Scotland, used as a first name since the 19th century, and apparently unrelated to Dallas, Texas, which was named for a U.S. vice president.

Dal, Dalles, Dallis, Delles

Dalton OE. Place name: "The settlement in the valley." Writer Dalton Trumbo.

Daleton, Dallton, Dalten

Daly Ir. Gael. "Assembly." Common Irish surname, used since the 1940s as a first name. Decathlon champion Daley Thompson.

Daley, Dawley

Dalziel Scot. Gael. Place name: "The small field."

Damek Slavic. Var. **Adam.** "Son of the red earth."

Adamec, Adamek, Adamik, Adamok, Adham, Damick, Damicke

Damian Gk. Meaning not clear: possibly "to tame," although the Greek root is also close to the word for "spirit." The name was revived in various forms (**Damon, Damien**) in the 1950s, having been neglected since the Middle Ages. As **Demyan,** it is currently very popular in Russia. Author Damon Runyon; ballet dancer Damien Woetzel.

Daemon, Daimen, Daimon, Daman, Damen, Dameon, Damian, Damiano, Damianos, Damianus, Damien, Damion, Damon, Damyan, Damyen, Damyon, Dayman, Daymian, Daymon, Demyan

Dan Dim. **Daniel.** Heb. "God is my judge." Used from time to time on its own. Actors Dan Ackroyd, Dan Blocker.

Dana OE. "From Denmark." Also possibly a place name referring to an English river. Surname first used as a boy's name in the 19th century, but now almost exclusively a girl's name, and a specifically American one. Artist Charles Dana Gibson; actor Dana Carvey.

Dane, Danie

Daniel Heb. "God is my judge." In the famous Old Testament story, Daniel is thrown into a den of lions because he insists on praying to his God while a captive in Babylon; he was, of course, rescued by the same God. The name has been used with moderate frequency until a spurt of popularity in the late 1950s, which endures still; the name is one of the top twenty in the U.S., England, and Ireland. Novelist Daniel Defoe; entertainers Danny Thomas, Danny Kaye; Senator Daniel Patrick Moynihan; actors Daniel Day-Lewis, Danny DeVito, Danny Aiello, Daniel Radcliffe.

Dan, Danal, Dane, Daneal, Danek, Dani, Danial, Daniele, Danil, Danilo, Danko, Dannel, Dannie, Danny, Danyal, Danyel, Deiniol

Dante Lat. "Lasting, enduring." Actually a nickname, since Italian poet Dante Alighieri's full name was Durante, and modern use of the name almost always refers to him. English artist Dante Gabriel Rossetti; football player Daunte Culpepper.

Dantae, Dantay, Dontae, Dontay, Donte

Darby OE. Place name: "Park with deer." Derived from **Derby**, a surname used as a first name. Darby is occasionally used for girls.

Darbey, Darbie, Derby

Darcy Ir. Gael. "Dark." Also Norman place name, "From Arcy." In Britain, more likely to be a boy's name, but in the U.S., more likely to be feminine.

D'Arcy, Darcey, Darsey, Darsy

Darius Gk. "Rich, kingly." Darius the Great was a renowned emperor of Persia in the 5th century B.C.

Darias, Dariess, Dario, Darious, Darrius, Derrius, Derry

Darnell OE. Place name: "The hidden spot."

Darnall, Darnel

Darrel Transferred surname, possibly originated as a French place name, like **Darcy**. There are many forms, of which **Darryl** is the favorite by a nose. In fact, that spelling, and the popularity of the name in the 1950s, may stem from the fame of film producer Darryl Zanuck. Baseball star Darryl Strawberry; musician Daryl Hall.

Darral, Darrell, Darrill, Darrol, Darroll, Darry, Darryl, Darryll, Daryl, Derrel, Derrell, Derril, Derrill, Deryl, Deryll

Darren Ir. Gael. "Great." Originally a surname, first used as a given name in this century. Its popularity was probably influenced by the TV series "Bewitched," in which the rather hapless leading man was named Darren.
Daren, Darin, Daron, Darran, Darrin, Darring, Darron, Darryn, Derrin, Derron

Darton OE. Place name: "Settlement of the deer."

Darwin OE. "Dear friend." Naturalist Charles Darwin.
Darwon, Darwyn, Derwin, Derwynn

David Heb. "Dear one." In the Old Testament, the young David used his slingshot to kill the mighty giant Goliath, and went on to become King of Israel and author of the Psalms. He has been a favorite subject of artists, notably sculptors of the Italian Renaissance, like Michelangelo and Donatello. Saint David is the patron saint of Wales, so the name is popular there, and in Scotland, where David was a royal name. In the U.S. the name is used by Jewish and Christian families alike, and was in the top ten boys' names from the 1950s through the 1990s. It has just recently been nudged a little farther down the charts. Explorer David Livingstone; actors David Niven, David Arquette, David Duchovny, David Schwimmer; baseball star Dave Winfield; TV host David Letterman; musician David Bowie; soccer player David Beckham.
Daffy, Daffyd, Dafydd, Dai, Dave, Davey, Davi, Davie, Davidde, Davide, Davidson, Davie, Davies, Davin, Davis, Daven, Davon, Davy, Davyd, Davydd

Davis OE. "David's son." Contraction of surname that cropped up in the Middle Ages. Confederate President Jefferson Davis; actor Brad Davis.
Dave, Davidson, Davies, Davison, Daviss, Davy

Dawson OE. "David's son." Another form of the medieval surname.
Daw, Dawe, Dawes

Dean OE. Place name, "Valley," or occupational name; "Church official." Surname used as a first name, mostly since the 1950s. Actor/singer Dean Martin; U.S. Secretaries of State Dean Acheson, Dean Rusk.
Deane, Deen, Dene, Deyn, Dino

Dearborn OE. Place name: "Brook of the deer."
Dearbourn, Dearburne, Deerborn

Decimus Lat. "Tenth," as in tenth child. Opportunities for use seem negligible today.
Decio

Declan Ir. Unknown meaning: name of a saint, popular in Ireland. The singer Elvis Costello was born Declan Patrick McManus.

Dedrick Var. **Theodoric**. OG. "The people's ruler." Also the source for the better-known **Derek**.
Dedric, Diederick, Dietrich

Deems OE. "Judge's child."

Delaney Ir. Gael. Meaning unclear: possibly "Offspring of the challenger."
Delaine, Delainey, Delainy, Delane, Delany

Delano OF. Surname of unclear origin: possibly "night-time" *(de la nuit)* or "nut tree" *(de la noix)*. It would be merely one of those odd family names if it had not been made famous by U.S. President Franklin Delano Roosevelt.

Delbert OE. "Day-bright."
Bert, Bertie, Dalbert, Dilbert

Delling ONorse. "Scintillating."

Delmore OF. "Of the sea." The more familiar form, at least as a place name, is the Spanish Delmar. Use is American only. Poet Delmore Schwartz.
Delmar, Delmer, Delmor

Delroy Fr. "The king." More common forms are **Elroy** and **Leroy**. Actor Delroy Lindo.
Delroi

Delwin OE. "Proud friend" or "bright friend."
Dalwin, Dalwyn, Delavan, Delevan, Dellwin, Delwyn, Delwynn

Demetrius Gk. "Follower of Demeter." It has been little used in English-speaking countries, though its Greek and Russian forms are well-known in those countries. Composer Dimitri Shostakovich.
Dametrius, Demetri, Demetrice, Demetris, Demitrios,

Dhimitrios, Dimetre, Dimitri, Dimitrios, Dimitrious, Dimitry, Dmitri, Dmitrios, Dmitry

Demos Gk. "The people." Also possibly homage to Greece's most famous orator, Demosthenes. Rare, even in Greece.
Demas

Dempsey Ir. Gael. "Proud." Boxer Jack Dempsey.
Dempsy

Dempster OE. "One who judges." Gossip columnist Nigel Dempster.

Denby Scan. Place name: "The Danes' village." Film critic David Denby.
Danby, Denbey, Denney, Dennie, Denny

Denham OE. Place name: "Village in a valley."

Denholm Scot. Place name. In the public eye currently because of the English actor Denholm Elliott.

Denley OE. Place name: "Meadow near the valley."
Denlie, Denly

Denman OE. Surname derived from place name: "Man who lives in the valley."

Dennis Gk. "Follower of Dionysius." Dionysos was the classical Greek god of wine, but the name also appears in the New Testament. Saint Denis is the patron saint of France. The name has had alternating centuries of favor and disfavor (16th out, 17th in), reaching the height of its 20th-century popularity around 1920. Actors Dennis Quaid, Dennis Christopher, Dennis Hopper, Dennis Franz, Denis Leary, Dennis Haysbert; sailor Dennis Conner.
Den, Denies, Denis, Dennes, Dennet, Denney, Dennie, Dennison, Denny, Dennys, Denys, Deon, Dion, Dionisio, Dionysius, Dionysus, Diot

Dennison OE. "Son of Dennis."
Den, Denison, Dennyson, Tennyson

Denton OE. Place name: "Settlement in the valley."
Denny, Dent, Denten, Dentin

Denver OE. Place name: "Green valley." Singer John Denver.

Denzel Cornish place name, used as a first name almost exclusively in Britain. Actor Denzel Washington.
Denzell, Denziel, Denzil, Denzill, Denzyl

Derek OG. "The people's ruler." Most common of the many anglicized forms of **Theodoric,** popular starting around 1890, peaking in the 1930s. Basketball player Derrick Coleman; baseball player Derek Jeter.

Darrick, Darriq, Dereck, Deric, Derick, Derik, Deriq, Derk, Derreck, Derrek, Derrick, Derrik, Derryck, Derryk, Deryk, Deryke, Dirk, Dirke, Dyrk

Dermot Ir. Gael. "Free man." Actor Dermot Mulroney.

Dermott, Diarmid, Diarmuid

Derry Ir. Gael. Place name: City in Northern Ireland formerly known as Londonderry. Also short form of **Derek, Dermot,** etc. Photographer Derry Moore.

Derrie

Derward OE. "Deer keeper."

Durward

Derwin OE. "Dear friend."

Darwin, Darwyn, Derwyn, Derwynn, Durwin

Desmond Ir. Gael. "From South Munster." Munster was an ancient kingdom in Ireland. Used in England since 1900, and briefly popular around 1920, but unusual now. South African cleric and activist Bishop Desmond Tutu.

Des, Desmund, Dezmond

Deverell OE. Place name: "Bank of the river."

Devine Ir. Gael. "Ox" or OF. "Divine."

Devlin Ir. Gael. "Fierce courage."

Delvin, Devland, Devlen, Devlon, Devlyn

Devon English and American place name. More common for girls than for boys.

Deven, Devin, Devonn, Devyn

Dewey Welsh. Var. **David.** Bookish parents may remember the Dewey Decimal System, invented by Melvil Dewey in 1876 and the organizing principle for the majority of American libraries until the Libary of Congress got in on the act and changed all the numbers.

Dewi, Dewie

DeWitt Flem. "Blond." Early American statesman De Witt Clinton.

Dewitt, Dwight, Witt

Dexter Lat. "Right-handed" or OE. "Woman dyer." Mod-

ern use, more common in Britain. Football player Dexter
Carter.
Dex

Diamond OE. "Bright guardian." Also, for girls, a jewel
name. Actor Lou Diamond Phillips.

Dick Dim. **Richard** (OG. "Dominant ruler"). Figure skater
Dick Button.

Didier Fr. "Much-desired." Male form of Désirée; currently
popular in France.

Diego Sp. Var. **James** (Heb. "He who supplants"). Painter
Diego Rivera.
Dago

Dieter OG. "Army of the people." Very fashionable in Germany.

Dietrich Ger. form of **Theodoric** (OG. "People's ruler").
See **Derek**.
Dedrick, Derek, Deke, Diederick, Dirk

Digby ONorse. "Town by the ditch." Like many English
surnames adapted from place names, became a first name
in the late 19th century without ever becoming very widespread.

Dillon Ir. Gael. "Loyal." Often confused with its popular
homonym, the Welsh **Dylan**. Actor Matt Dillon.
Dillan, Dilon, Dyllon, Dylon

Dinsmore Ir. Gael. Place name: "The hill fortress."
Dinnsmore

Dirk Var. **Derek** (OG. "The people's ruler"). Actor Dirk
Bogarde.

Dixon OE. "Son of Dick." Scottish surname transferred to
first name. Author Dixon Wecter.
Dickson, Dix

Doane OE. Place name: "Low, rolling hills."
Doan

Doherty Ir. Gael. "Harmful." Surname common in Ireland,
transferred occasionally to first-name status.
Docherty, Dougherty, Douherty

Dolan Ir. Gael. "Black-haired."

Dolph Dim. **Adolph**. Actor Dolf Lundgren.
Dolf, Dollfus, Dollfuss, Dollphus, Dolphus

Dominic Lat. "Lord." A name popular among Catholic families, possibly because of the fame of Saint Dominic, founder of an important monastic order. Use has spread since the 1950s. Still more common in Britain than the U.S. Clever for a child born on Sunday, "the Lord's day." Opera star Placido Domingo; basketball player Dominique Wilkins; writer Dominick Dunne.

Demenico, Demingo, Dom, Domenic, Domenico, Domenique, Domingo, Domini, Dominick, Dominie, Dominik, Dominique, Domino, Dominy, Nick

Donahue Ir. Gael. "Dark fighter." TV host Phil Donahue.

Donahoe, Donohoe, Donohue

Donald Scot. Gael. "World mighty." Common in Scotland for centuries, and popular elsewhere for some 50 years, peaking in 1925 but less popular since the 1950s, perhaps because Disney preempted the name by giving it to a cartoon duck. Actors Donald Sutherland, Don Cheadle, Donal Logue; real estate tycoon Donald Trump; singer Donny Osmond.

Donal, Donaldo, Donall, Donalt, Donaugh, Donel, Donelson, Donnel, Donnell, Donnie, Donny

Donato Lat. "Given."

Donatien, Donatus

Donnelly Ir. Gael. "Brown-haired fighter."

Donnell

Donovan Ir. Gael. "Dark." Surname become first name or, in the case of the pop singer who recorded "Mellow Yellow" in the late 1960s, only name. Football player Donovan McNabb.

Donavon, Donevin, Donevon, Donoven, Donovon

Dooley Ir. Gael. "Dark hero."

Doran Ir. Gael. "Fist" or "stranger, exile."

Dore, Dorian, Doron, Dorran, Dorren

Dorian Gk. Place name: "From Doris," an area in Greece. Introduced by Oscar Wilde in *The Picture of Dorian Gray;* the hero of the tale is a beautiful young man who succumbs to a life of vice. Notwithstanding this discouraging precedent, the name has had some popularity in the U.S.

Dore, Dorien, Dorrian, Dorrien, Dorryen

Dougal Celt. "Dark stranger." Most common in Scotland.

Doyle, Dougall, Dugal, Dugald, Dugall

Douglas Scot. Gael. Place name: "Black water." The name of a hugely powerful Scots clan. Though it was originally a girl's name, by the 19th century Douglas was used for boys. Its period of great popularity, which peaked in the 1950s, seems to have been inspired by the actors Douglas Fairbanks, father and son. Fairly steadily used, though not fashionable. Author Douglas Adams; Gen. Douglas MacArthur.

Douglass, Dugaid

Dow Ir. Gael. "Dark-haired."

Dowan, Dowe, Dowson

Doyle Ir. Gael. "Black stranger." Var. **Dougal**. Authors Paddy Doyle, Arthur Conan Doyle.

Drake Middle English. This is an unusually specific name, for it derives from the word *draca,* which was the medieval term for "dragon." Originally Drake designated the man who kept the inn with the dragon trademark, or the "Sign of the Dragon." It followed the usual route of becoming a surname, and thence a first name. English explorer Sir Francis Drake.

Drew Welsh. "Wise." Dim. **Andrew**. Used as an independent name since the 1960s. Football player Drew Bledsoe.

Dru

Drummond Celt. Meaning unclear. Use as a first name is concentrated in Scotland.

Drury OF. "Loved one." Drury Lane is a famous street in London's theater district, and also the home of the Muffin Man in a well-known children's song.

Drew, Drewry, Dru

Dryden OE. Place name: "Dry valley." Poet John Dryden.

Duane Ir. Gael. "Swarthy." Used primarily since the 1940s, predominantly in the U.S. **Dwayne** is the most popular spelling.

Dewain, Dewayne, Duwain, Duwaine, Duwayne, Dwain, Dwaine, Dwayne

Dudley OE. Place name: "People's field." Aristocratic family name in England, used as a first name since the 19th century. The absurd Canadian Mountie Dudley Doright was a staple character in the 1960s "Rocky and Bullwinkle Show." Actor Dudley Moore.

Duff Gael. "Swarthy." There are many English surnames turned first names that derive from the Gaelic *dubh,* which means dark. They may describe places (i.e., **Douglas**), or personal characteristics, as in this case.
Duffey, Duffie, Duffy

Dugan Ir. Gael. "Swarthy."
Doogan, Dougan, Douggan, Duggan

Duke Lat. "Leader." Last name transferred to first name, or possibly an abbreviation of the highly unusual **Marmaduke**. Current use is probably inspired either by John Wayne (who was nicknamed "Duke"), or the great jazz musician Duke Ellington.

Duncan Scot. Gael. "Brown fighter." A royal name in early Scotland: There was a King Duncan in 11th-century Scotland whose cousin Macbeth murdered him. Shakespeare later picked up the tale in his tragedy *Macbeth.* The name disappeared until a spell of 19th-century use in Scotland and a flurry of mostly English popularity in the 1950s and 1960s. Never a big hit in the U.S. Cabinetmaker Duncan Phyfe.
Dunc, Dunn

Dunham Gael. "Brown man."

Dunley OE. Place name: "Meadow with the hill."
Dunlea, Dunleigh, Dunlie, Dunly, Dunnlea, Dunnleigh, Dunnley

Dunlop Scot. Gael. Place name: "Muddy hill."

Dunmore Scot. Gael. Place name: "Big fortress on the hill."

Dunn Gael. "Brown." Writers Dominick and John Gregory Dunne.
Dunne

Dunstan OE. Place name: "Brown hill with stones." Name of an English saint who was Archbishop of Canterbury in the 10th century. Rarely used, even in Britain.
Dunsten, Dunstin, Dunston

Dunton OE. Place name: "Hill settlement."

Durant Lat. "Enduring." Much more common as a last name. **Dante** is an abbreviated version. The 19th-century historians Will and Ariel Durant; American painter Asher Durand; entertainer Jimmy Durante.

Dante, Durand, Durante

Durward OE. Occupational name: "Warder at the gate."

Derward

Durwin OE. "Dear friend."

Derwin, Derwyn, Durwyn

Dustin OG. "Brave warrior," or OE. place name: "Dusty area." Use of the name, which is quite substantial, is almost certainly influenced by the fame of actor Dustin Hoffman.

Dustan, Dusten, Duston, Dusty, Dustyn

Dwight Flemish. "White or blond." Var. **DeWitt**. Some sources claim Dwight is a contraction of a surname derived from Dionysius. Given fame in the U.S. by two Yale University presidents, and by President Dwight Eisenhower. Its moderate use as a first name was probably inspired by him, and had trailed off by the 1970s. Baseball star Dwight Gooden.

Dyer OE. Occupational name: "Dyer." Curiously enough, **Dexter** refers to a female dyer.

Dylan Welsh. "Son of the sea." Welsh legend tells of a sea-god named Dylan , but modern use of the name, which has spread well beyond Wales, is probably homage to poet Dylan Thomas. Though the name is extremely popular in Ireland, it is also quite frequently used in the U.S. The best-known example of this tribute is singer Bob Dylan, whose last name was originally Zimmerman. Some of the variant spellings given below are more closely related to homonym Dillon. Actor Dylan McDermott.

Dillan, Dillon, Dyllan, Dylon, Dylonn

Dyson OE. Last name that is probably a contraction of **Dennison**. Transferred to first-name use in the 19th century.

Eamon Ir. Var. **Edmund** (OE. "Wealthy protector"). Irish President Eamon de Valera may have been the inspiration behind the spurt of popularity between the 1950s and the 1970s. The name is rare in America.

Amon, Aimon, Aymon, Eamonn

Earl OE. "Nobleman, leader." The most popular of the English titles of nobility to be used as a first name, though **Baron** and **Duke** also occur. In the democratic U.S. it is probably a transferred surname rather than an allusion to the hereditary aristocracy. Author Erle Stanley Gardner; actor Errol Flynn; basketball star Earl ("the Pearl") Monroe; musician Earl Scruggs; Chief Justice of the U.S. Supreme Court Earl Warren.

Earle, Earlie, Early, Erl, Erle, Errol, Erroll, Erryl, Rollo

Eaton OE. Place name: "Settlement on the river."

Eatton, Eton, Eyton

Ebenezer Heb. "Rock of help." In the Old Testament, Samuel created a memorial to his victory over the Philistines, and called the stone Ebenezer. The name came to America with the Puritans, and was, improbably enough, at one point almost as popular a name as John. It was fading by the 19th century, and Ebenezer Scrooge in Charles Dickens's *A Christmas Carol* probably hastened its disappearance.

Eb, Ebbaneza, Eben, Ebeneezer, Ebeneser, Ebenezar, Eveneser, Evenezer

Eberhard OG. "Courage of a boar." Var. **Everett**. Pencil magnate Eberhard Faber.

Eberardo, Eberhardt, Eberdt, Ebert, Everard, Everhardt, Evrard, Evreux

Edbert OE. "Wealthy and bright."

Edel OG. "Noble." Unusual as a name in itself, but the first syllable of many combined forms such as **Adalric** and **Adelaide**. Biographer Leon Edel.

Adel, Adlin, Edelin, Edlin

Eden Heb. "Pleasure, delight." It is a short step from the Hebrew meaning of the word to its general association with Paradise. The name is used for girls as well as boys. English statesman Sir Anthony Eden.

Eaden, Eadin, Edin, Ednan, Edyn

Edgar OE. "Wealthy spearman." A royal name in Anglo-Saxon England which, like **Edmund,** endured through the Norman invasion and the resulting influx of Norman names. In Shakespeare's *King Lear,* Lear's son is called Edgar. Revived, like many Anglo-Saxon names, at the turn of the century, but the revival was short-lived. Poet Edgar Allan Poe; puppeteer Edgar Bergen; artist Edgar Dégas; author Edgar Rice Burroughs.

Eadgar, Eadger, Ed, Eddie, Edgard, Edgardo, Ned, Neddy, Ted, Teddie

Edison OE. "Son of Edward." Inventor Thomas Edison.

Eddison, Eddy, Edson

Edmund OE. "Wealthy protector." A popular, and sainted, king of the East Angles in the 9th century gave the name enough popularity to survive the Norman Conquest. Astronomer Edmund Halley; poet Edmund Spenser; explorer Sir Edmund Hillary; Governor Edmund "Pat" Brown; Senator Edmund Muskie.

Eadmund, Eamon, Eamonn, Ed, Eddie, Edmon, Edmond, Edmonde, Edmondo, Ned, Neddie, Ted, Teddy

Edric OE. "Wealthy ruler." Anglo-Saxon name that was pushed out of fashion by the Normans in the 11th century but revived briefly at the end of the 19th.

Ederic, Ederick, Edrich, Edrick

Edsel OE. Place name: "Wealthy man's house." Linked in most minds to automotive pioneer Edsel Ford, and the ill-fated car named after him. The name is still used in the Ford family.

Edward OE. "Wealthy defender." A name with long-lasting

popularity throughout the English-speaking world. Used by kings of England (including the saint Edward the Confessor) since before the Norman Conquest, and still a staple in the royal family. Though less of an obvious choice since the 1930s, it is still popular. Photographer Edward Steichen; ballet dancer Edward Villella; U.S. Senator Edward Kennedy; poet Edward Lear; artist Edouard Manet; Edward, Duke of Windsor; actors Edward Norton, Edward Burns.

Eadward, Ed, Eddie, Eddy, Edik, Edouard, Eduard, Eduardo, Edvard, Edvardas, Ewart, Lalo, Ned, Neddie, Ted, Teddie

Edwin OE. "Wealthy friend." Anglo-Saxon name revived at the end of the 19th century, and used with some frequency since then. Astronaut Edwin "Buzz" Aldrin; Attorney General Edwin Meese III.

Eadwinn, Ed, Eddy, Edlin, Eduino, Edwyn, Ned, Neddy, Ted

Efrem Var. **Ephraim**. Actor Efrem Zimbalist, Jr.

Efi, Efraim, Efrayim, Efren, Efrim

Egan Gael. "Burning." Irish use predominates.

Eagan, Eagen, Egann, Egon

Egbert OE. "Brilliant sword." Another 19th-century Anglo-Saxon revival, now little heard.

Egerton OE. Place name: possibly "Edgar's settlement." Occurs as a surname in the English aristocracy. Transferred to first-name use mostly in Britain.

Edgerton

Egidio It. "Kid, young goat." The anglicized version is Giles.

Eginhard Ger. "Sword power."

Eginard, Eginhardt, Einhard, Einhardt, Enno

Egor Rus. "Farmer." Currently popular in Russia, but very exotic in English-speaking countries.

Igor, Ygor

Einar ONorse. "Battle leader." Refers to the heroes of Valhalla, in the Old Norse legends.

Ejnar, Inar

Eion Ir. Var. **John** (Heb. "the Lord is gracious") by way of **Ian**.
Ean, Ion

Elbert Var. **Albert** (OE. "Highborn/shining"). The long form is **Ethelbert,** but it is virtually obsolete.

Elchanan Heb. "God is gracious." Old Testament name.
Elchana, Elhanan, Elhannan, Elkanah

Elden Var. **Alden** (OE. "Old friend"). Also possibly "valley of the elves." Surname changed to first name.
Eldin, Eldon, Eldwin, Eldwyn, Elton

Elder OE. Place name: "Elder trees." Also, in U.S., may denote a forebear who had high standing in one of the Protestant churches that are governed by councils of elders.
Eldor

Eldon OE. Place name: "Sacred hill." Used since the 19th century.

Eldred OE. "Old counsel." Anglo-Saxon name lost in the onslaught of Norman names, and brought back in the 19th-century craze for the picturesque remnants of the past.
Aldred, Eldrid

Eldridge Ger. "Sage ruler." Civil rights activist Eldridge Cleaver.
Eldredge, Eldrege, Eldrich, Eldrick, Eldrige

Eleazer Var. **Lazarus** (Heb. "The Lord will help"). The 19th-century fondness for obscure biblical names (Eleazer among them) tends to confirm the stereotype of the repressed religious Victorians. If nothing else, they must have read their Bibles carefully to come up with these names.
Elazar, Eleasar, Eleazaro, Eli, Elie, Eliezer, Ely

Eli Heb. "On high." In the Old Testament, Eli was Israel's high priest. This was a very holy name to the Hebrews. The Puritans used it freely, and it persisted through the 19th century but faded after the 1930s. American inventor Eli Whitney; author Elie Wiesel; actor Eli Wallach.
Elie, Eloi, Eloy, Ely

Elias Gk. Var. **Elijah**. Most common in the 17th century, but currently very popular in Spain.
Elice, Ellice, Ellis, Elyas

Elihu Heb. "God, the Lord." Like **Eleazer**, occasionally used in the 19th century.

Elijah Heb. "The Lord is my God." A great prophet in the Old Testament. Felix Mendelssohn, reputedly Queen Victoria's favorite composer, wrote an oratorio about him in 1846. The name was most popular in the early 19th century. Film director Elia Kazan; actor Elijah Wood.
Eli, Elia, Elias, Elie, Elihu, Eliot, Eliyahu, Eljah, Elliot, Ellis, Ely, Elyot, Elyott

Elisha Heb. "The Lord is my salvation." The successor to Elijah, as recounted in the Old Testament. Puritan name in the 17th century, a bit more widespread in the 19th, and all but obsolete now.
Eli, Elisee, Eliseo, Elisher, Eliso, Lisha

Ellard OG. "Noble and valorous."
Allard, Allerd

Ellery OE. Place name: "Island with elder trees." Some sources propose a relationship to **Hilary**. The famous fictional detective Ellery Queen is probably the best-known user of the name.
Ellary, Ellerey

Elliott Anglicization of **Elijah** or **Eli**. Surname first used as a given name in modern Scotland, quite popular in the U.S. Poet T. S. Eliot; actor Elliott Gould; Attorney General Elliot Richardson.
Eliot, Eliott, Elliot, Elyot, Elyott

Ellis Anglicization of **Elias**. Surname transferred to first name. Ellis Bell was the pseudonym used by Emily Brontë; when they first began publishing, each of the Brontë sisters chose a name that could be considered masculine. Anne was Acton Bell, and Charlotte was Currer Bell.
Elliss, Ellyce

Ellison OE. "Son of Ellis." Author Ralph Ellison.
Elison, Elisson, Ellson, Ellyson, Elson

Ellsworth OE. Place name: "Nobleman's estate" or possibly "Ellis's estate." Painter Ellsworth Kelly.
Ellswerth, Elsworth

Elmer OE. "Highborn and renowned." Anglo-Saxon name that has been much more popular in the U.S. than in Britain, especially in the late 19th century. Sinclair Lewis's well-known novel *Elmer Gantry,* published in 1927, was about a compelling charlatan of a minister. It was shocking, successful, and discouraging to parents who were considering Elmer as a name for their babies. Cartoon character Elmer Fudd.
Aylmar, Aylmer, Aymer, Ellmer, Elmir

Elmo Lat. from Gk. "Amiable" or It. "Godly helmet." Var. **Anselm**. Saint Elmo is the common name for Saint Erasmus, a 4th-century bishop-martyr who is patron saint of sailors. Saint Elmo's fire (also the name of a popular movie in the early 1980s) refers to the electrical discharges occasionally sighted at the top of a ship's mast. Parents who already have children may know Elmo as a furry red toddler-monster featured on "Sesame Street."

Elmore OE. Place name: "Moor with elm trees." Author Elmore Leonard.

Elroy Var. **Leroy** (Fr. "King").
Elroi, Elroye

Elsdon OE. Place name: "Hill of the nobleman."
Elsden, Ellsdon

Elston OE. Place name: "Settlement of the nobleman."
Ellston

Elton OE. Place name: "Old Settlement" or "Ella's town." Musician Elton John.
Alton, Eldon, Ellton

Elvin OE. "Elf friend" or "highborn friend." Var. **Alvin**.
Elven, Elwin, Elwinn, Elwyn, Elwynne

Elvio Sp. from Lat. "Blond, fair."

Elvis Scan. "All-wise." Variants are rare, since use, as in the case of singer Elvis Costello (né Declan Patrick McManus), is almost always influenced by the fame of Elvis

Presley. Figure skater Elvis Stojko; football player Elvis Grbac.

Alvis, Alvys, Elvio, Elviss, Elvo, Elvys

Elwell OE. Place name: "Old well."

Elwill

Elwin Var. Elvin.

Elvin, Elvis, Elvyn, Elwin, Win, Wynn

Elwyn Welsh. "Fair brow." Easily confused with **Elwin**, but more likely to be found in Wales, where it has a different meaning altogether.

Elwin, Elwynn

Elwood OE. Place name: "Old wood."

Ellwood, Woody

Ely OE. Place name (a river in South Wales and a cathedral and town in Cambridgeshire, England) turned surname. Or, more likely, a variant of **Eli**.

Emerson OG. "Emery's son." First-name use may be tribute to Ralph Waldo Emerson, the transcendentalist philosopher and "sage of Concord."

Emery OG. "Home ruler." Saw 19th-century use as a first name, predominantly American rather than British.

Amerigo, Amery, Amory, Emerey, Emeri, Emerich, Emmerich, Emmery, Emmory, Emory

Emil Lat. "Eager to please." The French form, **Emile**, took root slightly earlier in English-speaking countries. Used only since the mid-19th century, without any great period of popularity. French author Emile Zola; actor Emilio Estevez.

Aimil, Aymil, Emelen, Emile, Emilian, Emiliano, Emilianus, Emilio, Emilion, Emilyan, Emlen, Emlin, Emlyn, Emlynn

Emlyn Welsh place name given some prominence by playwright and actor Emlyn Williams.

Emmanuel Heb. "God is among us." Used in both the Old and the New Testaments, and as another name for Jesus. Slight use in the 17th century grew gradually right through the 19th, then tailed off. In the U.S. **Manuel** is fairly common among Catholics of Hispanic descent, who also use **Jesus** quite freely. Fashion designer Emmanuel Ungaro; pianist Emmanuel Ax.

Eman, Emanual, Emanuel, Emanuele, Emmanual,
Emmonual, Emmonuel, Emonual, Emonuel, Imanuel,
Immanuel, Immanuele, Manny, Manual, Manuel, Manuelo

Emmett Various derivations are possible, including OG. "Energetic, powerful," OE. "An ant," or even a last name relating to **Emma**. Famous clown Emmett Kelly; football player Emmitt Smith.

Emmet, Emmit, Emmitt, Emmot, Emmott

Engelbert OG. "Angel-bright." Entertainer Engelbert Humperdinck (whose original name, less memorable if more euphonious, was Gerald Dorsey).

Bert, Berty, Engelbert, Ingelbert, Inglebert

Ennis Var. **Angus** (Ir. Gael. "Sole or only choice").

Enoch Heb. "Vowed, dedicated." Old Testament name for the father of Methuselah. Briefly popular from the 1860s to 1880s, inspired by Tennyson's famous and sentimental poem "Enoch Arden." Now scarce.

Enock

Enos Heb. "Man." Old Testament name for one of Adam and Eve's great-grandsons. Mildly revived, not by the Puritans, but in the 19th century. Obscure in this century.

Enrico It. Var. **Henry** (OG. "Estate ruler"). Use by English-speaking families probably reflects the fame of operatic tenor Enrico Caruso. **Enrique** is the Spanish version of the name. Singer Enrique Iglesias.

Erico, Errico

Enzo It. Var. **Henry** (OG. "Estate ruler").

Enzio

Ephraim Heb. "Fertile, productive." Old Testament name used mostly in the 18th and 19th centuries.

Efraim, Efrain, Efrayim, Efrem, Efren, Efrim, Efrym,
Ephraem, Ephream, Ephrem, Ephrim, Ephrym

Erasmus Gk. "Loved, desired." The 16th-century Dutch humanist philosopher Geert Geerts wrote as Desiderius Erasmus. (**Desiderius** is the Latin form of Erasmus.) He may have been thinking of Saint Erasmus, who is more popularly known as Saint Elmo. Use of the name was greatest in the latter half of the 19th century, and probably refers to the philosopher rather than the saint.

Erasme, Erasmo, Ras

Erastus Gk. "Beloved."

Eraste, Rastus

Ercole It. "Splendid gift."

Ercolo

Erhard OG. "Strong resolve."

Erhardt, Erhart

Eric Scan. "All-ruler." In spite of the renown of Viking explorer Eric the Red (who colonized Iceland around A.D. 985) and his son Leif Ericsson, who reputedly discovered North America half a millennium before Columbus, Eric was little used until the turn of the 19th century. It caught on, however, becoming fashionable in Britain in the 1920s, in the U.S. some 50 years later. The German form, **Erich,** is currently popular in that country. Author Erich Segal; musician Eric Clapton; skater Eric Heiden; actors Eric Roberts, Eric McCormack.

Aeric, Aerick, Aerric, Aerrick, Aerricko, Arreck, Arric, Arrick, Erek, Erich, Erick, Erik, Eriq, Erric, Errick, Eryk, Rick, Rikky

Erin Ir. Gael. Name for Ireland. Mostly used by girls, and not in Ireland itself.

Erland OE. "Noble's land" or ONorse. "Foreigner, stranger." Actor Erland Josephson.

Arlan, Erlend

Erling OE. "Noble's son."

Ernest OE. "Sincere." Its great popularity at the turn of the 20th century was only confirmed by Oscar Wilde's play, *The Importance of Being Earnest.* Fell out of use after the 1930s. Author Ernest Hemingway; actor Ernest Borgnine; entertainer Ernie Kovacs.

Earnest, Ernesto, Ernestus, Ernie, Erno, Ernst

Errol Origin unclear, though most sources consider it a variation of **Earl.** It may also derive from a Scottish place name; there have been Scottish Earls of Erroll for more than 600 years. The most famous modern Errol was dashing movie actor Errol Flynn.

Erroll, Erryl, Erryle, Eryle, Rollo

Erskine Scot. Gael. Place name: "High cliff." Transference from last name to first occurred only in this century. Novelist Erskine Caldwell.

Erv, Erve, Ervine, Ervyn, Erwin, Erwyn, Erwynn, Irvin

Ervin Scot. Gael. Place name, or "Beautiful." Var. **Irving** (OE. "Sea friend"). General Erwin Rommel.

Esau Heb. "Hairy." In the Old Testament the story is told how Esau came out of the womb covered with hair, while his twin brother, Jacob, was hairless. The name was used somewhat in the 19th century.

Escot

Esmé Fr. "Esteemed." Originally a male name brought to Scotland by a French cousin of James VI. Now used mostly for girls, though scarce.

Esmay, Esmeling, Ismay, Ismé

Esmond OE. "Protected by grace." Survived the Norman Conquest as a last name, but was not rediscovered as a first name until the late 19th century, and was never widely used.

Ethan Heb. "Firmness, steadfastness." An Old Testament name given fame in the U.S. by Revolutionary War leader Ethan Allen, who captured Fort Ticonderoga with only eighty-three men. Currently fashionable in Wales. Actor Ethan Hawke.

Aitan, Eitan, Etan, Ethen

Etienne Fr. Var. **Stephen** (Gk. "Crowned").

Ethelbert OE. "Highborn, shining." The original form of **Albert**. A 6th-century king of Kent whom Saint Augustine converted to Christianity. The name was revived in the 19th century but is now extremely scarce.

Ethelwin OE. "Highborn friend." Anglo-Saxon name that followed the same cycle of 19th-century revival and 20th-century disuse.

Ethelwyn, Ethelwynne

Ettore It. "Loyal."

Eugene Gk. "Wellborn." In use since the early Christian era, and chosen by four popes. After centuries of disuse, it was dusted off in the 19th century and became very popular in the U.S. No longer in the first rank, but still occurs. Senator Eugene McCarthy; playwrights Eugene O'Neill, Eugène Ionesco; artist Eugène Delacroix.

Efigenio, Efigenios, Efigenius, Ephigenio, Ephigenios,
Ifigenio, Ifigenios, Iphigenios, Iphigenius, Eugen,
Eugenio, Eugenius, Evgeny, Gene

Eusebius Gk. "Devout." Name of a number of saints, the
best-known of whom was a 4th-century Italian bishop.

Esabio, Esavio, Esavius, Esebio, Eusabio, Eusaio,
Eusebio, Eusebios, Eusavio, Eusevio, Eusevios

Eustace Gk. "Fertile." Brought to Britain with the Normans, but never hugely popular there. Most common in
the late 19th century, little used in the U.S. The last names
Stacey and **Stacy** come from Eustace. (As girls' names,
they are diminutives of **Anastasia**.)

Eustache, Eustachios, Eustachius, Eustachy,
Eustaquio, Eustashe, Eustasius, Eustatius, Eustazio,
Eustis, Eustiss

Evan Welsh. Var. **John** (Heb. "The Lord is gracious"). Most
common in Wales, but also quite well-used in the U.S.

Euan, Euen, Evans, Even, Evin, Evyn, Ewan, Ewen,
Owen

Evelyn Surname transferred to first name, and more common for girls than boys. Author Evelyn Waugh's first wife
was also called Evelyn.

Evelin

Everard OE. "Boar hardness." Norman name more common as a surname, but revived in the 19th century. German form is **Eberhard**. Now rare.

Eberhard, Everardo, Evered, Everhart, Evrard, Evraud

Everett OE. "Boar hardness." Surname deriving from
Everard, used as a first name in the 19th century. Senator
Everett Dirksen; actor Rupert Everett.

Averett, Averitt, Eberhard, Eberhardt, Everard,
Evered, Everet, Everitt, Evrard, Eward, Ewart

Everley OE. Place name: "Boar meadow." Singing group
the Everly Brothers.

Everlie, Everly

Everton OE. Place name: "Boar settlement." Used as a first
name only in this century.

Ewald OE. "Law-powerful."

Evald, Evaldo, Euell, Ewell

Ewan Scot. Gael. Unclear origin: perhaps "Young man" or a variant of **Eugene**. Use confined to Scotland until the mid-20th century, but now spreading. Actor Ewan McGregor.
Euan, Euen, Ewen

Ewert OE. Occupational name: "Shepherd." Literally, "ewe-herder."
Evart, Evarts, Evert, Ewart

Ewing OE. "Law-friend." Unusual, though some families may have been inspired to use it in the 1980s by the Ewing family on the popular TV series "Dallas." Basketball player Patrick Ewing.
Ewin, Ewynn

Ezekiel Heb. "Strength of God." An important Old Testament prophet. Since the end of the 19th century, very scarce.
Esequiel, Ezechiel, Eziechiele, Eziequel, Zeke

Ezra Heb. "Helper." Old Testament prophet. The Puritans brought the name to America, where it was most used in the 19th century. Poet Ezra Pound.
Azariah, Azur, Esdras, Esra, Ezer, Ezri

Fabian Lat. Clan name, possibly meaning "one who grows beans." Name of a 3rd-century saint/pope, and latterly of a 1960s pop star. Not much used in the intervening 1700 years. Art director Fabien Baron.
Fabe, Fabek, Faber, Fabert, Fabianno, Fabiano, Fabianus, Fabien, Fabio, Fabion, Faebian, Faebien, Fabius, Fabiyus, Fabyan, Fabyen, Faybian, Faybien, Faybion, Faybionn

Fabrice Fr. from Lat. "Works with the hands."
Fabriano, Fabricius, Fabritius, Fabrizio, Fabrizius

Fabron Fr. "Young blacksmith."
   Fabre, Fabroni

Fagan Ir. Gael. "Little ardent one." The wily con artist Fagin in Dickens's *Oliver Twist* has probably put an indelible stamp on this name, particularly given the fame of the musical and movie versions.
   Fegan, Feggan, Fagin

Fairfax OE. "Blond."

Faisal Arab. "Resolute."
   Faysal, Feisal

Falkner OE. Occupational name: "Falcon trainer." Author William Faulkner.
   Falconer, Falconner, Faulconer, Faulconner, Faulkner, Fowler

Fane OE. "Happy, joyous."
   Fain, Faine

Farley OE. Place name: "Meadow of the sheep" or "Meadow of the bulls." Surname transferred occasionally to first name. Actor Farley Granger; author Walter Farley.
   Fairlay, Fairlee, Fairleigh, Fairlie, Farlay, Farlee, Farleigh, Farlie, Farly, Farrleigh, Farrley, Lee, Leigh

Farnell OE. Place name: "The fern hill." Originally a surname.
   Farnall, Fernald, Furnald

Farnham OE. Place name: "Meadow with ferns." Common surname with a little spurt of late-19th-century use as a first name.
   Farnam, Farnum, Fernham

Farnley OE. Place name: "Field with ferns."
   Farnlea, Farnlee, Farnleigh, Farnly, Fernleigh, Fernley

Farold OE. "Mighty voyager."

Farouk Arab. "Discerning truth from falsehood."
   Faruq, Faruqh

Farquhar Scot. Gael. "Very dear one." First-name use is occasional, and mostly Scottish.
   Farquharson, Farquar, Farquarson

Farr OE. "Voyager."

Farrell Ir. Gael. "Hero, man of courage."
   Farrel, Farrill, Farryll, Ferrel, Ferrell, Ferrill, Ferryl

Faust Lat. "Fortunate, enjoying good luck." Very rare as a first name, no doubt owing to the literary connotations, for the legendary Faust sells his soul to the devil. His story was retold by Marlowe, Goethe, Wagner, and Thomas Mann, among others.
Faustino, Fausto, Faustus

Favian Lat. "Man of wisdom."

Fay Ir. Gael. "Raven." Extremely rare as a boy's name, though somewhat popular for girls.
Faye, Fayette

Fedor Ger. Var. **Theodore** (Gk. "Gift from God"). Author Fyodor Dostoevsky.
Faydor, Feodor, Fyodor

Felix Lat. "Happy, fortunate." Not common in America, possibly because of a strong association with Felix the Cat and, more recently, "The Odd Couple's" Felix Unger. American physicist Felix Bloch.
Fee, Felic, Felice, Felicio, Felike, Feliks, Felizio, Felyx

Felton OE. Place name: "Settlement on the field."
Felten, Feltin

Fenton OE. Place name: "Settlement on the marsh." First used as a given name in the 19th century, but never widespread.

Ferdinand OG. "Bold voyager." A name that has always been more popular in Southern Europe than in the English-speaking countries. Explorers Ferdinand Magellan, Hernando Cortez; Former Philippines president Ferdinand Marcos.
Ferd, Ferdie, Ferdinando, Ferdo, Ferdynand, Fernand, Fernandas, Fernando, Hernando, Nando

Fergus Ir. Gael. "Highest choice." Mostly Scottish use.
Fearghas, Fearghus, Feargus, Fergie, Ferguson, Fergusson

Fermin Sp. "Strong."
Firmin

Fernley OE. Place name: "Fern meadow." Used since the late 19th century as a first name for children of both sexes, though primarily in Britain.
Farnlea, Farnlee, Farnleigh, Farnley, Fernlea, Fernlee, Fernleigh

Ferrand OF. "Gray-haired."
Farand, Farrand, Farrant, Ferrant

Ferris Ir. Gael. Possibly derived from **Fergus,** or else, via **Pierce,** an Irish variant of **Peter** (Gk. "Rock").
Farris, Farrish, Ferriss

Fidel Lat. "Faithful." The Puritans named boys Faithful, but Fidel is the modern form. However, since Fidel Castro's rise in Cuba, it is unlikely to be used by today's parents.
Fadelio, Fedele, Fidele, Fedelio, Fidal, Fidalio, Fidelio, Fidelis, Fidelix, Fidelo, Fido

Fielding OE. Place name: "The field." Author Henry Fielding.
Feilding, Field, Fielder

Filbert OE. "Very brilliant." Saint Philibert was a 7th-century monk who gave his name to a nut, since his feast day falls at the time when the nuts are ripe. In the U.S. filberts are more usually known as hazelnuts. The name is uncommon in any of its forms.
Bert, Filberte, Filberto, Philbert, Philibert, Phillbert

Filmore OE. "Very famous." Historically best-known under the presidency of Millard Fillmore (1850–53), but nostalgic rock fans may also remember the famous rock and roll venue in San Francisco.
Fillmore, Filmer, Fylmer

Finian Ir. Gael. "Fair." Perhaps familiar from the 1968 film *Finian's Rainbow* (Fred Astaire's last musical), but little used as a first name.
Finan, Finnian, Fionan, Fionn, Phinean, Phinian

Finlay Ir. Gael. "Fair-haired courageous one." Most often used in Scotland, where it is a common last name. Author Finley Peter Dunne.
Findlay, Findley, Finlea, Finlee, Finley, Finn, Finnlea, Finnley, Lee, Leigh

Finn Ir. Gael. "Fair" or OG. "From Finland."
Fin, Fionn, Fingal, Fingall

Finnegan Ir. Gael. "Fair." Common Irish surname. Given some prominence by James Joyce's last novel, *Finnegan's Wake.*
Finegan

Fiorello It. "Little flower." Would be almost unknown in the U.S. without the fame of New York mayor Fiorello La Guardia.

Fisk ME. "Fish." Probably an occupational name, indicating an ancestor who was a fishmonger.
Fiske

Fitch ME. Animal name: A fitch is a mammal related to the ferret or ermine. Use as a name probably goes back to an ancestor who hunted or kept fitches, rather than relating to the late-19th-century fashion for nature names.

Fitz OF. "Son of . . ." Usually short for one of the "Fitz-" names below. Derives from the Norman *filz* or "son."

Fitzgerald OF./OG. "Son of the spear-ruler." In the U.S., famous as the middle name of John F. Kennedy, and the last name of his grandfather, who was known as "Honey Fitz."

Fitzhugh OF./OG. "Son of intelligence." American painter Fitzhugh Lane.

Fitzpatrick OF./Lat. "Son of the nobleman."

Fitzroy OF. "Son of the king."

Flaminio Sp. "Roman priest."
Flamino

Flann Ir. Gael. "Ruddy, red-haired."
Flainn, Flannan, Flannery

Flavian Lat. "Yellow hair." Originally a Latin clan name, and common enough in the Roman Empire, but never revived in an English-speaking country.
Flavel, Flavelle, Flaviano, Flavien, Flavio, Flavius, Flawiusz

Fleming OE. "Man from Flanders." Flanders is now Belgium. Author (and James Bond creator) Ian Fleming.
Flemming, Flemmyng, Flemyng

Fletcher ME. Occupational name: "Arrow-maker."
Flecher, Fletch

Flint OE. Place name: "Stream." Denotes an ancestor who lived near a stream. In the U.S., "flint" is a kind of stone. Publisher Larry Flynt.
Flynt

Florent OF. "In flower." Impresario Florenz Ziegfeld.
  Fiorentino, Florentin, Florentino, Florentz, Florenz, Florinio, Florino, Floris, Florus

Florian Lat. "Blooming." Most common in Middle European countries, and currently popular in Germany.
  Florien, Florrian, Floryan

Floyd Welsh. "Gray-haired." Anglicization of **Lloyd**. Boxing star Floyd Patterson.

Flynn Ir. Gael. "Son of the ruddy man."
  Flin, Flinn, Flyn

Folke Scan. "People's guardian."
  Folker, Volker, Vollker

Forbes Scot. Gael. "Field." Used mostly in Scotland. Magazine founder Malcolm Forbes.

Ford OE. Place name. "River crossing." Most Americans will automatically associate the name with the car. Author Ford Madox Ford; automotive pioneer Henry Ford.
  Forden, Fordon

Forest OF. Occupational name: "Woodsman," or place name: "Woods." Most common in the U.S., spelled "Forrest." Novelist E. M. Forster; actor/director Forrrest Whittaker.
  Forester, Forrest, Forrester, Forster, Foster

Fortune OF. "Lucky."
  Fortunato, Fortunatus, Fortune, Fortunio, Fortuny

Foster OE. Occupational name: "Woodsman." Var. **Forest**.

Fowler OE. Occupational name: "Bird trapper."

Franchot Fr. Var. **Francis**. Actor Franchot Tone.

Francis Lat. "Frenchman" or "Free man." France was originally the Kingdom of the Franks. Saint Francis of Assisi gave the name its first fame; though he was named John, he had been nicknamed Francis because his father had him taught French as a boy. The name traveled to England via France, and was popular in the 17th and 19th centuries. **Frank** is more often used now probably owing to the rise of the feminine version and homonym, **Frances**. As **Francois,** this is currently a very popular name in France. Philosopher Sir Francis Bacon; composer Franz Josef Haydn; King Francois I of France; playwright Fer-

enc Molnar; French president Francois Mitterrand; film
director Francis Ford Coppola; "Star Spangled Banner"
author Francis Scott Key; football players Fran Tarkenton,
Franco Harris.

**Chico, Ferenc, Feri, Fran, Franco, Francesco,
Franche, Franchesco, Franchesko, Franchot,
Francisco, Franciscus, Franciskus, Francois, Franio,
Frank, Frankie, Franko, Frann, Frannie, Frans,
Fransisco, Frants, Frantz, Franz, Franzel, Franzen,
Franzin, Frasco, Frascuelo, Frasquito, Paco, Pacorro,
Panchito, Pancho, Paquito**

Frank Dim. Francis or Franklin. Used as an independent
name since the 17th century, and very popular at the turn
of the 20th century right through the 1930s. Now less
used, despite the durable popularity of its most famous
bearer, Frank Sinatra. Astronaut Frank Borman; actors
Frank Langella, Franco Nero, Frankie Muniz; architect
Frank Lloyd Wright; musician Frank Zappa.

Franc, Franco, Franck, Francke, Frankie

Franklin ME. "Free landholder." Surname transferred to
first name, popular in the U.S., especially in the 1930s and
1940s as homage to President Franklin Delano Roosevelt.
President Franklin Pierce apparently made less of an im-
pression, as his term (1853–57) did not inspire a surge of
infant Franklins.

**Francklin, Francklyn, Frank, Franklinn, Franklyn,
Franklynn**

Frazer Derivation unclear, possibly OE. "Curly hair" or an
old French place name. (Relationship to the French *fruise*
{charcoal} is debated.) Used mostly in Scottish families.

Fraser, Frasier, Frazier

Frayne ME. "Foreign."

Fraine, Frayn, Frean, Freen, Freyne

Frederick OG. "Peaceful ruler." Taken by the Hanoverian
kings to Britain, where it began a steady ascent to great
popularity that only faded in the 1930s. No longer fashionable, but sufficiently common so that it doesn't sound
outlandish. Actor Fred MacMurray; dancer Fred Astaire;
cartoon character Fred Flintstone; children's TV personal-

ity Fred Rogers; composer Frédéric Chopin; abolitionist Frederick Douglass; philosopher Friedrich Nietzsche; rock musician Fred Durst.

Eric, Erich, Erick, Erico, Erik, Eryk, Federico, Federigo, Fred, Fredd, Freddie, Fredek, Frederic, Frederich, Frederico, Frederigo, Frederik, Fredi, Fredric, Fredrick, Fredrik, Frido, Friedel, Friedrich, Friedrick, Fridrich, Fridrick, Fritz, Fritzchen, Fritzi, Fritzl, Fryderyk, Ric, Rich, Rick, Ricky, Rik, Rikki

Freeborn OE. Use of the descriptive term. May date back to slave days, or to the era of widespread serfdom, when to be born free was worthy of commemoration.

Freedom Use of the word as a given name is more common than one might think.

Freeman OE. See **Freeborn**.

Free, Freedman, Freeland, Freemon, Friedman, Friedmann

Fremont OG. "Protector of freedom." Explorer John Fremont.

Frewin OE. "Free friend."

Frewen

Frick OE. "Brave man." Industrialist and philanthropist Henry Clay Frick.

Fridolf OE. "Peaceful wolf."

Freydolf, Freydulf, Friedolf, Fridulf

Fritz Ger. Dim. **Frederick**. Film director Fritz Lang.

Frits

Fulbright OG. "Very bright." See **Filbert.**

Fulbert, Philbert, Philibert, Phillbert

Fuller OE. Occupational name: "One who shrinks cloth." The woolen fabric that was such a staple of the medieval English economy needed to be treated by fullers before it was made into clothes. The surname was most often used as a first name in the 19th century.

Fulton OE. Place name: "Settlement of the fowl" or "People's estate." Surname used as first name: in the U.S., possibly a compliment to Robert Fulton, inventor of the steamboat. Catholic bishop Fulton J. Sheen.

Fyfe Scot. Gael. Place name: Fifeshire is an area of Scotland. American cabinetmaker Duncan Phyfe.
Fife, Fyffe, Phyfe

Fyodor Rus. from Gk. "Divine gift." Var. **Theodore**. Author Fyodor Dostoyevsky.
Fedor, Feodor, Fyodr

Gable OF. Dim. **Gabriel**. When used, is probably influenced by the fame of actor Clark Gable, who was often known by just his last name.

Gabriel Heb. "Hero of God." Gabriel is an archangel who appears in Christian, Jewish, and Muslim texts. The name was uncommon in English-speaking countries, except for a spell of use in the 18th and 19th centuries, but is now used quite steadily in the United States, perhaps because of the universality of Gabriel's story. As **Gavriel,** very popular in Russia. Musician Peter Gabriel; writer Gabriel García Márquez; football player Roman Gabriel; actor Gabriel Byrne.
Gab, Gabbi, Gabbie, Gabby, Gabe, Gabi, Gabie, Gabriele, Gabrielli, Gabriello, Gabrielo, Gaby, Gavriel, Gavril, Gavrilo

Gadiel Arab. "God is my fortune."
Gaddiel

Gaetan It. Place name: Gaeta is a region in Southern Italy; the Gulf of Gaeta is just north of Naples.
Cajetan, Cajetano, Gaetano, Gaeton, Kajetan, Kajetano

Gage OF. "Oath."
Gaige

Gair Ir. Gael. "Small one."

Gaer, Geir

Galbraith Ir. Gael. "Foreign Briton." In Ireland, the name would have been used most commonly to describe a Scot. Economist John Kenneth Galbraith.

Galbrait, Galbreath, Gallbraith, Gallbreath

Gale Ir. Gael. "Foreigner"; OE. "Cheerful, happy." Much more common now as a girl's name, when it is usually a diminutive of **Abigail**. Football player Gale Sayers.

Gael, Gaell, Gaelle, Gail, Gaill, Gaille, Gaile, Gayle

Galen Gk. "Healer" or "Tranquil." A 2nd-century Greek physician named Galen was for centuries the only authority on the emergent practice of medicine. The name is seeing a flicker of trendy use among intellectuals.

Gaelan, Gaillen, Gaillen, Galeno, Galin, Gaylen, Gaylin, Gaylinn, Gaylon, Jalen, Jalin, Jalon, Jaylen, Jaylon

Gallagher Ir. Gael. "Foreign helper." Actor Peter Gallagher.

Galloway Old Gael. "Foreign Gael." Another name for a Scot. The Irish population includes a strong Scottish strain.

Gallway, Galway

Galton OE. "Owner of a rented land."

Galt, Galten, Gallton

Galvin Ir. Gael. "Sparrow" or "brilliantly white."

Gallven, Gallvin, Galvan, Galven, Galvon

Galway Irish place name: a city in Western Ireland. Critic Galway Kinnell; flutist James Galway.

Gamal Arab. "Camel."

Gamali, Gamul, Gemal, Gemali, Gemul, Jamal, Jammal, Jemaal, Jemal

Gamaliel Heb. "Recompense of God." An obscure biblical name probably brought to the U.S. by the Puritans. Little used since the 19th century. President Warren Gamaliel Harding.

Gamliel, Gmali

Gannon Ir. Gael. "Fair-skinned."

Gardner ME. Occupational name. In the eastern U.S., reminiscent of two distinguished families, known as the "blind" Gardners (the name has no *i*) or the "sighted" Gardiners. The former are famous for the Isabella Stewart Gardner Museum in Boston; the latter for Gardiner's Island on Long Island Sound.

Gardell, Gardener, Gardenner, Gardie, Gardiner, Gardnar, Gardnard

Gareth Welsh. "Gentle." The name of one of King Arthur's knights. Used in Britain since the 1930s, but rare elsewhere.

Garith, Garreth, Garret, Garyth

Garfield OE. "Spear field." Use as a first name probably honored President James Garfield, though indignation at his untimely death outweighed admiration for his skills, since his term lasted only a few months before he was assassinated in 1881. More recently the president has been upstaged by a fat orange cartoon cat who has made the name his own.

Garland OE. Place name: "Land of the spear." OF. "Wreath." Musician Garland Jeffries.

Garlan, Garlen, Garlend, Garlin, Garlind, Garllan

Garman OE. "Spearman."

Garmann, Garmen, Garmin, Garmon, Garrman

Garner ME. "To gather grain." Possibly a place name or occupational name originally, denoting an ancestor who lived near a granary, or who helped harvest grain. Actor James Garner.

Garnar, Garnier

Garnett OE. "Spear" or OF. "Red like a pomegranate." Although the girl's name is more likely to be a jewel name in the tradition of **Pearl** or **Ruby,** for boys, Garnett is usually a transferred last name. In England, boys may have been named for a famous Victorian soldier, Sir Garnet Wolseley. Basketball player Kevin Garnett.

Garnet

Garnock Old Welsh. Place name: "River of alder trees."

Garrett Var. **Gerard** dating from the Middle Ages.

Gareth, Garrard, Garret, Garreth, Garretson, Garrith, Garritt, Garrot, Garrott, Garyth, Gerrit, Gerritt, Gerrity, Jared, Jarod, Jarret, Jarrett, Jarrot, Jarrott

Garrick OE. "Spear-rule." Newscaster Garrick Utley.
  Garek, Garreck, Garrik, Garryck, Garryk
Garrison ME. "Protection, stronghold." Author Garrison
  Keillor; football player Garrison Hearst.
Garroway OE. "Spear-fighter."
  Garraway
Garson OE. "Gar's son." Gar in this case may be a diminu-
  tive of **Garrett, Gareth, Garland,** etc, or even a shorten-
  ing of **Garrison.**
Garth Scan. Occupational name: "Keeper of the garden."
  Used as a first name in this century, but never widely. Il-
  lustrator Garth Williams.
Garton OE. Place name: "Triangle-shaped settlement."
  Gorton
Garvey Ir. Gael. "Rough peace."
  Garrvey, Garrvie, Garvie, Garvy
Garvin OE. "Spear-friend."
  **Garvan, Garven, Garvyn, Garwen, Garwin, Garwyn,
  Garwynn**
Garwood OE. Place name: "Wood with fir trees."
  Garrwood, Woody
Gary OE. "Spear." Popularized by film idol Gary Cooper,
  whose name was originally Frank. Very fashionable from
  the 1950s to the 1970s, and still steadily used. Cartoonists
  Garry Trudeau, Gary Larson; actors Gary Cooper, Gary
  Oldman, Gary Sinise.
  Gari, Garey, Garrie, Garry
Gaspar Var. **Caspar.** Possibly Per. "He who guards the
  treasure."
  **Caspar, Casper, Gaspard, Gasparo, Gasper, Jaspar,
  Jasper, Kaspar, Kasper**
Gaston Fr. "Man from Gascony." Gascony is a region in the
  south of France whose inhabitants are reputed to be hot-
  tempered.
  Gascon
Gauthier Teut. "Strong ruler." Fashion designer Jean-Paul
  Gaultier.
  Galtero, Gaultier, Gautier, Gualterio, Gualtiero
Gavin Welsh. "White falcon" or "Little falcon." As

Gawain, this was the name of one of King Arthur's knights. The Scottish form, Gavin, has spread from Scotland to broad acceptance in Britain, especially in the last 30 years. Still rare in the U.S. Actor Gavin MacLeod.

Gavan, Gaven, Gavyn, Gavynn, Gawain, Gawaine, Gawayn, Gawayne, Gawen, Gawaine, Gwayn

Gaylord OF. "Lively, high-spirited." Author Gayelord Hauser.

Gaillard, Gallard, Galliard, Gay, Gayelord, Gayler, Gaylor

Gaynor Ir. Gael. "Son of the fair-skinned one." From a different root than the feminine version; for male children, this is strictly a transferred last name, and unusual at that.

Gaine, Gainer, Gainor, Gay, Gayner, Gaynnor

Geary ME. "Variable."

Gearey, Gery

Gene Dim. **Eugene** (Gk. "Well-born"). Used as an independent name since the late 19th century, especially in America. Actors Gene Kelly, Gene Wilder, Gene Hackman; drummer Gene Krupa.

Genio, Geno, Jeno

Geoffrey Var. **Jeffrey** (OG. Meaning unclear, something to do with "peace"). Norman name popular through the Middle Ages in Britain, and revived in the mid-19th century after a 350-year rest. The peak of its popularity was the 1970s in the U.S., and it is no longer a favorite. Performer Geoffrey Holder; medieval poet Geoffrey Chaucer; fashion designer Geoffrey Beene.

Geoff, Geoffery, Geoffroy, Geoffry, Geofrey, Jefery, Jeff, Jefferey, Jefferies, Jeffery, Jeffree, Jeffrey, Jeffry, Jeffrie, Jeffries, Jefry, Jeoffroi, Jephers, Jepherson, Jephrey, Jephry

George Gk. "Farmer." The popularity of the dragon-killing Saint George (patron of Boy Scouts, soldiers, and England) is undimmed by the fact that little proof of his existence can be found. George was a royal name in England, and admiration for George Washington in the U.S. gave the name a parallel popularity in the renegade colonies from the 18th century until the middle of the

20th. Now less common but still a steady presence. Singer George Michael; fashion designer Giorgio Armani; comedians George Burns, George Carlin; baseball legend George "Babe" Ruth; U.S. President George Bush; actor George Clooney.

Egor, Georas, Geordie, Georg, Georges, Georgi, Georgie, Georgios, Georgius, Georgiy, Georgy, Gheorghe, Giorgi, Giorgio, Giorgios, Giorgius, Goran, Gyorgy, Gyuri, Igor, Jerzy, Jiri, Jorgan, Jorge, Jorgen, Jurgen, Jurek, Jurik, Yorick, Yorik, Yurik, Ygor

Geraint Lat. "Old." From the same root as "geriatric." A Sir Geraint figures in certain Arthurian legends; the name is sparingly used in Britain in this century.

Gerant, Jerant, Jeraint

Gerald OG. "Spear ruler." Old name revived in the 19th century. Most popular in the middle of this century, but now less common. U.S. President Gerald Ford; TV journalist Geraldo Rivera.

Garald, Garold, Gary, Gearalt, Geralde, Geraldo, Gerard, Geraud, Gerek, Gerhard, Gerik, Gerold, Gerolld, Gerolt, Gerollt, Gerrald, Gerrard, Gerri, Gerrild, Gerrold, Gerry, Geryld, Giraldo, Giraud, Girauld, Girault, Jerald, Jerold, Jerri, Jerrold, Jerry

Gerard OE. "Spear brave." Closely related to **Gerald**, and its use follows a similar pattern. Particularly popular in Ireland. Poet Gerard Manley Hopkins.

Garrard, Garrat, Garratt, Garrett, Gearard, Gerardo, Geraud, Gerhard, Gerhardt, Gerhart, Gerrard, Gerri, Gerry, Girard, Girault, Giraud, Gherardo, Jarard, Jared, Jerard, Jerardo, Jerarrd, Jerrott

Geremia It. Var. **Jeremiah** (Heb. "The Lord exalts").

Germain Fr. "From Germany." There were several early saints called "Germanus" for their national origin, the most famous of whom gave his name to a church in Paris, Saint Germain-des-Prés. Singer Jermaine Jackson.

Germaine, German, Germane, Germanicus, Germano, Germanus, Germayn, Germayne, Germin, Jermain, Jermaine, Jermane, Jermayn, Jermayne

Geronimo It. Var. **Jerome** (Gk. "Sacred name"). Famous as the name of an Apache Indian chief and also as the cry with which American parachutists in World War II would leap from airplanes. Nobody knows why.

Heronimo, Herinomos, Hieronimo, Hieronymus, Jeronimo, Jeronimus

Gershom Heb. "Exile." Old Testament name, appearing, appropriately enough, in Exodus. The Puritans adopted it and brought it to the U.S., where it is rare, but like many Hebrew names, kept alive by Orthodox Jewish families.

Gersham, Gershon, Gershoom, Gerson

Gervase OG. Meaning unclear; possibly "With honor." Because of the popularity of a Saint Gervase, the name has been steadily used by English Catholics, but is otherwise unusual.

Garvey, Gervais, Gervaise, Gervasio, Gervasius, Gervaso, Gervayse, Gerwazy, Jarvey, Jarvis, Jervis

Giacomo It. Var. **Jacob** (Heb. "He who supplants").

Gibson OE. "Son of Gilbert." Actor Mel Gibson.

Gibb, Gibbes, Gibby, Gibbons, Gibbs, Gillson, Gilson

Gideon Heb. "Feller of trees" or "Mighty warrior." A biblical judge and hero who, with an army of only 300 men, liberated the Israelites from the Midianites. The latter-day Gideons are the group responsible for placing Bibles in hotel bedrooms.

Gideone, Gidi, Gidon, Hedeon

Gifford OE. Either "Brave giver" or "Puffy-faced." It is astonishing how rarely the derivations of names mean anything negative; this exception to that rule is used as a first name from time to time. Sports figure Frank Gifford; U.S. conservation pioneer Gifford Pinchot.

Giffard, Gifferd, Gyfford

Gilad Arab. "Hump of a camel"; Heb. "Monument, site of testimony."

Giladi, Gilead

Gilbert OG. "Shining pledge." Norman name much used in the Middle Ages, but use tapered away to mostly local favor in Scotland and Northern England. Very unusual in the U.S. Author Gilbert (G.K.) Chesterton.

Bert, Bertie, Burt, Gib, Gibb, Gil, Gilberto, Gilburt, Gill, Giselbert, Giselberto, Giselbertus, Guilbert

Gilby ONorse. "Estate of the hostage"; Ir. Gael. "Blond boy."

Gilbey, Gillbey, Gillbie, Gillby

Gilchrist Ir. Gael. "Christ's servant."

Gillchrist

Giles Gk. "Kid, young goat." The link with a shield or shield-bearer (sometimes the translation given for Giles) probably comes from the kidskin that ancient shields were made of. In modern times the name, a particular favorite in Scotland, was popular in Britain in the 1970s.

Egide, Egidio, Egidius, Gide, Gil, Gilles, Gillis, Gilliss, Gyles, Jiles, Jyles

Gillean Ir. Gael. "Servant of Saint John." Related to Gilchrist, Gillespie, Gilmore, etc., which all use the "Gil-" particle, meaning "servant."

Gilean, Gilian, Gillan, Gillen, Gilleon, Gillian, Gillion, Gillon

Gillespie Ir. Gael. "Son of the bishop's servant."

Gillaspie, Gillis

Gillett OF. "Young Gilbert." Poet Gelett Burgess.

Gelett, Gelette, Gillette

Gilmer OE. "Renowned hostage."

Gilmore Ir. Gael. "Servant of the Virgin Mary."

Gillmore, Gillmour, Gilmour

Gilroy Ir. Gael. "Servant of the redhead."

Gilderoy, Gildray, Gildroy, Gillroy, Gillray, Gilray

Gino It. Dim. **Ambrogino** (Gk. "Ever-living") or **Luigino** or possibly **Eugene** (Gk. "Well-born").

Geno, Jeno, Jino

Giovanni It. Var. **John** (Heb. "The Lord is gracious"). Artist Giovanni Bellini; author Giovanni Boccaccio; actor Giovanni Ribisi.

Geovanney, Geovanni, Gian, Gianni, Giannino, Giovan, Giovanno, Giovel, Giovell, Jovan, Jovanney, Jovanni, Jovanno

Girvin Ir. Gael. "Small rough one."

Girvan, Girven, Girvon

Giulio It. Var. **Julius** (Lat. "Youthful").
  Giuliano

Giuseppe It. Var. **Joseph** (Heb. "The Lord increases").
  Composer Giuseppe Verdi.

Giustino It. Var. **Justin** (Lat. "Just, fair").
  Giustinian, Giustiniano, Giusto

Gladwin OE. "Lighthearted friend."
  Gladwinn, Gladwyn, Gladwynne

Glanville OF. Place name: "Settlement of oak trees."

Glen Ir. Gael. Place name: "Glen." A glen is a narrow valley between hills. As a surname, Glen would indicate an
  ancestor who lived in such a valley. Singer Glen Campbell; band leader Glenn Miller; pianist Glenn Gould;
  hockey player Glen Murray.
  **Gleann, Glenn, Glennard, Glennie, Glennon, Glenny,
  Glin, Glinn, Glyn, Glynn**

Glendon Scot. Gael. Place name: "Settlement in the glen."
  Glenden, Glendin, Glenton

Glenville Gael. Place name that has been used occasionally
  as a first name. Along with **Glendon,** it has probably gained
  legitimacy from the popularity of **Glen** as a given name.
  Glanvill, Glanville, Glenvill

Goddard OG. "God-hard." Film director Jean-Luc Godard.
  **Godard, Godart, Goddart, Godhart, Godhardt,
  Gothart, Gotthard, Gotthardt, Gotthart**

Godfrey OG. "God-peace." Popular medieval name that
  faded very gradually to its near-disuse today. The fact that
  it was the name of a valet in the 1936 comic film *My Man
  Godfrey* might indicate that there was something indefin-
  ably buffoonish about the name by that date.
  **Giotto, Godefroi, Godfry, Godofredo, Goffredo,
  Gottfrid, Gottfried**

Godwin OE. "Friend of God" or "Good friend." Anglo-
  Saxon name that, though it did outlast the Norman Conquest in England, did not benefit from the 19th century
  revival that resuscitated many ancient names, so it is almost unknown in the U.S.
  **Godden, Godding, Godewyn, Godin, Godwinn,
  Godwyn, Goodwin, Goodwyn, Goodwynn, Goodwynne**

Golding OE. "Little golden one." *Lord of the Flies* author William Golding.
Golden, Goldman

Goldwin OE. "Golden friend." Film pioneer Samuel Goldwyn.
Goldewin, Goldewyn, Goldwinn, Goldwyn, Goldwynn

Goliath Heb. "Exile." Though babies are frequently named for David, the Old Testament bard, very few are given the name of the giant he killed with his slingshot. Even Cain, the first assassin, has inspired more parents. Nevertheless, the name is used from time to time.
Golliath, Golyath

Gomer OE. "Famous battle" or "Good fight." Also an Old Testament name. Grown-up fans of the goofy marine depicted by Jim Nabors in the 1960s TV series "Gomer Pyle" may have trouble taking the name seriously.

Gonzalo Sp. "Wolf." Currently a very fashionable name in Spain. Tennis star Pancho Gonzales.
Consalvo, Goncalve, Gonsalve, Gonzales

Gordon OE. Meaning unclear, possibly a place name meaning "Hill near meadows" or "Triangular hill." Historically associated with Scotland, but principal use has been 20th century. Balladeer Gordon Lightfoot; photographer Gordon Parks; hockey player Gordie Howe.
Gordan, Gorden, Gordie

Gore OE. "Spear" or "Wedge-shaped object." "Gore" is also an old term for a small, triangular-shaped piece of land, so this may be considered a place name, denoting an ancestor who lived on or near such a piece of land. Author Gore Vidal; politician Al Gore.
Goring

Gorman Ir. Gael. "Small blue-eyed one."

Gower Old Welsh. "Pure."

Grady Ir. Gael. "Renowned." A transferred Irish last name.
Gradea, Gradee, Gradey, Graidey, Graidy

Graham OE. "Gray homestead." Mostly Scottish name that was popular in Britain in the 1950s, without ever being much used in America. Author Graham Greene; inventor Alexander Graham Bell.
Graeham, Graeme, Grahame

Granger Middle French. "Farmer."
  Grainger, Grange

Grant Fr. "Tall, big." Another Scottish name, but one that has been more popular in the U.S. as a first name, probably inspired by President Ulysses S. Grant. Painter Grant Wood; actor Hugh Grant.
  Grantham, Grantley

Grantland OE. Place name: "The large fields," or possibly "Granta's fields." Sportswriter Grantland Rice.
  Grantleigh, Grantley, Grantly

Granville OF. Place name: "Big town." Though never frequent, use of the name has diminished since the 1960s, possibly because its slightly aristocratic sound has seemed too undemocratic for the age of equality.
  Granvil, Granvile, Granvill, Grenville

Gray OE. "Gray-haired." Poet Thomas Gray.
  Graye, Grey

Grayson OE. "Son of the gray-haired man."
  Graydon, Greydon, Greyson

Greeley OE. Place name: "Gray meadow" or perhaps "Green meadow." American use of the name (which is far from widespread) may reflect admiration for 19th-century journalist and politician Horace Greeley.
  Greelea, Greeleigh, Greely

Greenwood OE. Place name: "Green wood."

Gregory Gk. "Watchful, vigilant." A staple name in the Middle Ages, used by 16 popes and ten saints. Modern popularity dates from the 1940s, which means it is probably linked to actor Gregory Peck's rise to stardom. Like most names that were very fashionable in the 1950s, it is now a bit out of style. Cyclist Greg LeMond; musician Gregg Allman; actors Gregory Hines, Greg Kinnear.
  Graig, Greer, Greg, Greger, Gregg, Greggory, Gregoire, Gregoor, Gregor, Gregori, Gregorio, Gregorius, Gregos, Grigor, Grigori, Grigorios, Grygor, Grzegorz

Gresham OE. Place name: "Village surrounded by pasture."

Greville OF. Place name used occasionally in Britain.
  Grevill

Griffin Lat. "Hooked nose." The name of a mythical beast, usually half eagle (hence the hooked nose), half lion. Use as a name may be connected to the frequent heraldic use of the animal. Actor Griffin Dunne.
Griff, Griffen, Griffon, Gryffen, Gryffin, Gryphon

Griffith Welsh. "Strong chief." Used most often as a first name in the 16th through 18th centuries. This is the kind of slightly nostalgic name that seems ripe for revival, except that it's hard to say in a hurry.

Grimshaw OE. Place name: "Dark woods."

Griswold OF./Ger. Place name: "Gray woods."
Griswald

Grosvenor OF. "Great hunter." Grosvenor is the last name of one of the richest families in Britain. Their stake in London real estate is commemorated in names like Grosvenor Square.
Grosveneur

Grover OE. Place name: "Grove of trees." American use was probably inspired by President Grover Cleveland, but has faded since mid-20th century. Parents of "Sesame Street" viewers are more likely to be reminded of the self-proclaimed "cute, furry, lovable little monster" Grover.

Guido It. Var. **Guy.**

Guildford OE. Place name: "Ford with yellow flowers."
Gilford, Guilford

Guillaume Fr. Var. **William** (OG. "Will-helmet"). Poet Guillaume Apollinaire.
Guglielmo, Guilherme, Guillermo, Gwillym, Gwilym

Gunther Scan. "Warrior." Author Gunter Grass.
Guenter, Guenther, Gun, Gunn, Gunnar, Gunner, Gunners, Guntar, Gunter, Guntero, Gunthar, Guntur

Gus Dim. **Augustus** (Lat. "Worthy of respect").
Guss, Gustav

Gustave Scan. "Staff of the gods." A royal name in Sweden, used elsewhere in Europe in the 17th century, and in England in the 19th century. American use (which is uncommon) tends to harken back to Scandinavian ancestry. Composer Gustav Mahler; writer Gustave Flaubert.
Gus, Guss, Gustaf, Gustaff, Gustaof, Gustav, Gustavo, Gustavus, Gustovo, Gustus, Gusztav

Guthrie Ir. Gael. Place name: "Windy spot." Folk singers Woody and Arlo Guthrie.

    Guthree, Guthrey, Guthry

Guy Unclear origin, though some sources make a case for French "Guide" or Old German "Warrior." Made infamous in 1605 by Guy Fawkes, scapegoat of a plot to blow up the Houses of Parliament; in Britain November 5th is still Guy Fawkes Day, when a dummy was traditionally burned in effigy. The English shunned the name for two hundred years, but it became acceptable again by the mid-19th century, and use was increasing by the 1950s. To Americans, it is still a very English-sounding name. Actor Guy Pearce; film director Guy Ritchie.

    Guido

Gwynn Old Welsh. "Fair."

    Guinn, Gwin, Gwyn, Gwynedd

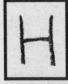

Habib Arab. "Loved one."

    Habeeb

Hackett OF./Ger. Occupational name: "Little hewer" (of wood).

    Hacket, Hackit, Hackitt

Hackman OF./Ger. Occupational name: "Hewer, hacker" (of wood). Actor Gene Hackman.

Hadden OE. Place name: "Hill of heather."

    Haddan, Haddon, Haddin, Haden, Hadon

Hadley OE. Place name: "Heather meadow." Interior designer Albert Hadley.

    Hadlea, Hadlee, Hadleigh, Hadly, Leigh

Hadrian Var. **Adrian** (Lat. "From Adria"). Adria was a north Italian city. A Roman Emperor Hadrian was responsible for the building of a vast wall across northern Britain, parts of which still stand.

Adrian, Adriano, Adrien, Hadrien

Hadwin OE. "Friend in war."

Hadwinn, Hadwyn, Hadwynne, Hedwin, Hedwinn

Hagen Ir. Gael. "Youthful one."

Hagley OE. Place name: "Enclosed meadow."

Haglea, Haglee, Hagleigh, Hagly

Haig OE. Place name: "Enclosed meadow."

Hal Dim. most commonly of **Henry**. In Shakespeare's plays about Henry IV, his son (to become Henry V) is affectionately known as "Prince Hal." Actors Hal Holbrook, Hal Linden; film director Hal Hartley.

Halbert OE. "Shining hero."

Halburt

Haldan Scan. "Half-Danish." The name takes on a certain significance when you consider that in ancient Britain, the Danes were fierce and frequent invaders.

Haldane, Halden, Halfdan, Halfdane, Halvdan

Hale OE. Either place name "from the hall," or "healthy hero." Revolutionary War hero Nathan Hale was hanged by the British as a spy. His famous last words on the scaffold were "I regret that I have but one life to lose for my country."

Hal, Hayle

Haley OE. Place name: "Hay meadow" or Ir. Gael. "Ingenious, clever." The widespread use of **Hayley** as a girl's name probably spells the end of its use as a boy's name. Football player Charles Haley; actor Haley Joel Osment.

Hailey, Haily, Haleigh, Halley, Hallie, Hayleigh, Hayley

Halford OE. Place name: "Valley ford" or "Hal's ford."

Hallford

Hall OE. Occupational name: "Worker at the hall." In this case, the hall would signify a large house or manor. Musician Darryl Hall.

Hallam OE. Place name: "The valley."

Hallem

Halliwell OE. Place name: "Holy well."

Hallewell, Hallowell, Hellewell, Helliwell

Hallward OE. Occupational name: "Guardian of the hall." Like many of these Anglo-Saxon names, it is unusual as a first name.
Halward, Halwerd, Hawarden

Halsey OE. Place name: "Hal's island."
Hallsey, Hallsy, Halsy

Halstead OE. Place name: "The manor grounds."
Hallstead, Hallsted, Halsted

Halton OE. Place name: "Estate on the hill."
Halten, Hallton, Halton

Ham Heb. "Heat." Old Testament name, one of the sons of Noah. Little used; the names of Noah's other two sons, Shem and Japheth, are even more rare.

Hamal Arab. "Lamb."
Amahl, Amal, Hamahl

Hamar ONorse. "Hammer."

Hamilton OE. Place name of several possible meanings such as "home-lover's estate" or "hill with grass." It was the surname of several aristocratic British families, and made the transition to a first name in the early 19th century. U.S. statesman Alexander Hamilton; figure skater Scott Hamilton.
Hamel, Hamelton, Hamil, Hamill

Hamill OE. "Scarred." May refer to the facial characteristic of a distant ancestor. Actor Mark Hamill; newspaper editor Pete Hamill.
Hamel, Hamell, Hammill

Hamish Scot. Var. **James** (Heb. "He who supplants"). Almost unknown outside of Scotland.

Hamlet OG./Fr. "Village: home." This name, like **Hamlin,** derives from a German root that means "home." Hamlet was a common first name until the beginning of the 19th century, but now its use would inevitably recall Shakespeare's tortured Danish prince. Author Dashiell Hammett.
Hammet, Hammett, Hammond, Hamnet, Hamnett

Hamlin OG. "Little home-lover." Actor Harry Hamlin; Abraham Lincoln's vice-president Hannibal Hamlin.
Hamblin, Hamelin, Hamlen, Hamlyn

Hanford OE. Place name: "High ford."

Hank Dim. **Henry** (OE. "Estate ruler"). Usually a nickname rather than a given name. Baseball star Hank Aaron.

Hanley OE. Place name: "High meadow."
Handlea, Handleigh, Handley, Hanlea, Hanlee, Hanleigh, Hanly, Henlea, Henlee, Henleigh, Henley

Hans Scan. Var. **John** (Heb. "The Lord is gracious"). Currently very popular in Germany. Writer Hans Christian Andersen.
Hannes, Hanns, Hansel, Hanss, Hanzel

Hanson Scan. "Son of Hans." Singing brothers Taylor, Isaac and Zac Hanson.
Hansen, Hanssen, Hansson

Harbin OF./Ger. "Little bright warrior."
Harben

Harcourt OF. "Fortified farm."
Harcort

Harden OE. Place name: "Valley of the hares."
Hardin, Hardon

Harding OE. "Son of the courageous one." This name is closely related to Hardy. U.S. President Warren G. Harding.
Hardinge

Hardwin OE. "Courageous friend."
Hardwen, Hardwinn, Hardwyn, Hardwynn

Hardy OG. "Bold, brave." Writer Thomas Hardy; fashion designer Hardy Amies.
Hardey

Harford OE. Place name: "Ford of the hares." Like many place names turned surnames, this was used as a first name in the nineteenth century.
Harfurd, Harrford, Harrfurd

Hargrove OE. Place name: "Grove of the hares." In modern times it seems curious that ancient names took such close note of the whereabouts of rabbits, but they might have constituted a significant portion of the average man's diet in those days.
Hargrave, Hargreaves

Harkin Ir. Gael. "Dark red."
Harkan, Harken

Harlan OE. Place name: "Army land."
　Harland, Harlen, Harlenn, Harlin, Harlyn, Harlynn

Harley OE. Place name: "The long field." Familiar to most people as half of the name of a great motorcycle, the Harley-Davidson.
　Arlea, Arleigh, Arley, Harlea, Harlee, Harleigh,
　Harlley, Harly

Harlow OE. Place name: "Army hill." Musician Arlo Guthrie.
　Arlo, Harlow, Harlo, Harloe

Harmon Var. **Herman** (OG. "Army man"). Actor Mark Harmon.
　Harman, Harmann, Harmonn

Harold Scan. "Army ruler." An Anglo-Saxon name revived to great popularity in the mid-19th century. It was greatly in vogue until the turn of the century, but is now rare. British Prime Minister Harold Macmillan; playwright Harold Pinter.
　Araldo, Aralt, Aroldo, Arry, Garald, Garold, Hal,
　Harald, Haralds, Haroldas, Haroldo, Harry, Herold,
　Herrold, Herrick, Herryck

Harper OE. "Harp player."
　Harpur

Harrison OE. "Son of Harry." Harrison is the more popular version of this name, but neither it nor Harris has been used much as a first name in the latter part of this century. Actor Harrison Ford.
　Harris, Harriss, Harrisson

Harry Dim. **Henry** (OE. "Home ruler"). Since about 1920, Harry has been used as an independent name about as frequently as **Henry**. In the U.S. this may have something to do with admiration for President Harry S. Truman. The cultural reach of Harry Potter may dim this name's utility for a while, though in England it is currently immensely popular. English parents may be thinking of Prince Henry of Wales, widely known as Harry. Actor Harry Belafonte; U.S. Supreme Court Justice Harry A. Blackmun; magician Harry Houdini.

Hart OE: "Stag." Poet Hart Crane; actor Hart Bochner.

Hartford OE. Place name: "Stag ford."

Hartley OE. Place name: "Stag meadow."
Hartlea, Hartlee, Hartleigh, Hartly

Hartman OG. "Hard, strong man."
Hartmann

Hartwell OE. Place name: "Well of the stags."
Harwell, Harwill

Harvey OF. "Burning for battle" or "Strong and ardent." Norman name revived in the 19th century, but now uncommon. Many people may recall the Jimmy Stewart movie *Harvey* in which he was upstaged by a giant invisible rabbit. Playwright and actor Harvey Fierstein.
Harvee, Harvie, Herve, Hervey

Harwood OE. Place name: "Wood of the hares."
Harewood

Hashim Arab. "Crusher of evil."
Hasheem, Hisham

Haskel Heb. "Intellect." Cinematographer Haskell Wexler.
Haskell

Haslett OE. Place name: "Headland with the hazel trees." Literary critic William Hazlitt.
Haslit, Haslitt, Hazel, Hazlett, Hazlitt

Hastings OE. "Son of the austere man."
Hastey, Hastie, Hasting, Hasty

Havelock Scan. "Sea competition." Author Havelock Ellis.

Haven OE. Place name: "Sanctuary, safe harbor."
Hagan, Hagen, Havin, Hogan

Hawley OE. Place name: "Hedged meadow."
Hawleigh, Hawly

Hawthorne OE. Place name: "Where hawthorn trees grow." Use in the U.S. may reflect admiration for the novelist Nathaniel Hawthorne.
Hawthorn

Hayden OE. Place name: "Hedged valley." Most commonly used in Wales. Actor Haden Christiansen.
Haden, Haydn, Haydon

Hayes OE. Place name: "Hedged area." U.S. President Rutherford B. Hayes; baseball player Charlie Hayes.
Hays

Hayward OE. Occupational name: "Keeper or guardian of the hedged enclosure."

Haywood OE. Place name: "Hedged forest." Writer Heywood Broun.
Heywood, Woody

Heath ME. Place name: "Heath." In Britain "heath" is the name for a large, open space that's not under cultivation. Football player Heath Shuler; actor Heath Ledger.

Heathcliff ME. Place name indicating a cliff near a heath. Most parents today would automatically associate it with the passionate hero of Emily Brontë's *Wuthering Heights*.

Heber Heb. "Togetherness." An Old Testament name used by the Puritans but rare in this century.
Hebor

Hector Gk. "Holds fast." One of the great heroes of the Trojan war, though today the verb form "to hector" means to bully or browbeat. Designer Ettore Sottsass; composer Hector Berlioz.
Ector, Ettore

Hedley OE. Place name: "Heathered meadow." Used in Britain in the late 19th century, but rare in the U.S.
Headleigh, Headley, Headly, Hedly

Hedeon Rus. Var. **Gideon** (Heb. "Feller of trees").
Eladio, Elado, Helado

Helmut Middle French. "Helmet." Photographer Helmut Newton.
Hellmut, Hellmuth

Henderson OE. "Son of Henry."
Hendrie, Hendries, Hendron, Henryson

Henry OG. "Estate ruler." Norman name that took root in Britain and became a royal name used by eight kings and, most recently, for the younger son of the Prince of Wales. This exposure may give new popularity to a name that was extremely common until the first quarter of this century and is now used less than unusual names like Dakota, Tristan, or Gavin. Explorer Henry Hudson; actor Henry Fonda; author Henry James; poet Henry Wadsworth Longfellow; artists Henri Matisse, Henri de Toulouse-Lautrec, Henri Rousseau; playwright Henrik Ibsen; singer Enrique Iglesias.

Arrigo, Enrico, Enrikos, Enrique, Enzio, Hal, Hank, Harry, Heike, Heindrick, Heindrik, Heiner, Heinrich, Heinrick, Heinrik, Heinz, Hendrick, Hendrik, Henerik, Henning, Henri, Henrik, Henrique, Henryk, Heriot, Herriot, Hinrich

Herbert OG. "Bright army" or "bright warrior." Norman name that faded in the Middle Ages, to be revived enthusiastically in the 19th century. Now unusual. U.S. President Herbert Hoover.

Bert, Bertie, Erberto, Harbert, Hebert, Herb, Herbie, Heribert, Heriberto

Hercules Gk. Meaning not quite clear: Possibly "glorious gift" or "glory of Hera." The legendary Greek hero who exhibited incredible strength. In modern times his physical strength might have been rivaled by the intellectual power of his namesake, Agatha Christie's fictional detective Hercule Poirot.

Ercole, Ercolo, Ercule, Herakles, Hercule, Herculie

Herman OG. "Army man." Another 19th-century revival of a Norman name, this one especially a U.S. favorite. Uncommon since the turn of the century. Authors Herman Hesse, Herman Melville.

Armand, Armando, Armin, Ermanno, Ermano, Ermin, Harman, Harmon, Hermann, Hermie, Herminio, Hermon

Hernando Sp. Var. Ferdinand. OG. "Bold voyager."

Herrick OG. "War ruler." The 17th-century poet Robert Herrick.

Herrik, Herryck

Hershel Heb. "Deer." As Herzl, this name is often used to commemorate Theodor Herzl, an early Zionist. Football player Herschel Walker; actor Herschel Bernardi.

Hersch, Herschel, Herschell, Hersh, Hertzel, Herzel, Herzl, Heschel, Heshel, Hirsch, Hirschel, Hirschl

Hesperos Gk. "Evening or evening star." The Greeks referred to Italy as Hesperia, since the sun set and the evening star rose there.

Hesperios, Hespero, Hesperus

Hewett OF. Dim. **Hugh** (Ger. "Small intelligent one").

Hewet, Hewie, Hewitt, Hewlett, Hewlitt

Hewson OE. "Hugh's son."

Hezekiah Heb. "God gives strength." Old Testament name little used since the 19th century.
Hezeki

Hieremias Gk. Var. **Jeremiah** (Heb. "Jehovah lifts up").

Hieronymos Gk. Var. **Jerome** (Heb. "Sacred name"). Painter Hieronymus Bosch.
Hierome, Hieronim, Hieronimos, Hieronymus

Hilary Gk. "Cheerful, happy." The name comes from the same root as the word "hilarious." Although it was used for boys (including a pope and a saint) until the 17th century, it was revived at the turn of the 20th century as a girl's name.
Helario, Hilaire, Hilar, Hilarid, Hilarie, Hilario, Hilarion, Hilarius, Hillary, Hillery, Hilliary, Hilorio, Ilario, Illario

Hildebrand OG. "Battle sword."
Hildebrandt, Hillebrand

Hillard OG. "Hard warrior."
Hilliard, Hillier, Hillyer

Hillel Heb. "Greatly praised." Sometimes used in honor of the celebrated 1st century Jewish scholar Rabbi Hillel.

Hilliard OG. "Battle guard" or OE. Place name: "Yard on a hill."
Hiller, Hillierd, Hillyard, Hillyer, Hillyerd

Hilton OE. Place name: "Hill settlement." Hotelier Conrad Hilton.
Hylton

Hippolyte Gk. Meaning not entirely clear, but alludes to horses. The Hippolytus in Greek legend, son of Theseus, was dragged to death by his bolting chariot-horses. Extremely rare.
Hippolit, Hippolitos, Hippolytus, Ippolito

Hiram Heb. Meaning not clear, possibly "most noble." Old Testament name little used in the 20th century, though fairly popular in the 19th. Sculptor Hiram Powers.
Hi, Hirom, Hy, Hyrum

Hobart A particularly American (though unusual) variant of **Hubert** (OG. "Bright or shining intellect").
Hobard, Hobert, Hobey, Hobie, Hoebart

Hobson OE. "Son of Robert."
   Hobbson
Hodgson OE. "Son of Roger."
   Hodge, Hodges
Hogan Ir. Gael. "Youth."
Holbrook OE. Place name: "Stream near the hollow."
Actor Hal Holbrook.
   Brook, Holbrooke
Holcomb OE. "Deep valley." "Combe" is a term, some-
times used in England, for a deep, narrow valley.
   Holcombe, Holcoomb
Holden OE. Place name: "Hollow valley."
Hollis OE. Place name: "Near the holly bushes" or "holly-tree
grove." Used as a girl's name with some frequency as well.
   Holliss, Hollister
Holmes ME. Place name: "Islands in the river." Arthur
Conan Doyle's fictional detective Sherlock Holmes.
Holt OE. Place name: "Woods, forest."
Homer Gk. "Security, pledge." The name of the classical
poet, author of the *Iliad* and the *Odyssey*. More popular in
the U.S. than elsewhere, especially in the 19th century.
Artist Winslow Homer.
   Homere, Homero, Homeros, Homerus, Omero
Honoré Lat. "Honored one." Familiar because of a fash-
ionable neighborhood and a shopping street in Paris called
the Faubourg Saint Honoré. French novelist Honoré de
Balzac.
   Honorius, Honoratus
Horace Lat. Clan name, possibly meaning "timekeeper."
Late 19th-century use may have been inspired in part by
the famous Roman poet Horace. British Admiral Horatio
Nelson; journalist Horace Greeley; basketball player Ho-
race Grant.
   Horacio, Horatio, Horatius, Horaz, Oratio, Orazio
Horst OG. "A thicket." Photographer Horst P. Horst.
   Hurst
Horton OE. Place name: "Gray settlement." Dr. Seuss char-
acter Horton of *Horton Hears a Who.*
   Horten, Orton

Hosea Heb. "Salvation." Name of an Old Testament prophet, but less popular, even in the 19th century, than other prophets' names like Joel or Amos.
Hoshea, Hoseia, Hosheia

Houghton OE. Place name: "Settlement on the headland."
Hough

Houston OE. Place name: "Settlement on the hill" or "Hugh's town." Sam Houston was the first president of the republic of Texas, before Texas entered the United States.
Hewson, Huston, Hutcheson, Hutchinson

Howard OE. Meaning unclear, possibly occupational name indicating a watchman of some kind. Millionaire Howard Hughes; sportscaster Howard Cosell.
Howie, Ward

Howe OG. "Lofty one" or ME. Place name: "Hill."
How

Howell Welsh. "Eminent, remarkable." The anglicized version of Hywel, a name mostly used in Wales. Author William Dean Howells.
Howel, Howells

Howland OE. Place name: "Land with hills."
Howlan, Howlen

Hubbard Var. Hubert.

Hubert OG. "Bright or shining intellect." An old European name that was popular around the turn of the century, but is now rare. U.S. Vice President Hubert Humphrey.
**Bert, Hobard, Hobart, Hubbard, Hube, Huberto,
Hubie, Humberto, Uberto, Ulberto**

Hudson OE. "Hugh's son." Explorer Henry Hudson.

Hugh OG. "Mind, intellect." Popular medieval name, steadily used (though at a diminishing rate) in the modern era. Its widespread use in the Middles Ages resulted in spin-off names like Hudson, Hewson, and Houston. **Hugo** is very fashionable in Spain. Film director Hugh Hudson; *Playboy* founder Hugh Hefner; U.S. Supreme Court Justice Hugo Black; actors Hugh Grant, Hugh Jackman; football player Hugh Douglas.
**Hew, Hewe, Huey, Hughes, Hughie, Hugo, Hugues,
Huw, Ugo**

Hulbert OG. "Bright grace."

  Bert, Hulbard, Hulburd, Hulburt

Humbert OG. "Renowned Hun." Made famous by the narrator of Vladimir Nabokov's *Lolita,* Humbert Humbert. Italian author Umberto Eco.

  Umberto

Humphrey OG. Meaning unclear, but alludes to peace. In the Middle Ages, the form **Humfrey** was used in England, but Humphrey was the usual form from 1700 on. Never immensely popular, especially since the 1960s. Actor Humphrey Bogart.

  Humfrey, Humfrid, Humfried, Humfry, Humph, Humphery, Humphry, Hunfredo, Onfre, Onfroi, Onofredo, Onofrio

Hunt OE. The word as a name, perhaps originally a shortening of **Hunter** or **Huntington**.

Hunter OE. Occupational name: "Hunter." Mostly Scots use. Journalist Hunter Thompson.

  Hunt

Huntington OE. Place name: "Hunter's settlement." Railroad magnate and philanthropist Henry Huntington.

  Hunt, Huntingdon

Huntley OE. Place name: "Meadow of the hunter."

  Huntlea, Huntlee, Huntleigh, Huntly

Hurlbert OE. "Shining army."

  Hulbert, Hurlburt, Hurlbutt

Hurley Ir. Gael. "Sea tide."

  Hurlee, Hurleigh, Hurly

Hurst ME. Place name: "Thicket of trees." Sometimes occurs as a place name in combination with the tree name, as in Elmhurst or Pinehurst.

  Hearst, Hirst, Horst

Hussein Arab. "Small handsome one." A royal name in Jordan.

  Husain, Husayn, Husein

Hutton OE. Place name: "Settlement on the bluff." Actor Timothy Hutton.

  Hutten

Huxford OE. Place name: "Hugh's ford."

Huxley OE. Place name: "Hugh's meadow." Author Aldous Huxley.

Huxlea, Huxlee, Huxleigh, Huxly

Hyacinthe Fr. "Hyacinth." Owing to the English-speaking tradition of flower names for girls, unlikely to be used as a boy's name, despite its origin as a male name. French painter Hyacinthe Rigaud.

Hyacinthos, Hyacinthus, Hyakinthos

Hyatt OE. Place name: "Lofty gate."

Hayatt, Hiatt

Hyde OE. Place name referring to a "hide," a measure of land current in the early Middle Ages. It amounted to about 120 acres.

Hyman Anglicized variant of **Chaim** (Heb. "Life").

Hayim, Hayyim, Hymie, Mannie

Iago Sp. Var. **James** (Heb. "He who supplants"). The Spanish name for Saint James, Santiago, was given to a number of geographical features (rivers, lakes, mountains) in South America, as well as being the capital city of Chile. Still, most English-speaking parents will remember the treacherous villain of Shakespeare's *Othello,* and pass this name by.

Jago, Yago

Ian Scot. Var. **John** (Heb. "God is gracious"). One of the few Scottish names that has achieved really broad popularity since the beginning of this century. James Bond's creator Ian Fleming; actor Ian McKellen.

Ean, Eann, Eion, Eon, Iain, Ion

Ib Dan. "Baal's pledge." Baal was an ancient god of the Semites. Ballet dancer Ib Andersen.

Ibrahim Arab. Var. **Abraham** (Heb. "Father of many"). This form of the name is more common in Muslim countries.

Ichabod Heb. "The glory is gone." An Old Testament name brought to the U.S. by the Pilgrims and given fame by Washington Irving, who named a character Ichabod Crane in *The Legend of Sleepy Hollow*.
Ikabod, Ikavod

Idris Welsh. "Eager lord." Mostly used in Wales around the turn of the century.

Ignatius Meaning unclear, though some sources suggest Latin "Ardent, burning" (from the same root as "ignite"). The most famous Ignatius is Saint Ignatius of Loyola, founder of the Society of Jesus, popularly known as the Jesuits. The name is rare in English-speaking countries.
Iggie, Ignac, Ignace, Ignacio, Ignacius, Ignatious, Ignatz, Ignaz, Ignazio, Inacio, Inigo

Igor Rus. Var. **Ingvar** (Scan. "Ing's soldier"). Composer Igor Stravinsky.
Inge, Ingemar, Ingmar, Yegor, Ygor

Ilario It. Var. **Hilary** (Gk. "Cheerful, merry").

Ilias Gk. Var. **Elijah** (Heb. "The Lord is my God").
Ilie

Imad Arab. "Support, mainstay."

Immanuel Var. **Emmanuel** (Heb. "God is among us"). German philosopher Immanuel Kant.
Imanoel, Imannuel, Imanuel

Ince Hung. "Innocent."

Ingemar Scan. "Ing's son." Ing, in Norse mythology, was a powerful god of fertility and peace. His name is an element in several modern names. Film director Ingmar Bergman.
Ingamar, Ingemur, Ingmar

Inglebert Var. **Englebert** (OE. "Angel-bright").
Ingbert, Ingelbert

Ingram OE. "Raven of Anglia." A first name until the 17th century, now more commonly a surname that is occasionally transferred.

Ingraham, Ingrahame, Ingrams, Ingrim, Yngraham, Yngraham

Ingvar Scan. "Ing's soldier."
Ingevar

Inigo OE. Var. **Ignatius**. In modern times, likely to be homage to the great English architect Inigo Jones.

Innis Scot. Gael. Place name: "Island."
Ennis, Innes, Inness, Inniss

Innocenzio It. "Innocent."
Innocent, Innocenty, Inocencio

Ioakim Rus. Var. **Joachim** (Heb. "God will judge").
Ioachim, Ioachime

Ira Heb. "Watchful." Old Testament name revived in the 19th century, but never very popular. Lyricist Ira Gershwin.

Irving OE. "Sea friend." Also a Scottish place name. Used as a first name since the middle of the last century. Composer Irving Berlin; author Irving Stone.
Earvin, Erv, Ervin, Irv, Irvin, Irvine

Irwin OE. "Boar friend." Revived from roughly 1860 to 1940s, but little used since. Author Irwin Shaw; actor Bill Irwin.
Erwin, Erwinn, Erwyn, Irwinn, Irwyn

Isaac Heb. "Laughter." In the Old Testament, Abraham's son, born when his father was 100 years old. The Puritans used the name enthusiastically, and it remained popular through the 18th century, fading very gradually. Less fashionable in the last 50 years. Scientist Isaac Newton; angler Izaak Walton; authors Isaac Bashevis Singer, Isaac Asimov; football player Isaac Bruce; singer Isaac Hanson.
Ike, Ikey, Ikie, Isaak, Isac, Isacco, Isak, Issac, Itzak, Izaak, Izak, Izik, Izsak, Yitzhak, Zack, Zak

Isaiah Heb. "The Lord helps me" or "Salvation of God." Like so many Old Testament names, popular with the Puritans in the 17th century, brought to America, and revived by the Victorians. Now rare. Basketball player Isiah Thomas.
Isa, Isaia, Isaias, Isia, Isiah, Issiah, Izaiah, Iziah

Isham OE. Place name: "Home of the iron one."

*Ishmael Heb. "The Lord will hear." Old Testament name immortalized in the first line of Herman Melville's *Moby Dick*: "Call me Ishmael."

Ismael, Ismail, Ysmael, Ysmail

Isidore Gk. "Gift of Isis." Isis was the principal goddess of ancient Egypt, and Isidore was a popular name among the ancient Greeks. There are several saints named Isidore, but the name is probably most famous in its feminine form, **Isadora.**

Dore, Dorian, Dory, Isador, Isadore, Isidor, Isidoro, Isidorus, Isidro, Issy, Izidor, Izydor, Izzy, Ysidro

Ismail Arab. A variant of **Ishmael.** Film director Ismail Merchant; football playing brothers Raghib and Qadry Ismail.

Ishmael, Ismaal, Ismael, Ismal, Ismayl, Izmail, Ysmal, Ysmail

Israel Heb. Meaning unclear, though some sources suggest "wrestling with the Lord," for this was the name given Jacob in the Old Testament after his three-day bout with his Lord. Came to be synonymous with the Jewish people, and was consequently used as the name for the new Jewish state founded in 1948. Author Israel Shenker.

Yisrael

Istvan Hung. Var. **Stephen** (Gk. "Crowned"). Film director Istvan Szabo.

Ivan Rus. Var. **John** (Heb. "God is gracious"). Used in English-speaking countries for the last hundred-odd years. Tennis star Ivan Lendl.

Ifan, Iwan

Ivo OG. "Yew wood." Since yew wood was used for bows, the name may have been an occupational one meaning "archer." The most famous form is probably **Ives** from the old nursery rhyme "As I was going to St. Ives/I met a man with seven wives . . ." Uncommon nevertheless.

Ivair, Ivar, Iven, Iver, Ives, Ivon, Yves, Yvo

Ivor Norse, meaning unclear. Possibly related to **Ivo** or to **Ingvar.** Used now and then in Britain, scarce in the U.S. Songwriter Ivor Novello.

Ifor, Ivar, Iver, Yvor

Jabez Heb. "Borne in pain." Old Testament name that lasted fairly well until around 1930.

Jabes, Jabesh

Jabir Arab. "Consolation."

Jacinto Sp. from Gk. **Hyacinth** (flower name). There was a 3rd-century Saint Hyacinth, and the name has been used for both sexes. In Greek legend, Apollo loved a beautiful youth of the name; the hyacinth flower sprang up from his blood when he died.

Giacintho, Giacinto, Jacindo

Jack Familiar form of **John** (Heb. "The Lord is gracious") or, less often, **Jacob** (Heb. "He who supplants"). Used as an independent name from the 1850s to the 1920s, then subsided. Currently experiencing quite a little renaissance, possibly because of its slightly rugged, down-home aura. Also very fashionable in England, Scotland, and Ireland. Actors Jackie Gleason, Jack Nicholson, Jack Black; comedian Jack Benny; exercise guru Jack LaLanne.

Jackie, Jackman, Jacko, Jacky, Jacq, Jacqin, Jak, Jaq

Jackson OE. "Son of Jack." May indicate an ancestor's admiration for U.S. President Andrew Jackson or, in Southern families, Civil War General Stonewall Jackson. Artist Jackson Pollock; singer Jackson Browne.

Jack, Jackie, Jacksen, Jacky, Jakson, Jaxen

Jacob Heb. "He who supplants." In the Old Testament, Jacob, Esau's brother, impersonates his brother at his blind father Isaac's deathbed by covering his hands with a goatskin ("for Esau was a hairy man"), securing the blessing meant for the elder son. One of the top five names in the U.S. for several years, though most boys officially

named Jacob will probably be called **Jake.** Senator Jacob
Javits; actor Jake Gyllenhall.

**Cob, Cobb, Cobby, Giacamo, Giacobo, Giacomo,
Giacopo, Hamish, Iacopo, Iacovo, Iago, Iakob,
Iakobos, Iakov, Jaco, Jacobo, Jacobi, Jacoby, Jack,
Jackie, Jacko, Jacky, Jacques, Jacquet, Jago, Jaime,
Jake, Jakie, Jakob, Jakov, Jakub, James, Jamesie,
Jamey, Jamie, Jamsey, Jay, Jayme, Jim, Jimmie,
Seamus, Shamus, Yakov**

Jacques Fr. Var. **James** via **Jacob.** Familiar from the well-
known song "Frère Jacques." Undersea explorer Jacques
Cousteau.

Jacot, Jacque, Jaq, Jaques

Jaden Modern invented name. Will Smith and Jada Pinkett
have a son named Jaden, probably formed from **Jada.**
Something about the ever-popular "J-" sound and the two-
syllable cadence (as well as the celebrity provenance?)
has made other parents choose this name as well.

Jael Heb. "Mountain goat." Also used for girls, although
rare in either case.

Yael

Jaime Sp. Var. **James.**

Jaimey, Jaimie, Jayme, Jaymie

Jake Dim. **Jacob.** Used independently since the 1960s, and
quite steadily chosen by today's parents.

Jamal Arab. "Handsome." Very popular in the U.S. among
black or Muslim families.

**Jamaal, Jamahl, Jamall, Jamaul, Jameel, Jamel,
Jamell, Jamil, Jamill, Jammal, Jemaal, Jemahl,
Jemall, Jimal, Jimahl, Jomal, Jomahl, Jomall**

James English variant of **Jacob** (Heb. "He who supplants"). In the New Testament there are two apostles
known as James, though the Old Testament version of the
name is always **Jacob.** The apostles are known a bit un-
fairly as James the Greater and James the Less. The name
was popularized by the Stuart kings James I and II, and
has been a stable favorite ever since, especially in the
British Isles. Writer James Joyce; actors James Mason,
James Caviezel, James Gandolfini, Jimmy Stewart; enter-

tainer Jimmy Durante; five U.S. presidents: James Buchanan, James Garfield, James Madison, James Polk, Jimmy Carter.

Diego, Giacomo, Giamo, Hamish, Iago, Jacques, Jago, Jaime, Jaimes, Jaimey, Jaimie, Jameson, Jamesie, Jamesy, Jamcy, Jamie, Jamison, Jaymes, Jaymie, Jaymz, Jim, Jimmie, Jimmy, Seamus, Seumas, Seumus, Shamus

Jameson OE. "Son of James."

Jaimison, Jamieson, Jamison

Jamie Dim. **James**. Traditionally mostly Scottish, but currently quite steadily used as an independent name. However, since it is very popular as a girl's name, this phenomenon may fade.

Jaime, Jaimie, Jamee, Jamey, Jayme

Jan Dutch. Var. **John** (Heb. "The Lord is gracious"). According to records maintained by the Social Security Administration, in 2001 Jan was the 483rd most popular name for boys. This is probably a testament to the poyglot nature of America; parents born abroad are unlikely to perceive this as a girl's name and probably even pronounce it with a "Y" rather than a "J." Painters Jan Van Eyck, Jan Vermeer.

Hans, Janek, Janos

Janson Scan. "Jan's son." Used as a first name only in this century.

Jansen, Janssen, Jansson, Jantzen, Janzen, Jenson, Jensen

Japheth Heb. "He expands." Along with Ham and Shem, one of Noah's sons. Little used, except by the Puritans.

Jareb Heb. "He will struggle."

Jared Heb. "He descends." Related to **Jordan**. Old Testament name used by the Puritans, and suddenly, inexplicably popular in the 1960s. Actor Jared Leto.

Jarad, Jarid, Jarod, Jarrad, Jarrard, Jarred, Jarrid, Jarrod, Jerad, Jerod, Jerrad, Jerred, Jerrod

Jarek Slavic. "January."

Jarman OG. "German." Film director Derek Jarman.

Jarmann, Jerman

Jaroslav Slavic. "Beauty of spring." A popular name in Czechoslovakia. Historian Jaroslav Pelikan.
Jarek, Jaroslaw

Jarrett Var. **Garrett** (OE. "Spear-brave").
Jarett, Jarret, Jarrot, Jarrott, Jerrett, Jerrot, Jerrott

Jarvis Var. **Gervase** (OG. Meaning unclear: possibly "with honor"). Musician Jarvis Cocker.
Jarvey, Jary, Jervey, Jervis

Jason Heb. "The Lord is salvation." The name is actually a variation of **Joshua,** formed by biblical translators. Jason was a legendary Greek hero who, after many adventures, recovered the Golden Fleece from an enemy kingdom. The name was phenomenally popular in the 1970s after centuries of sporadic use, and is still very well used. Actors Jason Robards, Jason Lee, Jason Priestley, Jason Patric, Jason Biggs.
Jace, Jacen, Jaisen, Jaison, Jase, Jasen, Jasin, Jasun, Jay, Jayce, Jaysen, Jayson

Jasper Eng. Var. **Caspar**. Possibly Persian "He who guards the treasure." Jasper is also a strikingly colorful variety of quartz. Painter Jasper Johns.
Gaspar, Gasper, Jaspar, Jesper

Javier Sp. Var. **Xavier**. Meaning obscure, but refers to Saint Francis Xavier.
Havier, Haviero, Javi, Javiero

Jay Lat. "Jaybird." A medieval name that has survived especially in the U.S., where it is given to boys and girls alike. Its use may be inspired by the first Chief Justice of the U.S. Supreme Court, John Jay. Financier Jay Gould; comedian Jay Leno; author Jay McInerney; actors Jaye Davidson, Jay Mohr.
Jae, Jaye, Jeh

Jean Fr. Var. **John** (Heb. "The Lord is gracious"). Author and artist Jean Cocteau; playwright Jean Molière; author Jean-Paul Sartre; actor Jean-Claude Van Damme.

Jed Dim. **Jedidiah**. Lent a certain rustic aura by Jed Clampitt, a character on the popular 1960s TV show "The Beverly Hillbillies."
Jedd, Jedediah

Jedidiah Heb. "Beloved of the Lord." Old Testament name that was used by the Puritans in the 17th century.
Jedd, Jedediah

Jeff Dim. **Jefferson, Jeffrey.** Used as an independent name in this century. Actors Jeff Daniels, Jeff Goldblum, Jeff Bridges.

Jefferson OE. "Son of Jeffrey." Surname used as a first name. A sterling example of this use is president of the Confederacy Jefferson Davis, who was born in 1808, during the presidency of Thomas Jefferson.
Jeff, Jeffers, Jeffersson, Jeffey, Jeffie

Jeffrey OG. Meaning unclear, but refers to "peace." Norman name popular through the Middle Ages in Britain and revived in the mid-19th century after a 350-year rest. The peak of its popularity was the 1970s in the U.S., with this form preferred to **Geoffrey.** Race-car driver Jeff Gordon.
Geoff, Geoffrey, Geoffroi, Geoffroy, Geoffry, Geofrey, Geofry, Godfrey, Godfry, Gottfried, Jefery, Jeff, Jefferey, Jefferies, Jeffery, Jeffree, Jeffries, Jeffry, Jeffy, Jefry, Jeoffroi, Joffre, Joffrey

Jem Dim. **James** or **Jeremiah.** Rare as nickname or independent name.

Jenkin Flemish. "Little John." A name as popular and well used as **John** has naturally produced numerous last names as well, some of which find their way back to first-name status.
Jenkins, Jenkyn, Jenkyns, Jennings

Jens Scan. Var. **John.**
Jensen, Jenson, Jensson

Jeremiah Heb. "The Lord exalts." Old Testament prophet who lived in Jerusalem when it fell to the Babylonians. The Book of Jeremiah is so relentlessly gloomy in outlook that "jeremiad" has become the term for a lengthy denunciatory complaint. The Puritans used Jeremiah somewhat, but **Jeremy** has eclipsed it in modern times.
Dermot, Dermott, Diarmid, Geremia, Jem, Jemmie, Jereme, Jeremia, Jeremias, Jeremija, Jeremiya, Jeremy, Jermyn, Jerry, Yeremia, Yeremiya, Yeremiyah

Jeremy Modern form of **Jeremiah.** One source suggests

that the modern penchant for Jeremy was sparked by a 1960s TV series called "Here Come the Brides." This may be true, since the Jeremy on the show had brothers named Jason and Joshua, names that were simultaneously fashionable. Actor Jeremy Irons; football player Jeremy Shockey.

Jem, Jemmie, Jemmy, Jeramee, Jeramey, Jeramie, Jere, Jereme, Jeremie, Jeromy, Jerry

Jermaine Var. **Jarman** (OG. "German") or **Germain** (Fr. "From Germany"). Made famous by Michael Jackson's older brother, Jermaine. Basketball player Jermaine O'Neal.

Germain, Germaine, Jermane, Jermin, Jermyn

Jerome Gk. "Sacred name." The 5th-century Saint Jerome was responsible for a Latin translation of the Bible. He is often portrayed with a lion, from the legend that he removed a thorn from the lion's pad and the beast rewarded him with lifelong fidelity. The name has been best used in the 16th and 19th centuries. Songwriter Jerome Kern; choreographer Jerome Robbins; football player Jerome Bettis.

Gerome, Geronimo, Gerrie, Gerry, Hierome, Hieronim, Hieronimo, Hieronimos, Hieronimus, Hieronymos, Hieronymus, Jairo, Jairome, Jeroen, Jeromo, Jeronimo, Jerrome, Jerron, Jerrone, Jerry

Jerry Dim. **Jeremy, Gerald**, etc. Actor Jerry Orbach.

Gerrey, Gerry, Jerre, Jerrey, Jerrie

Jerzy Pol. Var. **George** (Gk. "Farmer"). Writer Jerzy Kozinski.

Jesse Heb. "The Lord exists." The biblical father of King David. In America the formidable athlete Jesse Owens (whose success at the 1936 Olympics chagrined the Nazis) has given the name great resonance for black families; the fame of politician Jesse Jackson may continue to do so. Outlaw Jesse James.

Jess, Jessie, Yishai

Jesus Heb. "The Lord is salvation." Used mostly by families of Latin American origin, but **Joshua,** from the same Hebrew derivation, is tremendously popular across the U.S.

Jesous

Jethro Heb. "Preeminence." Old Testament name that occurred from time to time until the late 19th century. A flicker of modern use may have been inspired by the rock group Jethro Tull.

Jeth, Jethroe

Jim Dim. **James** (Heb. "He who supplants"). Used occasionally as an independent name. Actors Jim Broadbent, Jim Carrey.

Jimi, Jimmee, Jimmey, Jimmie, Jimmy, Jimson

Joab Heb. "Praise Jehovah."

Joachim Heb. "God will judge." Composer Josquin Des Pres; actor Joaquin Phoenix.

Akim, Ioakim, Jachim, Jakim, Joacheim, Joaquim, Joaquin, Josquin, Yachim, Yakim

Job Heb. "The afflicted." In the Old Testament, the Book of Job recounts the trials of an innocent man who was sorely tried by his God but remained faithful: hence "the patience of Job." Revived by the Puritans and used fairly steadily since the 17th century.

Joab, Jobe

Jock Familiar var. **Jacob** (Heb. "He who supplants") or **John** (Heb. "The Lord is gracious"). A slang term for a Scotsman, probably because the local accent turns **Jack** into Jock. Not actually used in Scotland, and in the U.S. avoided because it is a slightly derogatory term for an athlete. Sportsman Jock Whitney.

Jocko

Jody Familiar var. **Joseph** (Heb. "Jehovah increases"). In Marjorie Kinnan Rawlings's Pulitzer Prize-winning novel *The Yearling,* the young hero is called Jody, but the name is more likely to be used for a girl.

Jodey, Jodi, Jodie

Joe Dim. **Joseph.** Sometimes given as an independent name. Baseball player Joe diMaggio; boxer Joe Louis; hockey player Joe Thornton.

Joel Heb. "Jehovah is the Lord." Along with **Amos,** the most common of the Old Testament prophets' names, though **Hosea** also occurs. Joel is currently very popular in Spain. For some reason the parents of the late 20th century who have scoured the Old Testament for names have had a strong predilection for those beginning with *J*. Actors Joel McCrea, Joel Grey.

Yoel

John Heb. "The Lord is gracious." Given a sound foundation by two crucial saints, John the Baptist and John the Evangelist. (There are another thirty-odd significant saints named John.) The name has been used by 25 popes, an English king, and endless numbers of parents all over the world. In the English-speaking countries it was the most popular boy's name for over 400 years, losing ground only in the 1950s. Now some of its variants, like **Ian** and **Sean,** are gaining. Actors John Gielgud, John Barrymore, John Wayne, John Cusack, John Leguizamo, Johnny Depp; four U.S. presidents: John F. Kennedy, John Tyler, John Adams, John Quincy Adams; poet John Donne; Beatle John Lennon; composer Johannes Bach; football player John Elway; lawyer Johnnie Cochrane.

Anno, Ean, Eian, Eion, Euan, Evan, Ewan, Ewen, Gian, Giannes, Gianni, Giannis, Giannos, Giovanni, Hannes, Hanno, Hans, Hanschen, Hansel, Hansl, Iain, Ian, Ioannes, Ioannis, Ivan, Ivann, Iwan, Jack, Jackie, Jacky, Jan, Jancsi, Janek, Janko, Janne, Janos, Jean, Jeanno, Jeannot, Jehan, Jenkin, Jenkins, Jens, Jian, Jianni, Joannes, Joao, Jock, Jocko, Johan, Johanan, Johann, Johannes, Johon, Johnie, Johnnie, Johnny, Jon, Jona, Jonnie, Jovan, Jovanney, Jovanni, Jovonni, Juan, Juanito, Juwan, Sean, Seann, Shane, Shaughn, Shaun, Shawn, Vanek, Vanko, Vanya, Yanni, Yanno, Zane

Johnson OE. "Son of John." Mostly 19th-century use. Playwright Ben Jonson; track star Michael Johnson; President Lyndon B. Johnson.

Jonson, Johnston

Jonas Gk. var. **Jonah** (Heb. "Dove"). Jonah is the biblical hero who was swallowed alive by a whale, in whose belly he lived for three days. He had been thrown overboard by sailors from the ship he was traveling on in order to calm a stormy sea; by extension, the term "Jonah" means someone who brings bad luck. The name, nevertheless, has been used with some frequency, though never immense popularity. Medical pioneer Jonas Salk.

Jonah, Jonaso

Jonathan Heb. "Gift of Jehovah." Related to **Nathan,** rather than to **John.** In the Old Testament, the great friend of King David. Used in the 17th century, then neglected from the 18th until the 1940s. Some of its current extensive use probably comes about because it resembles John. English author Jonathan Swift; actors Jon Voight, Jonathan Lipnicki.

Johnathan, Johnathon, Jon, Jonathon

Jones Surname derived from John. Particularly popular in Wales.

Jordan Heb. "Descend." Named after the River Jordan. First used in the Middle Ages by Crusaders returning from the Holy Land. Revived slightly in the 19th century. Unusual in that it is quite popular for both boys and girls. Male use has the edge at the moment.

Giordano, Jared, Jarred, Jarod, Jarrod, Jarrot, Jarrott, Jerad, Jerred, Jerrod, Jerrot, Jerrott, Jordaan, Jordao, Jordon, Jori, Jory, Jourdain, Jourdan, Jud, Judd

Jorge Sp. Var. **George** (Gk. "Farmer"). Baseball player Jorge Posada.

Jorgen Dan. Var. **George** (Gk. "Farmer").

Jeorg, Jerzy, Jorg, Jori, Joris, Jurgen, Juri

José Sp. Var. **Joseph.** Opera singer José Carreras; baseball player José Canseco; jockey José Santos.

Joseph Heb. "Jehovah increases." Name that occurs for principal figures in both the Old and the New Testaments of the Bible. It has been less widely used than **John** and has fewer international variants. Currently a top-ten name in England. Actors Josef Sommer, Joseph Fiennes; writers Joseph Conrad, Joseph Wambaugh; revolutionary Che Guevara; painter Joseph M.W. Turner.

Che, Giuseppe, Giuseppino, Iosep, Iosef, Iosif, Iosip, Jessop, Jessup, Jo, Jodi, Jodie, Jody, Joey, Joop, Joos, Jose, Josef, Joseito, Josep, Josip, Josif,

Josephe, Josephus, Joss, Josue, Joszef, Jozef, Osip,
Pepe, Pepito, Peppi, Pino, Pipo, Sepp, Seppi, Yousef,
Yusif, Yussuf, Yusuf, Yusup, Yuszef

Joshua Heb. "The Lord is salvation." An Old Testament
hero, Moses' successor. Passed over by the Puritans, revived somewhat in the 18th century, and currently immensely fashionable in the U.S. and Britain alike. Painter
Joshua Reynolds; director Joshua Logan; actors Josh
Lucas, Josh Hartnett.

Josh, Joshuah, Josua, Josue, Joushua, Jozua,
Yehoshua

Josiah Heb. "The Lord supports." An Old Testament king
of Judah. Most common in the 18th century, now rare.
Porcelain entrepreneur Josiah Wedgwood.

Josia, Josias

Juan Sp. Var. **John** (Heb. "The Lord is gracious"). Basketball player Juwan Howard; baseball player Juan Gonzales;
King Juan Carlos of Spain.

Juwan

Judah Heb. "Praise." **Jude** is the more common form.

Jud, Judas, Judd, Jude

Jude Lat. Var. **Judah.** Very unusual, probably because of
the traitorous apostle Judas Iscariot. There was, however,
another apostle named Jude who now enjoys some popularity as the patron saint of lost causes. Actor Jude Law.

Jud, Judah, Judas, Judd, Judsen, Judson

Jules Fr. Var. **Julius.** Author Jules Verne; playwright and
cartoonist Jules Feiffer.

Julian Lat. Var. **Julius.** First took hold in the 18th century,
and became fashionable in the 1950s through 1970s. The
French form, **Julien,** is currently popular in France.
Steadily used today. Musician Julian Lennon; activist Julian Bond.

Jolyon, Julyan, Julianus, Julien

Julius Lat. Clan name: "Youthful." Common in Christian
Rome and revived in the 19th century. Now scarce.
Singers Julio Iglesias, Julius La Rosa; basketball player
Julius Erving.

Giulio, Jolyon, Jule, Jules, Julio

Juri Slavic. Var. **George** (Gk. "Farmer").

    Jaris, Yuri

Justin Lat. "Fair, righteous." Another name well used by Roman Christians, but unusual elsewhere until very recently. It is now extremely fashionable, right up there with **Joshua, James,** and **John**. Actor Justin Henry; singer Justin Timberlake.

    Giustino, Giusto, Joos, Joost, Just, Juste, Justen, Justinas, Justinian, Justinius, Justino, Justinus, Justis, Justo, Justus, Justyn

Kaiser Var. **Caesar** (Lat. Possibly "hairy"). The connotations, of course, are of imperial rule, as in Germany's Kaiser Wilhelm.

Kalil Arab. "Friend." Writer Kahlil Gibran.

    Kahil, Kahleel, Kahlil, Kaleel, Khaleel, Khalil

Kamal Arab. "Perfection, perfect."

    Kameel, Kamil

Kane Welsh. "Beautiful" or Ir. Gael. "Warrior's son." Surname transferred occasionally to first name in this century.

    Cahan, Cahane, Cain, Kahan, Kahane, Kain, Kaine, Kayne, Keane

Kareem Arab. "Highborn, generous." Basketball star Kareem Abdul-Jabbar.

    Karam, Karim

Karl OG. "Man." Var. **Charles**. The Germanic form of the name; as **Carl,** it was fairly well used in the U.S. 1850–1950. *K* spellings are not as readily adopted for boys' names as they are for girls'. Fashion designers Karl Lagerfeld, Karl Kani; economist Karl Marx; basketball player Karl Malone.

Carl, Kale, Karel, Karlan, Karlens, Karli, Karrel, Karol, Karoly

Kaspar Var. **Caspar** (Possibly Per. "He who guards the treasure"). Originally **Jasper**. Traditionally one of the Three Kings (perhaps the one carrying the gold) was named **Caspar**.

Kasper

Kavan Ir. Gael. "Handsome."

Cavan, Kayvan, Kayven

Kavanagh Ir. Gael. "Follower of Kevin." Principally an Irish surname.

Cavanagh, Cavanaugh, Kavanaugh

Kay Old Welsh. "Rejoicing." Ancient name borne, in legend, by one of the knights of the Round Table. Now all but obliterated as a male name by the women's name **Kay,** which is a diminutive of **Katherine.**

Kai, Keh

Kazimierz Var. **Casimir** (Slavic. "Bringing peace"). Associated with Poland for her famous 11th-century king who brought peace to the nation.

Kaz, Kazimir, Kazmer

Keane OE. "Sharp." As in a "keen wit" or a "keen eye." Actor Edmund Kean.

Kean, Keen, Keene

Kearney Var. **Carney** (Ir. Gael. "The winner").

Karney, Karny, Kearny

Kedar Arab. "Powerful."

Kadar, Keder

Keefe Ir. Gael. "Handsome; lovable, loved."

Keeffe

Keegan Ir. Gael. "Small and ardent." Historian John Keegan.

Keagan, Keagen, Keegen, Keeghan, Kegan

Keelan Ir. Gael. "Small and slim."

Kealan, Keallan, Keallin, Keilan, Keillan, Kelan

Keeley Ir. Gael. "Handsome." Also possibly a variant of **Kelly** (Ir. Gael. "Eager for battle").

Kealey, Kealy, Keelie, Keely

Keenan Ir. Gael. "Small and ancient." Football player

Keenan McCardell; actors Keenan Ivory Wayans, Keenan Wynn.
Keen, Keenen, Kienan, Kienen

Keir Gael. "Dark-skinned, swarthy." Actor Keir Dullea.

Keith Scot. Gael. "Forest." Originally a place name, adopted as a first name for non-Scots in the 19th century. Peaked in the 1960s in the U.S., but still fairly steadily used. Baseball player Keith Hernandez; Rolling Stone Keith Richard; actor Keith Carradine.

Kelby ONorse. Place name: "The farm near the spring."
Kelbey, Kelbie, Kellby

Kell ONorse. Place name: "Spring."

Kelly Ir. Gael. "Warrior." Originally a very common Irish last name, and very popular as a girl's first name from the 1950s. Use for boy babies has diminished accordingly. TV producer David E. Kelley.
Kelley, Kellie

Kelsey OE. Place name, incorporating a word particle that means "island." Until ten years ago this was a boy's name, but by 1995, it was one of the top twenty girl's names in the U.S. Actor Kelsey Grammer.
Kelsie, Kelsy

Kelton OE. Place name: "Town of the keels." Probably originally referred to a town where ships were built.
Keldon, Kelltin, Kellton, Kelten, Keltin, Keltonn

Kelvin Meaning and origin unclear; possibly OE. "Keel friend" (keel, in this case, standing in for ship) or a place name alluding to a river. Brief spurt of use in the 1920s was mostly British.
Kelvan, Kelven, Kellven, Kelvon, Kelvyn, Kelwin, Kelwinn, Kelwyn

Kemp ME. "Fighter, champion." Basketball player Shawn Kemp.

Kempton ME. Place name: "From the warrior's settlement."

Ken Dim. **Kenneth** and other "Ken-" names. Used independently, but parents who played with Barbie dolls may be hard put to name a baby after Barbie's boyfriend Ken. Baseball player Ken Griffey, Jr.; singers Kenny Rogers,

Kenny Loggins; saxophone player Kenny G; writer Ken Kesey.

Kenney, Kennie, Kenny

Kendall OE. Place name: "The valley of the Kent," a river in western England. Some sources also suggest "the bright river valley." In either case, a transferred surname used as a first name since the 19th century.

Kendal, Kendel, Kendell, Kendill, Kendle, Kendyl, Kendyll, Kenny

Kendrick OE. "Royal ruler." Revived as a first name in the 19th century, but unusual.

Kendricks, Kendrik, Kendryck, Kenric, Kenrick, Kenricks, Kenricks, Kenrik

Kenelm OE. "Brave helmet."

Kenhelm, Kennelm

Kenley OE. Place name: "The king's meadow."

Kenlea, Kenlee, Kenleigh, Kenlie, Kenly

Kenn Welsh. "Bright water." Also a variant of **Kenneth**.

Kennard OE. "Brave and strong."

Kennaird

Kennedy Ir. Gael. Some sources suggest "Helmet/head," while "Ugly/head" is also offered, which would make this one of the rare names to refer to negative characteristics or habits possessed by ancestors. Use of Kennedy as a first name may be inspired by President John F. Kennedy. Violinist Nigel Kennedy.

Canaday, Canady, Kennedey

Kenneth Ir. Gael. "Handsome" or "sprung from fire." Originally a favorite Scottish name that spread starting in the late 19th century. Very popular in the U.S. in the 1950s and 1960s. Art historian Kenneth Clark; actor Kenneth Branagh.

Ken, Kennet, Kennett, Kennith, Kenny

Kent OE. Place name: a county in England. Familiar as a surname, and used in the U.S. as a first name. In the 1930s and 1940s monosyllabic names (**Clark, Burt, Kirk**) seemed to project a manly aura and enjoyed a consequent burst of popularity. Football player Kent Graham; artist Rockwell Kent.

Kennt, Kentt

Kenton OE. Place name: "The royal settlement." In use as a first name since the 1950s.

Kentan, Kentin, Kenton

Kenward OE. "Brave or royal guardian."

Kenway OE. "Brave or royal fighter."

Kenyon Ir. Gael. "Blond."

Kermit Ir. Gael. "Without envy." A variant of **Dermot,** made famous (and virtually unusable) by the popular green Muppet Kermit the Frog.

Kern Ir. Gael. "Small swarthy one."

Curran, Kearn, Kearne, Kearns

Kernaghan Ir. Gael. "Victorious."

Carnahan, Kernohan

Kerr Scan. Place name: "The swampy place." Used basically in Scotland as a first name.

Carr, Karr

Kerry Irish place name: Kerry is a county in southwestern Ireland. Also, according to some sources, "dark-haired." Used more often for girls. Football player Kerry Collins; basketball player Kerry Kittles.

Kearie, Keary, Kerrey, Kerrie

Kerwin Possibly OE. "Swamp friend" or Ir. Gael. "Little dark one."

Kervin, Kervyn, Kerwinn, Kirwan, Kirwen

Kevin Ir. Gael. "Handsome" (a meaning that certainly applies to two famous Kevins, actors Kline and Costner). Originally an Irish name that spread to wider use in the 20th century. Most popular in the 1960s, but still fairly standard. Makeup artist Kevyn Aucoin; basketball player Kevin Garnett.

Kevan, Keven, Kevon, Kevyn

Khalid Arab. "Never-ending."

Kieran Ir. Gael. "Dark, swarthy." Becoming popular in Ireland, and showing some signs of spreading farther afield. Actor Kieran Culkin.

Ciaran, Keiran, Keiron, Kernan, Kieren, Kiernan, Kieron, Kierren, Kierrin, Kierron

Kidd Middle English. "Kid, young goat." Probably an occupational name, possibly indicating an ancestor who kept goats. Pirate Captain William Kidd.

Kidder

Killian Ir. Gael. "Small and fierce." From the same root as **Kelly.** Mysteriously enough, this name is currently very popular in France.

Kilean, Kilian, Killean

Kimball OE. "Bold war-leader."

Kimbal, Kimbel, Kimbell, Kimble

Kimberly OE. Place name: The "-ly" suffix indicates a meadow. *The Facts on File Dictionary of First Names* traces the masculine use of the name to the Boer War, when many English soldiers were fighting in the South African town of Kimberley. It has been virtually taken over by girls, however, and was a great favorite in the 1960s.

Kim, Kimbo, Kimberleigh, Kimberley

Kincaid Celt. "Battle leader." Artist Thomas Kinkade.

Kinkade

King OE. "King." A last name since the Middle Ages. Modern use may be homage to Martin Luther King.

Kingman OE. "King's man." U.S. Ambassador Kingman Brewster.

Kingsley OE. Place name: "King's meadow." Surname transferred to first name, particularly in Britain. Novelist Kingsley Amis; actor Ben Kingsley.

Kingslea, Kingslie, Kingsly, Kinsey, Kinslea, Kinslee, Kinsley, Kinslie, Kinsly

Kingston OE. Place name: "King's settlement."

Kingswell OE. Place name: "King's well."

Kinnard Ir. Gael. Place name: "The tall hill."

Kinnaird

Kinnell Ir. Gael. Place name: "Top of the cliff."

Kipp OE. Place name: "Pointed hill."

Kip, Kyp

Kirby OE. Place name: "Church village." Mostly 19th-century use. Baseball player Kirby Puckett.

Kerbie, Kerbey, Kirbey, Kirbie, Kirkby

Kiril Gk. "The Lord." As **Cyril,** used in Britain around the turn of the century.

Cyril, Cyrill, Kirill, Kirillos, Kyril, Kyrill

Kirk ONorse. "Church." Some 19th-century use in Britain, but it was really brought into circulation by actor Kirk Douglas.

Kerk, Kirke

Kirkley OE. Place name: "Church meadow." Like the following names, this became a last name after being a place name, and is only occasionally used as a first name.

Kirklea, Kirklee, Kirklie, Kirkly

Kirkwell OE. Place name: "Church spring."

Kirkwood OE. Place name: "Church forest." Author James Kirkwood.

Kit Dim. **Christopher** (Gk. "Bearer of Christ"). A nickname for Christopher long before **Chris** was thought of. Christopher Columbus named the Caribbean island of Saint Kitts for himself and Saint Christopher, the patron of travelers.

Kitt

Klaus Var. **Claus** (dim. **Nicholas**; Gk. "Victorious people"). Even spelled with the more anglicized "C," unusual in English-speaking countries. Actor Klaus Maria Brandauer.

Klaas, Klaes

Klemens Var. **Clement** (Lat. "Mild, giving mercy").

Klemenis, Klement, Kliment

Knox OE. Place name. May be a variant of **Knoll.** Religious reformer John Knox founded the Scottish Presbyterian church in the mid-16th century.

Knut Scan. "Knot." Brought to Britain by the 11th century King Canute of Denmark, who became the King of England in 1016. Very rare, except in those of Scandinavian descent. Football coach Knute Rockne; author Knut Hamsun.

Canute, Cnut, Knute

Konrad Var. Conrad (OG. "Courageous advice"). Despite occasional increases in numbers, a name that has never been widely popular in English-speaking countries. Anthropologist Konrad Lorenz.

Kord, Kort, Kunz

Konstantin Var. **Constantine** (Lat. "Steadfast"). The form **Constant** was popular among the Puritans (as a virtue name) and was revived in the 19th century to occasional modern use. Constantine, the Latin form, was the name of the first Christian Roman emperor, and a royal name in Greece.

Konstant, Konstantio, Konstanty, Konstanz, Kostas

Kornel Var. **Cornelius** (Lat. "Like a horn"). Comes from a Latin clan name and, as Cornelius, was often used under the Roman Empire. Painter Kees Van Dongen.

Kees, Kornelisz, Kornelius, Kornell

Krispin Var. **Crispin** (Lat. "Curly-haired"). Saint Crispin, supposedly a 3rd-century martyr, is patron of shoemakers. The name was somewhat popular in Britain in the 17th and 18th centuries, and was revived in the 1960s, but has not spread to the U.S. in any significant numbers.

Kristian Var. **Christian** (Gk. "Anointed, Christian"). A girl's name that (contrary to the usual movement) became a male name, possibly after the huge success of John Bunyan's *Pilgrim's Progress* (1684), whose hero is called Christian.

Krist

Kristofer Var. **Christopher** (Gk. "Carrier of Christ"). The much-loved story of Saint Christopher is that he lived alone by a river, carrying travelers across the ford on his back. A child whom he was carrying became almost too heavy to bear, and proved afterward to be the Christ child. Actually the tale has little basis in fact, and probably springs from the literal translation of the name, which originally alluded to carrying Christ in one's heart. Actor Kris Kristofferson.

Kristoffer, Kristofor, Kristopher, Kristophor, Krzysztof

Kurt Ger. Var. **Conrad** (OG. "Courageous advice"). Actor Kurt Russell; author Kurt Vonnegut; musician Kurt Cobain; football player Kurt Warner.

Kyle Scot. Place name: "Narrow spit of land." Well-traveled parents may have crossed the Kyle of Lochalsh to reach the Isle of Skye. Kyle is one of the two dozen most popular names in the U.S. for boys, and a "feminine" version of the name, **Kylie,** is almost as hot for girls. Actor Kyle MacLachlan.

Laban Heb. "White." Old Testament name revived by the Puritans. Has appeared sporadically since.
Lavan

Lachlan Scot. Gael. Either "Belligerent" or "From the fjord-land," which would refer to Norway, thus indicating a Viking ancestor. The name is unusual, even in Scotland. Media magnate Lachlan Murdoch.

Lacy OF. Place name of obscure meaning, used as a boy's name in the 19th century more commonly for girls today, and only occasionally for either gender.
Lacey, Lacie

Ladd ME. "Manservant or young man." Most likely to be a transferred surname. Actor Alan Ladd.
Lad, Laddey, Laddie, Laddy

Laird Scot. "Lord of the land."

Lamar OG. "Land famous." Plutocrat Lamar Hunt.
Lamarr, Lemar, Lemarr

Lambert OG. "Land brilliant." Medieval and Renaissance use was encouraged by veneration for the Belgian martyr Saint Lambert, but in the more secular times since, nothing has occurred to save it from neglect. Actor Christopher Lambert.
Lambart, Bert, Lamberto, Lambirt, Landbert

Lamont Scan. "Man of law." Mostly U.S. use around the 1940s. Bicycle racer Greg LeMond.
Lammond, Lamond, Lemond

Lance Var. **Lancelot**. Mildly popular on its own in the middle of this century. Parents may have erroneously thought it referred to the medieval jousting weapon. Bicycle racer Lance Armstrong; singer Lance Bass.
Lantz, Lanz, Launce

Lancelot OF. "Servant." Most famous, of course, for the knight of the Round Table who seduced King Arthur's wife, Guinevere. Used as a first name in the romantic 19th century, rare since the middle of this century.
Launcelot

Lander ME. Occupational name: Possibly "Laundry-man" or "Landowner." More probably the latter, since the laundering trade, in medieval Britain, was unlikely to provide much of a career.
Land, Landers, Landis, Landiss, Landor, Landry

Landon OE. Place name: "Grassy plain."
Land, Landan, Landen, Landin

Lane ME. Place name. More common for boys than for girls, though still unusual for both. This is the kind of name that is likely to be a mother's maiden name transferred to a first name.
Laine, Layne

Lang ONorse. "Tall one."
Lange

Langdon OE. Place name: "Long hill."
Landon, Langden

Langford OE. Place name: "Long ford." Many English place names are just compounds of familiar elements that still exist in our spoken language.

Langley OE. Place name: "Long meadow."
Langlea, Langlee, Langleigh, Langly

Langston OE. Place name: "Long town" or "Tall man's town." The "Lang-" element could have two meanings in this instance. Poet and writer Langston Hughes.
Langsden, Langsdon, Langton

Langward OE. Descriptive/occupational name: "Tall guardian."

Langworth OE. Place name: "Long paddock."

Lanny Dim. **Roland**. OF. "Famous land." More common as a nickname.

Larkin Ir. Gael. "Rough, fierce." Poet Philip Larkin.

Larrimore OF. "Armorer."
  Larimore, Larmer, Larmor, Lorimer

Larry Dim. **Lawrence**. Given as an independent name in this century, and with some regularity today. Basketball player Larry Bird; actor/writer Larry David.

Lars Scan. Var. **Lawrence**. Artist Carl Larsson.
  Larsen, Larson, Larsson

Laszlo Hung. "Famous ruler."
  Laslo, Lazlo

Latham Scan. Place name: "The barn."
  Lathom

Lathrop OE. Place name: "Farmstead with barns."

Latimer ME. Occupational name: "Interpreter." Possibly one who could translate into Latin.
  Lattemore, Lattimore, Latymer

Lawford OE. Place name: "The hill-ford." Actor Peter Lawford.

Lawler Ir. Gael. "Mutterer."
  Lawlor, Loller, Lollar

Lawrence Lat. "From Laurentium." Laurentium was a city south of Rome known for its numerous laurel trees. Though the place no longer exists, the name endures, at first given staying power by the popularity of Saint Lawrence (who was martyred by being grilled alive). Brought to Britain with the Norman Conquest, and after an eventual 19th-century decline, was soundly revived in the U.S. in this century. Popularity began to tail off after the 1970s. Actors Laurence Olivier, Laurence Fishburne; bandleader Lawrence Welk; football player Lawrence Taylor; author Laurens Van Der Post; opera singer Lauritz Melchior; impresario Lorenz Ziegfeld.

Larance, Laranz, Lärenz, Larrance, Larrence, Larrens, Larrey, Larry, Lars, Laurance, Lauren, Laurence, Laurens, Laurent, Laurentios, Laurentius, Laurenz, Laurie, Laurits, Lauritz, Lavrans, Lavrens, Lawrance, Lawrey, Lawrie, Lawry, Lenci, Lon, Lonny, Lorant, Loren, Lorenc, Lorencz, Lorens, Lorentz, Lorenz, Lorenzen, Lorenzo, Lorin, Loritz, Lorrence, Lorrenz, Lorry, Lowrance

Lawson OE. "Son of Lawrence." Used as a first name mostly since 1850. Author Robert Lawson.

Lawton OE. Place name: "Hill-town." Actor Charles Laughton.

Laughton, Loughton

Lazarus Heb. "The Lord will help." Biblical name: Lazarus was the man whom Jesus raised from the dead. Little used, perhaps since in the Middle Ages it became a synonym for "leper."

Eleazer, Lazar, Lazare, Lazarillo, Lazaro, Lazear, Lazer, Lazzaro

Leander Gk. "Lion-man." The mythical Greek Leander swam across the Hellespont to visit his beloved, Hero. This was a saint's name as well, but has never been very widely used.

Ander, Leandre, Leandro, Leandros, Leanther, Lee, Leiandros, Leo, Liander, Liandro

Lee OE. Place name: "Pasture or meadow." One of the few truly unisex names. Usually a name becomes exclusively feminine once it is used for girls (**Ashley, Leslie**). The tenacious masculine hold on Lee may have been helped by tough-guy actor Lee Marvin. U.S. use seems to have been sparked by admiration for Confederate General Robert E. Lee. Peaked in the 1950s. Chrysler chairman Lee Iacocca; actor Lee Majors.

Lea, Leigh

Leggett OF. "One who is sent; delegate."

Legate, Leggitt, Liggett

Leif Scan. "Loved." Explorer Leif Ericsson.

Lief

Leighton OE. Place name: "Meadow settlement." Used as

a first name starting in the 19th century. Artist Frederick Leighton.

Layton, Leyton

Leith Scot. Gael. "Broad river."

Leland OE. Place name: "Meadow land." Philanthropist Leland Stanford; dramatic agent Leland Hayward.

Le, Leeland, Leighland, Leyland

Lemuel Heb. "Devoted to God." Old Testament name passed over in the wholesale Puritan revival of biblical names, but given new life from around 1840 into the 1930s. Currently extremely rare.

Lem, Lemmie

Lennon Ir. Gael. "Small cloak or cape."

Lennox Scot. Gael. "With many elm trees."

Lenox

Leo Lat. "Lion." Common in Roman times, and the name of 13 popes, but little used in the 18th and early 19th centuries. Perhaps it was the historical appeal of the name that made it more popular at the turn of the century. Astrological appeal notwithstanding, it is only moderately used today. Author Leo Tolstoy; actor Leo G. Carroll.

Lee, Leon, Leoncio, Leonel, Leonello, Leontios, Lev, Lion, Lyon

Leon Gk. Var. **Leo.** Very popular in the U.S. 1870–1890, and currently more familiar than Leo, but still very unusual. Author Leon Uris.

Leoncio, Leone, Lioni, Lionisio, Lionni

Leonard OG. "Lion-bold." Name of a saint who was much venerated in the Middle Ages (as patron of prisoners, among others), but did not inspire many parents until the 18th century. Use grew gradually to 1930, has diminished since. Artist Leonardo Da Vinci; composer Leonard Bernstein; actors Leonard Nimoy, Leonardo DiCaprio.

Lee, Len, Lenard, Lenn, Lennard, Lennart, Lennerd, Lennie, Lenny, Leo, Leon, Leonardo, Leondaus, Leone, Leonerd, Leonhard, Leonid, Leonidas, Leonides, Leonis, Lonnard, Lonny

Leopold OG. "People brave." Use mainly British and European. The fact that it has been a royal or aristocratic

name in Belgium, Austria, and Britain has not increased its sparse use.
Leo, Leupold

Leroy OF. "The king." Occupational name: One of the servants or pages of a king. Revived in the late 19th century, especially in America, but use today is minimal. Poet Amiri Baraka was originally named Everett LeRoi Jones.
Elroi, Elroy, Lee, Leeroy, Leroi, Roy

Leslie Scot. Gael. Place name: Some sources suggest "The gray castle." Became a last name, then (in the 18th century) a first name used for boys and girls. Boys' use has been tied to admiration for actor Leslie Howard, and is more common in Britain. Infrequent for boy babies in the U.S., as Leslie has become a girl's name. Actor Leslie Nielsen.
Leslea, Leslee, Lesley, Lesly, Lezly

Lester OE. Place name: "From Leicester," an area in central England. First-name use dates from the mid-19th century, and its popularity lasted about 100 years.
Leicester, Les

Lev Rus. Var. Leo.

Leverett OF. "Baby rabbit." May indicate an ancestor who hunted or trapped rabbits.
Leveret, Leverit, Leveritt

Leverton OE. "From the rush-farm."

Levi Heb. "Joined, attached." In the Old Testament, one of Jacob's sons, whose descendants (known as the Levites) were Israel's tribe of priests. After its revival by the Puritans, the name has been steadily used.
Levey, Levin, Levon, Levy

Lewis Anglicization of **Louis** (OG./OFr. "Renowned warrior"). Briefly popular in the late 19th century, but now takes a back seat to Louis, which is not particularly fashionable. In Britain, though, this version is very much in style. Author Lewis Carroll.
Lew, Lewes, Lou, Louis

Liam Ir. Var. **William** (OG. "Will-helmet"). Actor Liam Neeson.

Liberio Port. "Freedom."
Liberato, Liberatus, Liberto

Lidio Port. "From Lydia." Lydia was an area of Asia famous for its two rich kings, Midas and Croesus. The female form, Lydia, is more common than the male.
Licio, Lydio

Lincoln OE. Place name: "Town by the pool." Surname transferred occasionally to a first name. The fame of Abraham Lincoln did not, surprisingly enough, encourage parents to use the name widely, and it is not a favorite today. Football player Lincoln Kennedy.
Linc, Link

Lindberg OG. Place name: "Linden tree mountain." Would probably be unknown as a first name without the career of flier Charles Lindbergh. Very scarce.
Lindbergh, Lindburg, Lindy

Lindell OE. Place name: "Linden tree valley."
Lindal, Lindall, Lindel, Lyndall, Lyndell

Lindley OE. "Linden tree meadow."
Lindlea, Lindlee, Lindleigh, Lindly

Lindsay OE. Place name: "Island of linden trees." Originally a surname, used for boys until the middle of this century, but now quite popular as a girl's name. Film director Lindsay Anderson; New York mayor John Lindsay.
Lind, Lindesay, Lindsee, Lindsey, Lindsy, Lindy, Linsay, Linsey, Linzy, Lyndsay, Lyndsey, Lyndsie

Linford OE. Place name: "Linden tree ford" or "Flax ford." The elements meaning flax ("Lin-") and linden tree ("Lind-") are so similar that they have probably been confused over the years. Track star Linford Christie.
Lindford, Lynford

Linley OE. Place name: "Flax meadow."
Linlea, Linlee, Linleigh, Linly

Linton OE. Place name: "Flax settlement."
Lintonn, Lynton, Lyntonn

Linus Gk. "Flax." May have originated as a descriptive name, applied to someone with flaxen or extremely pale hair. This description does not apply to today's best-known Linus, the famous *Peanuts* character who is lost without his blanket. Actor Linus Roache.
Lino

Lionel Lat. "Young lion." Used in the Middle Ages and never resoundingly revived beyond a twinge of popularity in the 1920s and 1930s. Actor Lionel Barrymore; pop star Lionel Richie.

Leonel, Leonello, Lionell, Lionelo, Lionello, Lionnel, Lionnell, Lionnello, Lyonel, Lyinell, Lyonelo, Lyonnel, Lyonnell, Lyonnello

Litton OE. Place name: "Settlement on the hill." Author Lytton Strachey.

Litten, Littonn, Lytten, Lytton

Llewellyn Welsh. "Resembling a lion." This is the generally accepted meaning, though some scholars think the origin relates to an element meaning "leader." Rare outside of Wales in any case.

Lew, Lewellen, Lewellyn, Llewellen, Llwewellin

Lloyd Welsh. "Gray" or "sacred." One of the most common Welsh names in general use, perhaps because it is one of the simplest. Particularly widespread in the 1940s. Actor Lloyd Bridges; Senator Lloyd Bentsen.

Floyd, Loyd

Locke OE. Place name: "Woods" or "Fortified place," or OG. "Pond." Philosopher John Locke.

Lock, Lockwood

Logan Ir. Gael. Place name: "Small hollow." Author Logan Pearsall Smith; playwright & director Joshua Logan.

Logen

Lombard Lat. "Long-bearded." May also have origins as a place name: Lombardy is an area in northern Italy. Very rare as a first name. Football coach Vince Lombardi; bandleader Guy Lombardo.

Lombardi, Lombardo

Lon Dim. Alonso (OG. "Ready for battle"). Mostly associated with sinister film actor Lon Chaney.

Lonn, Lonnie, Lonny

Loren Var. Lawrence via **Lorenzo**. A purely modern form, in use since the 1940s but not common.

Lorin, Lorren, Lorrin, Loron

Lorenzo It. var. **Lawrence** (Lat. "From Laurentium"). Sub-

stantially used in the U.S., most likely in Latino communities. Actor Lorenzo Lamas.
Laurencio, Loreno, Lorent, Lorento, Lorentz, Lorenzino, Nenzo

Lorimer Lat. Occupational name: "Harness maker."
Lorrimer, Lorymer

Loring OG. "Renowned warrior's son." Related to **Louis.**
Lorring

Lorne Var. **Lawrence** (Lat. "From Laurentium"). Also a Scottish place name, and more common in Scotland. Actor Lorne Green; TV producer Lorne Michaels.
Lorn

Louis OG./Fr. "Renowned warrior." The German form is **Ludwig,** and an early French variant was **Clovis,** a name borne by several Frankish kings. The later French kings (18 of them) who chose Louis as their name were no doubt harking back to those early monarchs, one of whom included the 13th-century saint. Lewis was the more common form in Britain until a mid-19th-century revival of Louis, which was very popular in the U.S. until the depression era. Musician Louis Armstrong; scientist Louis Pasteur; archaeologist Louis Leakey; authors Louis L'Amour, Robert Louis Stevenson; actor Lou Gossett, Jr.
Aloysius, Lew, Lewes, Lewis, Lodewick, Lodovico, Lou, Louie, Lucho, Ludovic, Ludovicus, Ludvig, Ludvik, Ludwig, Luigi, Luis

Lowell OF. "Young wolf." Mostly 19th-century use. Poet Robert Lowell.
Lovel, Lovell, Lowe, Lowel

Lucas Var. **Luke.** Generally a transferred last name, but gaining popularity in Britain as a first name, and quite popular in the U.S. as well. In Germany, this is a top-ten name. Actor Lukas Haas.
Loucas, Loukas, Lukas

Lucian Lat. "Light." More unusual form of Lucius, which itself is quite rare. Artist Lucian Freud; opera star Luciano Pavarotti.

Luciano, Lucianus, Lucien, Lucio, Lucjan, Lukianos, Lukyan

Lucius Lat. "Light." Used by the Romans, but extremely scarce in the 20th century.

Luca, Lucas, Luccheus, Luce, Lucias, Lucio, Lukas, Luke, Lukeus

Ludlow OE. Place name: "Ruler's hill."

Ludlowe

Ludoslaw Polish "Glorious people."

Ludwig Ger. "Renowned in battle." Very unusual in English-speaking countries, where **Louis** or **Lewis** are used instead. Composer Ludwig van Beethoven.

Ludo, Ludovic, Ludovico

Luke Gk. "From Lucanus," a region of southern Italy. Not, strictly speaking, a nickname for **Lucius** and **Lucian**, though it may be used that way. The most famous Luke is, of course, the author of the Gospel and of Acts. He was a physician, and is patron saint of doctors and artists. After medieval use it was rather neglected, but the name is turning up quite frequently in preschools and hospital nurseries. Actors Luke Perry, Luke Wilson.

Loukas, Luc, Lucas, Lucian, Lucien, Lucio, Lucius, Luck, Lucky, Lukacs, Lukas

Lundy Scot. Place name "Grove near the island," or possibly Fr. "Monday's child." Generally a transferred surname.

Lunn Ir. Gael. "Strong, warlike."

Lon, Lonn

Luther OG. "Army people." Generally homage to Martin Luther, the German religious reformer, or to Martin Luther King, Jr., the civil rights activist. Botanist Luther Burbank; singer Luther Vandross.

Lotario, Lothair, Lothar, Lothario, Louther, Lutero

Lyle OF. Place name: "The island." First-name use was mostly in the middle of this century.

Lisle, Lyall, Lyell, Lysle

Lyman OE. "Meadow-dweller."

Leaman, Leyman

Lynch Ir. Gael. "Mariner." One of the most common Irish

last names, occasionally transferred for first-name use. Film director David Lynch; actor John Lynch.

Lyndon OE. Place name: "Linden tree hill." First-name use coincides with the 19th-century fondness for transferred surnames, but has been given extra renown by President Lyndon Baines Johnson.

Lin, Linden, Lindon, Lindy, Lyn, Lynden

Lysander Gk. "Liberator."

Lesandro, Lisandro, Lizandro

Mac Scot. Gael. "Son of." Also used as a nickname for given names that begin with "Mac-," many of which are transferred last names.

Mack, Mackey, Mackie

Macadam Scot. Gael. "Son of Adam." The 19th-century engineer John McAdam gave his name to a method of paving roads that became very widespread.

MacAdam, McAdam

Macallister Scot. Gael. "Son of Alistair." Alistair is the Scottish version of **Alexander**.

MacAlister, McAlister, McAllister

Macardle Scot. Gael. "Son of great courage."

MacArdell, McCardell

Macbride Ir. Gael. "Son of the follower of Saint Brigid," who was an influential 5th-century Irish nun.

Macbryde, McBride

Maccoy Ir. Gael. "Son of Hugh." The phrase "the real McCoy" came from Scotland, where it referred to something of the highest quality.

MacCoy, McCoy

Maccrea Ir. Gael. "Son of grace." Actor Joel McCrea.

MacCrae, MacCray, MacCrea, Macrae, McCrea

Macdonald Scot. Gael. "Son of Donald." The McDonalds were a powerful Scottish clan.
MacDonald, McDonald

Macdougal Scot. Gael. "Son of Dougal." Since Dougal means "dark foreigner," this may refer to an ancestor who was a Viking invader (not all of whom were blond).
MacDougal, MacDowell, McDougal, McDowell

Macgowan Ir. Gael. "Son of the blacksmith."
MacCowan, MacCowen, MacGowan, Magowan, McGowan, McGowen, McGown

Mackenzie Ir. Gael. "Son of the wise ruler."
MacKensie, McKenzie, McKensie

Mackinley Ir. Gael. "Learned ruler." U.S. President William McKinley.
MacKinlay, McKinlay, McKinley

Macmahon Ir. Gael. "Son of the bear." TV host Ed McMahon.
MacMahon, McMahon

Macmurray Ir. Gael. "Son of the seafarer." Actor Fred McMurray.
MacMurray, McMurray

Macy OF. Place name: "Matthew's estate." Department store founder R.H. Macy; actor William Macy.
Macey

Maddock Old Welsh. "Benevolent, charitable."
Madoc, Madock, Madog

Maddox Anglo-Welsh. "Benefactor's son." A contracted form of "Maddock's son." Novelist Ford Madox Ford.
Madocks, Maddocks, Madox

Madison OE. "Son of the mighty warrior." More common than many of these "son of" names, possibly because of admiration for U.S. President James Madison. However, since this name has been in the top ten girls' names since 1997, parents of boys are unlikely to use it. Novelist Madison Smartt Bell.
Maddison, Maddy, Madisson

Magee Ir. Gael. "Son of Hugh."
MacGee, MacGhee, McGee

Magnus Lat. "Great." Appropriately enough, a royal name

in Norway and Denmark. It was transferred from Scandinavia to Scotland, where it is used somewhat.

Magnes, Magnusson, Manus

Maguire Ir. Gael. "Son of the beige one."

MacGuire, McGuire, McGwire

Major Lat. "Greater." Use (which is sparing) probably harks back to the military title used in the British and American armies.

Majer, Mayer, Mayor

Makarios Gk. "Blessed."

Macario, Macarios, Macarius, Maccario, Maccarios, Mackario, Mackarios, Makar, Makkarios

Malachi Heb. "Angel, messenger." Name of one of the minor prophets in the Old Testament, but not widely used. Author Malachi Martin.

Malachie, Malachy, Malaki, Malakie, Malaquias, Malechy, Maleki, Makequi

Malcolm Scot. Gael. "Devotee of St. Columba." The name of the prince of Scotland who became king after Macbeth murdered his father, Duncan. Shakespeare's play was based on historical fact. The name has been used primarily in Scotland, but spread more widely in the middle of the 20th century. Black families may use it in honor of Malcolm X who, upon his conversion to Islam, took the name El-Hajj Malik El-Shabazz. Publisher Malcolm Forbes.

Malcolum, Malkolm

Malik Arab. "Master." Actor Art Malik.

Maleek, Maleeq, Mallik, Maliq

Malin OE. "Little strong warrior."

Mallen, Mallin, Mallon

Mallory OF. "Unhappy, unlucky." Literally, *malheureux.* Originally a nickname, transferred to a last name and thus to a first name. Used quite often for girls now, though it was originally a man's name. Poet Sir Thomas Malory.

Mallery, Mallorie, Malory

Maloney Ir. Gael. "Pious, disciple of Sunday worship."

Malone, Malonee, Malonie, Malony

Malvin Var. Melvin. Could come from a number of sources:

possibly Ir. Gael. "Polished chief," OE. "Council-friend," or an adaptation of **Melville**.

Malvinn, Malvyn

Mandel Ger. "Almond."

Mandell, Mandelson

Manfred OE. "Man of peace." Seldom found in real life, but used by Byron for an antihero in an eponymous epic poem.

Manfredo, Manfrid, Manfried, Mannfred, Mannfryd

Manley OE. Place name: "Man's meadow." Or originally a descriptive term meaning "masculine." Poet Gerard Manley Hopkins.

Manlea, Manleigh, Manly

Manning OE. "Son of the man." Football player Peyton Manning.

Mannyng

Mansel OE. "From the manse." A manse is a house occupied by a clergyman.

Mansell

Mansfield OE. Place name: "Field by the little river."

Manton OE. Place name: "Man's or hero's town."

Manten, Mannton

Manuel Dim. **Emanuel** (Heb. "God be with us"). Most widely used in Spanish-speaking countries, but it has a considerable presence in the U.S. as well. Shoe designer Manolo Blahnik; artist Manuel Ocampo; baseball player Manny Ramirez.

Mano, Manolo, Manny

Manville OF. Place name: "Great town."

Mandeville, Manvel, Manvile, Manvill

Marcel Fr. Dim. **Marcellus** (Lat. "Little warrior"). One of the less common of a group of names that all have their root in the Roman god of war, Mars. Author Marcel Proust; pantomime artist Marcel Marceau; football player Marcellus Wiley.

Marceau, Marcelin, Marcellin, Marcellino, Marcello, Marcellus, Marcelo, Marcely

Marcus Lat. "Warlike." The root of such names as **Mark** and **Marcel,** and based on the name of the Roman war god, Mars. Common enough in Roman times, but unknown in English-speaking countries until the 19th century. When Mark was hugely popular in the 1970s, **Marcus** also crept up the charts possibly boosted by the hit TV series "Marcus Welby, M.D." Retailer Stanley Marcus; hockey player Markus Naslund.

Marc, Marco, Marko, Markus

Marden OE. Place name: "The valley with the pool." Painter Brice Marden.

Mario It. Var. **Mark.** New York Governor Mario Cuomo; chef Mario Batali.

Marianus, Marius, Meirion

Marion Fr. Var. **Mary** (Heb. "Bitter or rebellious"). Almost always a girl's name, and likely to cause some confusion if given to a boy. The most famous male Marion, Marion Morrison, chose the unmistakably masculine "John Wayne" when he changed his name. Revolutionary war soldier Francis "Swamp Fox" Marion.

Mariano

Mark Lat. "Warlike." The anglicized version of **Marcus,** and the most popular in this country. In spite of the automatic exposure given the name by the evangelist Saint Mark, it was not widely used in the Middle Ages, nor indeed was it really common until a sudden inexplicable flurry of use in the 1950s. The popular author Mark Twain (whose real name was Samuel Clemens) took his pseudonym from the call of Mississippi River boatmen: "Mark twain!" meant that the water they were navigating was two fathoms deep. Explorer Marco Polo; choreographer Mark Morris; swimmer Mark Spitz; baseball player Mark McGwire; fashion designer Marc Jacobs; actors Mark Harmon, Mark Wahlberg.

Marc, Marco, Marcos, Marcus, Marek, Mario, Marius, Marko, Markos, Markus, Marq, Marquus

Marland OE. Place name: "Land near the lake." Some sources suggest that the name means "famous land" and is the source of **Marlon** as well.

Marlin, Marlon, Marlond, Marlondo

Marley OE. Place name: "Meadow near the lake." Musician Bob Marley.
Marlea, Marleigh, Marly

Marlon OF. "Little hawk," or possibly a variation of **Merlin**. Current use, which is scanty, is inspired by the career of actor Marlon Brando.
Marlen, Marlin, Marlinn, Marlonn

Marlow OE. Place name: "Hill near the lake." Rare as a first name, though classic film lovers might be reminded of Humphrey Bogart as Philip Marlowe in *The Big Sleep*. English playwright Christopher Marlowe.
Marloe, Marlowe

Marmion OF. "Tiny one." Extremely rare, though used by Sir Walter Scott in a popular narrative poem of that title.
Marmeon, Marmionn, Marmyon

Marsden OE. Place name: "Swampy valley." Painter Marsden Hartley.
Marsdin, Marsdon

Marsh OE. Place name: "Swamp or marsh." Like **Marsden** and **Marston,** more generally a last name, occasionally used as a first name. Nineteenth-century parents were particularly fond of transferring surnames as given names. Painter Reginald Marsh.

Marshall OF. Occupational name: "Horse-keeper." Also a military title of great honor, as in "field marshal." As a last name, common in Scotland, and used rather widely as a first name since the early 19th century. Department store founder Marshall Field; media theorist Marshall McLuhan; actor David Marshall Grant; Supreme Court Justice Thurgood Marshall; football player Marshall Faulk; pop singer Marshall Mathers.
Marchall, Marischal, Marischall, Marschal, Marsh, Marshal, Marshell

Marston OE. Place name: "Town by the marsh."

Martin Lat. "Warlike." Like **Marcus** and its variants, Martin originates with the Roman war god, Mars. The 4th-century Saint Martin (most famous for dividing his cloak in two and giving half to a beggar) was much venerated, making his name popular in the Middle Ages. The influence of Protestant reformer Martin Luther may have added to the name's appeal, since it was used very steadily right into the 19th century, though there are comparatively few variants. The pattern since then has been of moderate use, except for a spurt of popularity in the 1950s. U.S. President Martin Van Buren; film director Martin Scorsese; actors Martin Short, Martin Lawrence.

Marinos, Mart, Martel, Martell, Marten, Martenn, Martie, Martijn, Martinien, Martino, Martinos, Martinus, Marton, Marty, Martyn

Marvin Origin obscure, though many sources suggest OE. "Sea lover," while others claim that it is Welsh. Popular in America starting in the 19th century, peaking in the 1920s, and now unusual. Actor Lee Marvin; songwriter Marvin Hamlisch; singer Marvin Gaye; football player Marvin Harrison.

Marve, Marven, Marwin, Marwynn, Mervin, Mervyn, Merwin, Merwyn, Murvin, Murvynn

Marwood OE. Place name: "Lake near the woods."

Maslin OF. "Little Thomas."

Maslen, Masling, Maslon, Masslen, Masslin, Masslon

Mason OF. Occupational name: "Stoneworker." Transferred from surname status starting in the mid-19th century. Actor James Mason.

Mather OE. "Powerful army." The surname of a dynasty of 17th- and 18th-century Massachusetts theologians, Richard, Increase, and Cotton Mather.

Maither, Matther

Matthew Heb. "Gift of the Lord." Like **Mark, Luke,** and **John,** given great exposure by the author of one of the four Gospels. In more religious eras, parents would hear these names over and over again in the course of a year. Matthew began to be neglected in the 19th century and was little used early in the 20th until an enthusiastic revival at midcentury. It is still one of the top ten boys' names in the United States and in Britain as well. Actors

Matthew Broderick, Matthew Modine, Matthew Perry, Matthew McConaughey, Matt Leblanc, Matt Damon; photographer Mathew Brady; poet Matthew Arnold; tennis star Mats Wilander.

Madteo, Madteos, Madtheos, Mat, Mata, Mateo, Mateusz, Mathé, Matheu, Mathew, Mathian, Mathias, Mathieu, Matias, Matico, Mats, Matt, Mattaeus, Mattaus, Matteo, Matthaus, Mattheus, Matthias, Matthiew, Mattias, Mattie, Mattieu, Matty, Matvey, Matyas, Matz

Matthias Ger. Var. **Matthew.** German painter Matthias Grunewald.

Mathias, Mattias

Maurice Lat. "Dark-skinned, Moorish." Roman name brought to Britain by the Normans and widely used into the 17th century. A 19th-century revival faded around 1900; the name still occurs. Actor Maurice Chevalier; writer Maurice Sendak; composer Maurice Ravel.

Mauricio, Maurids, Maurie, Maurise, Maurits, Mauritius, Mauritz, Maurizio, Maury, Maurycy, Morey, Morice, Moricz, Moris, Moritz, Moriz, Morrel, Morrey, Morrice, Morrill, Morris, Morriss, Moss, Mo

Max Dim. **Maxwell, Maximilian.** Appeared at the turn of the 20th century, fashionable by the 1930s, then faded, but today's parents are showing interest in it again. Writer Max Beerbohm; actor Max von Sydow.

Maks, Maxence, Maxson

Maximilian Lat. "Greatest." Appropriately enough, used by the emperor of Mexico and the Holy Roman emperor, though a bit of a mouthful for a child. German parents apparently don't see it that way, for the name is extremely popular there. Actor Maximilian Schell.

Mac, Mack, Maks, Maksim, Maksym, Maksymilian, Massimiliano, Massimo, Max, Maxey, Maxemilian, Maxemilion, Maxie, Maxim, Maxime, Maximiliano, Maximilianus, Maximilien, Maximillian, Maximino, Maximo, Maximos, Maxy, Maxymilian, axymillian

Maxwell OE. Place name: Maybe "Maccus's well," though some sources also suggest "large well" or "important man's well." Mostly Scottish last name, fairly common as a first name. Editor Maxwell Perkins; playwright Maxwell Anderson.

Maxwelle

Mayer Lat. "Larger." Var. **Major**. Also Ger. "Farmer," Heb. "Bright, shining." Banker Mayer Rothschild.

Maier, Meir, Meyer

Mayfield OE. Place name: "Strong one's field."

Mayhew OF. Var. **Matthew** (Heb. "Gift of the Lord").

Maynard OE. "Hard strength." See **Meinhard**. Economist John Maynard Keynes.

Mayne, Maynhard, Meinhard, Meinhardt, Menard

Mayo Ir. Gael. Place name: "Yew tree plain." Mayo is a county in western Ireland. It is also most commonly the short name for a condiment used in sandwiches, a fact parents should bear in mind.

Mead OE. Place name: "Meadow." Architect William Rutherford Mead.

Meade, Meed

Medwin OG. "Strong friend."

Medvin, Medwinn, Medwyn

Meinhard Ger. "Hard strength." **Maynard** is the anglicized form.

Mainard, Maynard, Meinhardt, Meino

Meinrad Ger. "Strong counsel."

Mel Dim. **Melvin** and other "Mel-" names. Actor Mel Gibson; filmmaker Mel Brooks.

Melbourne OE. Place name: "Mill stream." Also the name of a prominent city in Australia. Occasional use.

Mel, Melborn, Melburn, Milbourn, Milbourne, Milburn, Millburn, Millburne

Melchior Pol. "King." Traditionally the name of one of the Three Kings, along with **Caspar** and **Balthasar**. Opera singer Lauritz Melchior.

Malchior, Malkior, Melker, Melkior

Meldon OE. Place name: "Mill hill."

Melden

Meldrick OE. "Mill ruler."

Melderick, Meldric

Melville OE./OF. Place name: "Industrious one's town." Author Herman Melville.

Melvin Could come from a number of sources: possibly Ir. Gael. "Polished chief," OE. "Sword friend," or an adaptation of **Melville**.

Malvin, Malvyn, Malvynn, Mel, Melvyn, Melwin, Melwyn, Melwynn, Vinnie

Menachem Heb. "Comforter." Israeli statesman Menachem Begin.

Menahem, Nachum, Nahum

Mendel Semitic. "Wisdom, learning."

Mendell, Mendeley

Mercer ME. Occupational name: "Storekeeper." Choreographer Merce Cunningham; musician Johnny Mercer.

Merce

Meredith Welsh. "Great ruler." More commonly a girl's name, but still clung to for boys in Wales. Composer Meredith Willson.

Meredyth, Merideth, Meridith

Merle Fr. "Blackbird." Very rare for boys. Singer Merle Haggard.

Merlin ME. "Small falcon." Also the name (via a mistranslation: see **Mervin**) of the wizard of the Arthurian legends. Use dates from the 20th century. Football player Merlin Olsen.

Marlin, Marlon, Merle, Merlen, Merlinn, Merlyn, Merlynn

Merrick Anglicization of a Welsh variant of **Maurice**. Used from time to time in this century. Theater producer David Merrick.

Merrik, Meyrick

Merrill Origin disputed, perhaps OF. "Famous" or a phonetic variation of the girl's name **Meryl**. Its status as a surname probably depends on the medieval use of its antecedent, **Muriel**. Poet James Merrill.

Meril, Merill, Merrel, Merrell, Merril, Meryl

Merritt OE. "Little renowned one."

Merrett, Merit, Meritt

Merton OE. Place name: "Town by the lake." Theologian Thomas Merton.

Merwyn, Murton

Mervin Old Welsh. "Sea hill." **Mervyn** is more common in Britain. Merlin the wizard of Arthurian legend was known in Welsh as Myrddin, translated into Latin as **Merlin**. The name was mildly popular around the turn of the century.

Merven, Mervyn, Mervynn, Merwin, Merwinn, Merwyn, Murvin, Murvyn

Meshach Heb. Meaning unknown. Old Testament name: one of three Hebrew men (along with the now scarce Shadrach and Abednego) thrown into a fiery furnace by King Nebuchadnezzar and rescued by an angel. Used sparingly in the 19th century, even more rare today. Actor Meshach Taylor.

Meyer Ger. "Farmer"; Heb. "Bringer of light." Architect Richard Meier; financier Mayer Rothschild.

Mayeer, Mayer, Mayor, Meier, Meir, Myer

Micah Heb. Var. **Michael**. Very easily confused with Michael when it is spoken.

Mike, Mikey, Mikal, Mycah

Michael Heb. "Who is like the Lord?" In the New Testament, Michael is the name of the archangel who defeats the dragon. Usage was steady until a period of neglect that lasted from the early 19th to the early 20th century. The subsequent revival was immense, and Michael was, according to many listings, the most popular name for American boys from the 1970s right through to 1997 when it was displaced by **Jacob**. Even as we move into the 21st century, this continues to be a favorite. In France, as **Michel,** and in Russia as **Mikhail,** it is also on the top-ten list. Baseball star Mickey Mantle; actors Mickey Rooney, Michael Caine, Michael J. Fox, Michael Chiklis, Michael Gambon, Michael Imperioli, Mike Meyers; singers Michael Jackson, Mick Jagger; cartoon star Mickey Mouse; Soviet statesman Mikhail Gorbachev; hockey player Mike Modano; fashion designer Michael Kors.

Micael, Mical, Michal, Micheal, Michel, Michele,

Michiel, Mickey, Micky, Miguel, Mihail, Mihaly,
Mikael, Mike, Mikel, Mikey, Mikhail, Mikhalis, Mikhos,
Mikkel, Miko, Mikol, Miky, Mischa, Misha, Mitch,
Mitchell, Mychal, Mykal, Mykell

Miles Several possible origins, including Lat. "Soldier," OG.
"Merciful," or variant of **Emil** (Lat. "Eager to please").
Since the end of the 18th century, it has been quite unusual.
Pilgrim leader Miles Standish; musician Miles Davis.

Milan, Milo, Myles

Milford OE. Place name: "Mill-ford."

Millford

Millard OE. "Guardian of the mill." U.S. President Millard
Fillmore.

Millerd, Millward, Milward

Miller OE. Occupational name. Use as a first name began in
the late 19th century, is now sparing. Playwright Arthur
Miller.

Millar, Myller

Mills OE. Place name "Near the mills," or possibly a contraction of "Miles's son."

Milo Ger. Var. **Miles**. Very unusual. Actor Milo O'Shea.

Milton OE. Place name: "Mill town" or perhaps "Middle
town." One of the more commonplace names transferred
to a first name, dating from the early 19th century. Poet
John Milton; comedian Milton Berle.

Milt, Millton, Milten, Miltin, Mylton

Minor Lat. "Younger." Photographer Minor White.

Menor, Miner, Meinor, Mynor

Misha Rus. Var. **Michael**. Given some modern exposure as
the nickname of superstar dancer Mikhail Baryshnikov.
Musician Misha Dicter.

Mischa

Mitchell Middle English. Var. **Michael**. The last name
evolved in the Middle Ages, when surnames began to be
regularly used, and it was transferred back to a first name
in the 19th century. It was popular in the middle of the
20th century, and is now steadily used without being fashionable. Bandleader Mitch Miller.

Mitch, Mitchel, Mitchill, Mytch

Modred OE. "Brave counselor." In the Arthurian legend, Modred is Arthur's illegitimate son who tries to claim his father's throne, and engineers his ultimate downfall.
Mordred

Mohammed Arab. "Highly praised." The name of the prophet and founder of Islam. There are many different forms of this name as it has been spelled in many different languages. Boxer Mohammed Ali.
**Mahmood, Mahmoud, Mahmud, Mahomet, Mehmood,
Mehmoud, Mehmud, Mohammad, Muhammad,
Muhammed**

Monahan Ir. Gael. "Monk."
Monaghan, Monoghan

Monroe Ir. Gael. Place name: May mean "Mouth of the Roe River" or possibly "The red marsh." U.S. President James Monroe; novelist H.H. Munro.
Monro, Munro, Munroe

Montague Fr. Place name: "Sharply pointed mount." More common as first name in the 19th century.
Montagew, Montagu

Montgomery OE. Place name: "Mount of the rich man." Unusual as a first name, and very likely to be shortened to **Monty**. Actor Montgomery Clift.
Monte, Montie, Montgomerie, Monty

Monty Dim. "Mont-" names like **Montague** and **Montgomery**, used rarely as a given name. Given slightly ridiculous connotations by TV master of ceremonies Monty Hall and British comedy troupe Monty Python.

Moore OE. Place name: "The moors" or OF. "Dark-skinned" (as in "Moorish"). Clement Clarke Moore was the author of the much-loved poem "'Twas the night before Christmas."
More

Mordecai Heb. Meaning not clear, but possibly "Follower of Marduk" (who was a god of the Babylonians). An Old Testament name revived by the Puritans and neglected since the 19th century.
Mordechai, Mordy, Mort

Moreland OE. Place name: "Moor-land." Moor is a British

term referring to a large, rolling expanse of scrubby, infertile wild land.
Moorland, Morland

Morgan Different sources give several meanings, including Welsh. "Great and bright" and OE. "Bright or white sea dweller." The name is most common in Wales as both a first and a last name. Actor Morgan Freeman; financier J.P. Morgan.
Morgen, Morgun, Morrgan

Morley OE. Place name: "Meadow on the moor." TV commentator Morley Safer.
Moorley, Moorly, Morlee, Morleigh, Morly, Morrley

Morris Anglicization of **Maurice** (Lat. "Dark-skinned, Moorish"). Now more common as a surname. Choreographer Mark Morris.
Morey, Morice, Moris, Morrey, Morrie, Morrison, Morrisson, Morry

Morse OE. "Son of Maurice." Contracted from Morrison. Inventor Samuel F.B. Morse.
Morrison

Mortimer OF. Place name: "Still water." Literally, "dead sea," *mort mer.* First-name use, as with so many of these place names, dates from the 19th century. Entrepreneur Mortimer Zuckerman.
Mort, Morty, Mortymer

Morton OE. Place name: "Moor town." Like **Mortimer,** used as a first name since the 19th century, though probably more common.
Morten

Morven Scot. Gael. "Huge mountain." First-name use is mostly Scottish, and generally confined to girls.
Morfin, Morfinn, Morfyn, Morvyn

Moses History unclear. Some sources suggest Heb. "Savior," while others claim it means "Taken from the water." The latter definition clearly comes from the biblical story of the infant Moses afloat in the bulrushes, whence he was rescued by Pharaoh's daughter, later to become the great leader of the exiled Israelites. Always current in Jewish families, adopted by the Puritans in the 17th century, now uncommon. Israeli defense minister Moshe Dayan.

Mioshe, Mioshye, Mo, Moe, Moise, Moises, Mose, Moshe, Mosheh, Mosie, Moss, Moyses, Mozes

Muhammad Arab. "Greatly praised." Name of the prophet and founder of Islam. There are some 500 variants of this name, and if they were all counted as one name, it would be the most popular name in the world.

Hamid, Hammad, Mahomet, Mehmet, Mihammad, Mohamet, Mohammad, Mohammed, Muhamet, Muhammed

Muir Scot. Gael. Place name: "Moor." Naturalist John Muir.

Murdock Scot. Gael. "Sea fighter" or "Sailor." Generally Scottish usage; in the U.S., occurs mainly as a transferred surname. Media magnate Rupert Murdoch.

Murdo, Murdoch, Murtagh, Murtaugh

Muriel Ir. Gael. "Sea bright." Usually a female name.

Murphy Ir. Gael. "Sea fighter." A quintessentially Irish last name, in occasional use as a first name.

Murfee, Murfey, Murfie, Murphee, Murphey, Murphie

Murray Scot. Gael. Place name, or possibly "Mariner." Somewhat common as a first name in the 1930s and 1940s, but now little used.

Moray, Murrey, Murry

Myron Gk. "Fragrant oil." Not, despite its sound, related to myrrh (as carried by the Three Kings). Like **Murray**, most common in the middle third of the 20th century.

Miron

Nabil Arab. "Highborn."
    Nabeel
Nachman Heb. "Comforter."
    Menachem, Menahem, Nacham,
Nachmann, Nahum
Nadim Arab. "Friend."
    Nadeem
Nairn Scot. Gael. Place name: "River with alder trees."
    Nairne
Najib Arab. "Of highborn parentage."
    Nageeb, Nagib, Najeeb
Naldo Sp. Dim. **Reginald** (OG. "Powerful advice").
Napoleon OG. Meaning unclear, though tradition says it
means "Lion of Naples." Another possibility is Greek
"New town." Napoleon Bonaparte (who obviously in-
spired its use) came not from Naples, but from Corsica.
    Leon, Leone, Nap, Napoleone
Narcisse Fr. "Daffodil." Not, as it would be in English, a
flower name, but the name of a beautiful Greek youth who
became enamored of his own reflection—hence "narcissism."
    Narciso, Narcissus, Narkissos, Narses
Nasser Arab. "The winner."
    Nasir, Naser, Nasr
Nat Dim. **Nathan, Nathaniel.**
Natal Sp. "Birthday." Referring, of course, to the birthday
of Jesus, or Christmas.
    Natale, Natalino, Natalio, Nataly
Nathan Heb. "Given." Old Testament name, revived in the
18th century and quite popular in the last 40 years. It has
been in the top fifty boys' names in the U.S. for a dozen
years. Nathan Hale was the American spy who declared,
just before he was hanged by the British in 1776, "I regret

that I have but one life to lose for my country." Critic
George Jean Nathan; actor Nathan Lane.

Nat, Natan, Nate, Nathen, Nathon

Nathaniel Heb. "Given by God." New Testament name of
one of the apostles (who was also called Bartholomew).
Used by the Puritans, and a steady presence ever since,
though quite a bit less popular than **Nathan**. Author
Nathaniel Hawthorne; musician Nat "King" Cole; slave
insurrectionist Nat Turner.

Nat, Natanael, Nataniel, Nate, Nathan, Nathaneal,
Nathanial, Nathanyal, Nathanyel, Natty, Nethanel,
Nethaniel, Nethanyel, Thaniel

Neal Ir. Var. Neil.

Neale, Neall, Nealle, Neel

Ned Dim. **Edward** (OE. "Wealthy defender"); **Edmund**
(OE. "Wealthy protector").

Nehemiah Heb. "The Lord's comfort." Old Testament
prophet, Puritan name, rare in this century.

Nechemia, Nechemiah, Nechemya

Neil Gael. "Champion." Although the name of the most famous Celtic king of Ireland (Niall of the Nine Hostages),
it has been used mostly in Scotland until the middle of
this century. Astronaut Neil Armstrong; singers Neil Diamond and Neil Young; playwright Neil Simon; actor
Sam Neill.

Neal, Neale, Neall, Nealle, Nealon, Neel, Neile, Neill,
Neille, Neils, Nels, Nial, Niall, Niel, Niles

Nels Scan. Var. **Nicholas** (Gk. "People of victory").

Nelson Eng. "Son of Neil." Established by parents who admired the exploits of English Admiral Nelson at the Battle of Trafalgar. Used consistently, if never widely, since
then. Actor Nelson Eddy; New York Governor and U.S.
Vice President Nelson Rockefeller; South African activist
Nelson Mandela.

Nealson, Neils, Neilson, Neillson, Nels, Nelsen, Niles,
Nils, Nilson, Nilsson

Nemesio Sp. "Justice."

Neptune Roman god of the sea, and a fanciful name for
sea-loving parents.

Nesbit OE. Place name: "Bend shaped like a nose." Refers to a bend in a road, or else to a plot of land.

Naisbit, Naisbitt, Nesbitt, Nisbet, Nisbett

Nestor Gk. "Traveler, voyager." Cinematographer Nestor Almendros.

Nester, Nesterio, Nestore, Nestorio

Neville OF. Place name: "New town." More common in Britain, but very rare in the U.S. Musical conductor Neville Marriner.

Nev, Nevil, Nevile, Nevyle

Nevin Anglicization of Gaelic names that mean "Holy, sacred," or "Little bone" or "Servant of the saint's disciple."

Nev, Nevan, Neven, Nevins, Nevon, Niven

Newell OE. Place name: "New hall." The "hall" was often a term for the local manor in early England.

Newall, Newel, Newhall

Newland OE. Place name: "New land."

Newlin Old Welsh. Place name: "New pond."

Newman OE. "Newcomer." Began to be used as a first name in England in the 19th century, perhaps influenced by the fame of reforming cleric John Henry (Cardinal) Newman. Now scarce. Actor Paul Newman.

Neuman, Neumann, Newmann

Newton OE. Place name: "New town." Like many place names turned last names, made the move to a first name in the 19th century, and has now drifted back to last-name status. Entertainer Wayne Newton; English mathematician Isaac Newton.

Niall Ir. Gael. "Champion." A less common variant of **Neil**, used chiefly in Ireland.

Nial

Nicholas Gk. "People of victory." A New Testament name given even greater fame by the 4th-century Saint Nicholas, patron saint of children and (via his Dutch name, Sinte Klaas) the original Santa Claus. The name was widespread in the Middle Ages through the 17th century, then had a long period of disuse that ended in the middle of the 20th century. This is now one of the top ten names for boys in the nation and is also extremely well used in Germany, Russia, and

- France. Theater director Nikos Psacharapolous; Dickens novel *Nicholas Nickleby;* actors Nicolas Cage, Nickolas Grace, Nicol Williamson; composer Nicolai Rimsky-Korsakov; political philosopher Niccolo Machiavelli.

Claas, Claes, Claus, Colas, Cole, Colet, Colin, Collin, Klaas, Klaes, Klaus, Nic, Nicanor, Niccolo, Nichol, Nichole, Nicholl, Nichols, Nick, Nickey, Nickie, Nicklas, Nickolas, Nickolaus, Nicky, Nicol, Nicola, Nicolaas, Nicolai, Nicolas, Nicolao, Nicolay, Nicolet, Nicollet, Nicolis, Nicoll, Nicolls, Nicolo, Nik, Niki, Nikita, Nikki, Nikkolas, Nikkolay, Nikky, Niklaas, Niklas, Nikolai, Nikolas, Nikolaus, Nikolay, Nikolos, Nikos, Nilos

Nicodemus Gk. "Victory of the people." New Testament name, very scarce.

Nicodemo, Nikodema

Niels Dan. Var. **Neil** (Gael. "Champion").

Niel, Niles, Nils

Nigel Ir. Gael. "Champion." Related not, as many sources claim, to the Latin *niger* ("black"), but to the Latin form of **Neil,** Nigellus. Almost exclusively a British name, popular in this century. Actor Nigel Havers.

Nissim Heb. "Wondrous things."

Nixon OE. "Son of Nicholas." A contraction of "Nicolas's son," or "Nick's son." After the disgrace of President Nixon in the early 1970s, unlikely to be used as a first name.

Noah Heb. Meaning unclear, possibly "rest" or "wandering." The latter would be appropriate for the patriarch who drifted in the ark for 40 days. Steadily but not widely used since the 17th century. Lexicographer Noah Webster; actor Noah Wyle.

Noach, Noak, Noé

Noble Lat. "Aristocratic." Use as a first name may derive from surnames, or from the use of the adjective as a name. Mostly 19th century.

Noel Fr. "Christmas." Used since the Middle Ages, but not very widespread. More likely to be chosen for girls. Playwright and actor Noel Coward.

Nata, Natal, Natale, Nowel, Nowell

Nolan Ir. Gael. "Renowned." A last name transferred to first name. Baseball star Nolan Ryan.
Noland, Nolen, Nolin, Nollan

Norbert OG. "Renowned northerner." Saint's name that was mildly popular in the middle of the 20th century.
Bert, Bertie, Berty, Norberto

Norman OE. "Northerner." The Normans of France were originally from Scandinavia, or the North, but the name was also used in England even before the Norman Conquest. After medieval use, it was neglected until a substantial 19th-century revival, which has long since faded. Artist Norman Rockwell; authors Norman Vincent Peale, Norman Mailer; TV producer Norman Lear.
Norm, Normand, Normen, Normie

Norris OF. "Northerner." May also derive from the French word for "nurse." Modern use dates from the 19th century. Novelist Frank Norris.

Northcliff OE. Place name: "Northern cliff."
Northcliffe, Northclyff, Northclyffe

Northrop OE. Place name: "Northern farm." Critic Northrop Frye.
Northrup

Norton OE. Place name: "Northern town." Revived as a first name in the mid-19th-century.

Norville Old Anglo/Fr. Place name: "Northern town."
Norval, Norvel, Norvell, Norvil, Norvill, Norvylle

Norvin OE. "Northern friend."
Norvyn, Norwin, Norwinn, Norwyn, Norwynn

Norward OE. "Warden of the north."
Norwerd

Norwell OE. "Northern well."

Norwood OE. "Woods in the north."

Nuncio It. "Messenger." Comes from the same root that gives us the word "announce."
Nunzio

Nuri Arab. "Light."
Noori, Nur, Nuriel, Nuris

Oakes OE. Place name: "Near the oak trees." Transferred surname.
Oak, Oaks, Ochs
Oakley OE. Place name: "Oak-tree meadow." The equally unusual **Ackerley** and **Acton** also refer to landmark oak trees.
Oak, Oakes, Oakleigh, Oaklee, Oakly

Obadiah Heb. "Servant of God." One of the lesser Old Testament prophets. The name has faded gradually from sight after its revival by the Puritans in the 17th century.
Obadias, Obadya, Obed, Obediah, Obie, Ovadiah, Ovadiach, Oved

Oberon OG. "Highborn and bearlike." This is its more famous (though little-used) form, as used by Shakespeare for the King of the Fairies in *A Midsummer Night's Dream.* It also occurs (very rarely) as **Auberon.** Author Auberon Waugh.
Auberon, Auberron, Oberron

Obert OG. "Wealthy and bright."

Octavius Lat. "Eighth child." In English-speaking countries the name had its heyday in the Victorian era of large families. It has survived slightly better in Latin countries. Mexican poet Octavio Paz.
Octave, Octavian, Octavien, Octavio, Octavious, Octavo, Octavus, Ottavio

Odell Derivation disputed. Some sources relate it to either German "Rich" or Greek "Song," but *The Facts on File Dictionary of First Names* claims that it derives from an Old English place name: "Woad hill." Woad is a blue dye reputedly used by the ancient Druids in their religious rites.
Dell, Odall, Odie

Odolf OG. "Prosperous wolf." In the Middle Ages, to allude to a man as a "wolf" was to compliment his fierceness and courage.

Odolff, Odulf

Ogden OE. Place name: "Oak valley." Launched as a first name in the 19th century, but never widely used. Poet Ogden Nash.

Ogdan, Ogdon

Olaf Scan. "Ancestor." A royal name in Norway, as well as a saint's name, but when it came to the British Isles with Norse invaders, it did not catch on. Novelist Ole Edvart Rolvaag.

Olaff, Olav, Olave, Ole, Olin, Olle, Olof, Olov

Oleg Rus. "Holy." Fashion designer Oleg Cassini.

Olin Eng. Var. **Olaf**. Actor Ken Olin.

Olen, Olyn

Oliver Lat. "Olive tree" is the most common meaning assigned, but some scholars suggest ONorse. "Kindly" or "Ancestor," among other possibilities. It came to Britain from France, and the controversial Lord Protector Oliver Cromwell made it unpopular for generations. A mild revival occurred in the late 19th century, and the name is infrequently used in the U.S. today. It is very fashionable in England, though. Charles Dickens's *Oliver Twist;* director Oliver Stone; actor Oliver Platt.

Noll, Oliverio, Olivero, Olivier, Oliviero, Olivio, Olivor, Olley, Ollie, Olliver, Ollivor

Omar Arab. "Elevated; follower of the Prophet." Heb. "Expressive." Currently popular in Arab countries and among Muslims in the U.S. Poet Omar Khayyam; actor Omar Sharif; General Omar Bradley.

Omer

Onslow OE. Place name: "Enthusiast's hill."

Onslowe, Ounslow

Oran Ir. Gael. "Green." Also Aramaic. "Light."

Oren, Orin, Orran, Orren, Orrin

Oren Heb. "Pine tree"; Ir. Gael. "Fair, pale-skinned." Very unusual. U.S. Senator Orrin Hatch.

Orin, Orren, Orrin

Orestes Gk. "Man of the mountain." An important figure in

Greek myth, the son of Agamemnon and the brother of Electra, with whose help he murdered his mother (to avenge his father, whom *she* had murdered). Orestes appears in eight of the classic Greek tragedies. Not a cheerful heritage, overall.

Aoresty, Aresty, Oreste

Orford OE. Place name: "Ford of cattle."

Orion Gk. "Son of fire or light." In Greek myth, Orion was a mighty hunter who was turned into the constellation of the same name.

Oryon

Orlando Sp. Var. **Roland** (OG. "Famous land"). Mostly literary and minor late-19th-century use. Composer Orlando Gibbons; football player Orlando Pace; actor Orlando Bloom.

Arlando, Land, Lanny, Orlan, Orland, Roland, Rolando

Orman OG. "Sea-man" or OE. "Spear-man."

Ormand

Ormond OE. place name "Mountain of bears," or "Spear or ship protector"; Ir. Gael. "Red." Irish last name, occasionally transferred.

Ormand, Ormonde

Oro Sp. "Golden."

Orrick OE. Place name: "Old oak tree." Poet Orric Johns.

Orric

Orson Lat. "Like a bear." In an old French story, a child named Orson is reared in the forest by a bear. The name is very unusual, though it may be used by ardent fans of director Orson Welles. Actor Orson Bean.

Orsen, Orsin, Orsini, Orsino, Orsis, Orsonio, Sonny, Urson

Orton OE. Place name: "Shore settlement." Playwright Joe Orton.

Orval OE. "Strength of a spear." Also variant of **Orville**.

Orville OF. Place name: "Town of gold." Though the name translates this way, it may actually have been coined by an 18th-century novelist. Never widespread. Flight pioneer Orville Wright.

Orv, Orval, Orvell, Orvil

Orvin OE. "Spear-friend."
   Orwin, Orwynn
Osbert OE. "Divine and bright." Anglo-Saxon name revived mildly with the antiquarian craze of the 19th century, but now extremely rare. Poet Osbert Sitwell.
Osborn OE. "Divine bear." The 19th-century revival of this Anglo-Saxon name was followed by another small spurt of use in the middle of the 20th century. Rock star Ozzy Osbourne.
   Osborne, Osbourn, Osbourne, Osburn, Osburne, Ozzie
Oscar Scan. "Divine spear." Anglo-Saxon name revived by 18th-century literary use, reaching substantial popularity by the late 19th century. Fans of "Sesame Street" might hesitate to name a baby for the curmudgeonly Oscar the Grouch, but some parents bravely persist. Lyricist Oscar Hammerstein II; playwright Oscar Wilde; fashion designer Oscar de la Renta.
   Oskar, Osker, Ossie, Ozzy
Osgood OE. "Divine Goth." The Goths were a Germanic ethnic group that took over various parts of Europe after the fall of the Roman Empire. Since the Goths were not Christian until well into the sixth century, the meaning of this name is puzzling.
Osmar OE. "Divine and wonderful."
Osmond OE. "Divine protector." Anglo-Saxon name revived in the 19th century, but scarcely found now. Henry James named one of his most sinister characters (Isabel Archer's suitor in *The Portrait of a Lady*) Gilbert Osmond. Singer Michael Osmond; actor Haley Joel Osment.
   Osman, Osment, Osmonde, Osmont, Osmund, Osmunde
Osred OE. "Divine counsel."
Osric OE. "Divine ruler."
   Osrick
Osten Var. Austin (Lat. "Worthy of respect").
   Austen, Austin, Ostin, Ostyn
Oswald OE. "Divine power." Another Anglo-Saxon name that endured partially because of the fame of two saints of

the name. Use has been mostly 19th century, though actor
Ozzie Nelson's real name was Oswald. Fashion designer
Ossie Clark.

**Ossie, Osvald, Osvaldo, Oswaldo, Oswell, Ozzie,
Waldo**

Oswin OE. "Divine friend."

Osvin, Oswinn, Oswyn, Oswynn

Othman OG. "Wealthy man."

Otis OE. "Son of Otto." Use is mostly American. Actor Otis
Skinner.

Oates, Otess

Otto OG. "Prosperous." German name that was fairly common in English-speaking countries until Otto von Bis-
marck's German armies became threateningly powerful at
the turn of the 20th century. The Second World War
against Germany further limited the name's use.

Odo, Othello, Otho

Oved Heb. "Worshiper, follower." Related to **Obadiah.**

Obed

Owen Welsh. Var. Eugene. Gk. "Wellborn." Fairly common
outside Wales since the 18th century. Now steadily used in
the U.S. Author Owen Wister; actor Owen Wilson.

Ewan, Ewen, Owain, Owin

Oxford OE. Place name: "Ford of the oxen." Once upon a
time this was either a kind of laced shoe (generally de-
tested by children) or a famous English university. Now
also a health-care company.

Oxxford

Pablo Sp. Var. **Paul** (Lat. "Little"). Artist Pablo Picasso; cellist Pablo Casals; poet Pablo Neruda.
Pablos

Paco Sp. Var. **Francis** (Lat. "From France"). A diminutive of **Francisco**. Fashion designer Paco Rabanne.
Pacorro

Paddy Ir. Var. **Patrick** (Lat. "Noble, patrician"). Unusual as a given name, though so common as a nickname that it used to be used as a generic term for Irishmen. Author Paddy Chayefsky.
Paddey, Paddie, Padraic, Padraig

Page Fr. A young boy in training as a personal assistant to a knight. Usually a transferred surname, possibly indicating an ancestor who was a page. In the U.S., this has become almost exclusively a girl's name, but some of the diminutives and variations, like **Padgett,** are still used for boys.
Padget, Padgett, Paget, Pagett, Paige, Payge

Palmer OE. "One who holds a palm." Usually indicates a pilgrim, who would have carried a palm branch on his pilgrimage.
Pallmer, Palmar, Palmerston

Paquito Sp. Dim. **Francis** (Lat. "From France").
Paco

Paris OE. Place name: "From Paris," the city. Also a figure in Greek myth who was Helen of Troy's lover. Use of the name is predominantly American and is beginning to cross over to use for girls.
Parris

Parker OE. "Park keeper." Occupational name turned surname, popular in the 19th century as a given name but now more unusual. Actor Parker Stevenson; musician Charlie Parker; historian Francis Parkman.

Parke, Parkes, Parkman, Parks

Parkin OE. "Little Peter."

Parken

Parnell OF. "Little Peter." Made famous by the 19th-century Irish politician Charles Parnell, who campaigned for home rule in Ireland.

Parrnell, Pernell

Parr OE. Place name: "Castle park."

Parrish OF. "Ecclesiastical locality." A parish is the area under the care of one pastor or priest. The name would originally have been a last name based on a place name.

Parish, Parris, Parriss

Parry Old Welsh. "Son of Harry." Composer Hubert Parry.

Parrey, Parrie

Pascal Fr. "Child of Easter." Used as a first name in English-speaking countries only since the 1960s, and very scarce. Philosopher Blaise Pascal.

Pascale, Pascalle, Paschal, Paschalis, Pascuale, Pasquale

Patrick Lat. "Noble, patrician." A Roman name made famous by the 5th-century missionary (and patron of Ireland) Saint Patrick, whose feast day on March 17 is celebrated with parades in the United States, an honor accorded to few other saints. The name spread outside of Ireland in the 18th century and was widely used by the middle of the 20th century. It is now steadily used and has lost its firm associations with Ireland. U.S. statesman Patrick Henry; actors Patrick Fugit, Patrick Swayze, Patrick Dempsey, Jason Patric; playwright John Patrick Shanley; basketball player Patrick Ewing.

Paddey, Paddie, Paddy, Padhraig, Padraic, Padraig, Padriac, Pat, Patrece, Patric, Patrice, Patricio, Patrik, Patrizio, Patrizius, Patryk, Pats, Patten, Patton, Patty

Patton OE. Place name: "Fighter's town." Almost too appropriate a meaning for the name of General George Patton. Author Alan Paton.

Paten, Patin, Paton, Patten, Pattin

Paul Lat. "Small." Popular Roman and medieval name whose tremendously widespread modern use dates from the 18th century. Paul is the name of the resilient Sir Paul McCartney, as well as of the pope who spearheaded Vatican II. It is not fashionable in the current vogue for original names, but steadily used by parents seeking a familiar name that everybody knows how to spell. Russian parents enthusiastically use **Pavel**. Artists Paul Cézanne, Paul Gauguin; actors Paul Newman, Paul Bettany; Revolutionary War hero Paul Revere; musician Paul Simon; hockey player Pavel Bure.

Paavo, Pablo, Paolo, Pauel, Paulie, Paulin, Paulinus, Paulus, Pauly, Pavel, Pawel, Pol, Poll, Poul

Paxton Lat./OE. Place name: "Peace town." Actors Paxton Whitehead, Bill Paxton.

Packston, Paxon, Paxten, Paxtun

Payne Lat. "Countryman." See **Paine**.

Paine

Pedro Sp. Var. **Peter** (Gk. "Rock"). Filmmaker Pedro Almodovar.

Pedrio, Pepe, Petrolino, Piero

Pell ME. "Skin, parchment." As in parchment that legal documents would be written on; this may be an occupational name, indicating an ancestor who was a clerk.

Pall

Pembroke Celt. Place name: "Bluff, headland."

Pembrook

Penley OE. Place name: "Enclosed meadow."

Penlea, Penleigh, Penly, Pennlea, Pennleigh, Pennley

Penn OE. "Enclosure." In the U.S., tied to the eminent Quaker and founder of Pennsylvania, William Penn.

Pen

Percival OF. "Pierce the vale." Invented by a medieval poet for one of King Arthur's knights, and its meaning is not completely clear. Adopted with some enthusiasm, however, and was particularly well used in the late 19th century, along with more genuinely ancient names. Now scarce.

Parsafal, Parsefal, Parsifal, Perce, Perceval, Percevall, Percey, Percivall, Percy, Purcell

Percy Fr. "From Percy." A Norman place name that became

associated with an immensely powerful aristocratic family in the North of England. Its greatest popularity coincided with that of **Percival,** and like that name, Percy is now widely neglected. Author Walker Percy; poet Percy Bysshe Shelley.

Pearcy, Percey, Percie

Peregrine Lat. "Traveler, pilgrim." "Peregrinations" is a synonym for "wanderings." Peregrine is also the name of a kind of falcon. The name persists in a small way in Britain. English writer Peregrine Worsthorne.

Peregrin, Peregrino, Peregryn

Perkin OE. "Little Peter."

Perkins, Perkyn, Perrin

Perry Dim. **Peregrine**; or OE. Place name: "Pear tree." Modern use seems mostly to be inspired by fictional detective Perry Mason. Singer Perry Como; designer Perry Ellis.

Parry, Perrie

Pesach Heb. "Spared." The Hebrew name for the great holiday of Passover, which commemorates the fact that Jehovah spared the Israelites in a plague that killed many Egyptians.

Pessach

Peter Gk. "Rock." New Testament name; the saint who, tradition has it, guards the gates to Heaven. The name's greatest popularity came in the first three-quarters of the twentieth century, prompted, some sources suggest, by the play *Peter Pan.* Artists Piero della Francesca, Peter Paul Rubens; Russian emperor Peter the Great; actors Peter O'Toole, Peter Krause; Peter Rabbit; film directors Peter Bogdanovich, Peter Jackson; tennis player Pete Sampras.

Peadar, Pearce, Peder, Pedro, Peerus, Peirce, Per, Perkin, Pero, Perrin, Perry, Pete, Petey, Peto, Petr, Pierce, Piero, Pierre, Pierson, Piet, Pieter, Pietrek, Pietro, Piotr, Pjotr, Pyotr

Peverell OF. "Piper."

Peverall, Peverel, Peveril

Peyton OE. Place name: "Fighting-man's estate." Probably related to **Patton.** Primarily American use, probably as a transferred last name, i.e., a mother's maiden name. Football players Walter Payton, Peyton Manning; basketball player Gary Payton.

Payton

Phelan Ir. Gael. "Wolf." Mostly Irish use.

Felan, Phelim, Felim

Phelps OE. "Son of Philip."

Philip Gk. "Lover of horses." The name of one of the twelve apostles, and a staple since early Christian times, though it receded somewhat in the 19th century. A 20th-century resurgence peaked in the 1960s and like **Peter,** Philip is familiar but not common. Britain's Prince Philip; Crown Prince Felipe of Spain; painter Filippo Lippi; playwright Philip Barry; talk show host Phil Donahue; actor Philip Seymour Hoffman; author Philip Roth; football player Phil Simms.

Felipe, Filip, Filippo, Fillip, Fyllip, Phil, Philipp, Philippe, Philippos, Philippus, Phillip, Phillips, Phyllip, Phyllip, Pip, Pippo

Philo Gk. "Loving."

Phineas Derivation and meaning unknown, though many sources offer Heb. "Oracle." Another possible meaning is "mouth of brass," which would be appropriate for showman Phineas T. Barnum. Violinist Pinchas Zuckerman.

Fineas, Phinehas, Pincas, Pinchas, Pinchos, Pincus, Pinhas, Pinkus

Pickford OE. "From the ford at the peak."

Pierce Var. **Peter** (Gk. "Rock"). One of a group of **Peter**-derived names along with **Piers, Pearson,** etc. Actor Pierce Brosnan.

Pearce, Pears, Pearson, Pearsson, Peerce, Peirce, Piers, Pierson, Piersson

Pierre Fr. Var. **Peter**. Currently well-used in France. Canadian Prime Minister Pierre Trudeau.

Piers Gk. "Rock." **Peter** is actually the Latin form of the name that the Normans took to Britain as Piers. This form, along with **Pierce,** has been an alternate form more popular in Britain than in America.

Pearce, Pears, Pearson, Pierce, Pierson, Piersson

Pio Lat. "Pious." A name used by twelve popes, but not found much among English-speaking children.
Pius

Pitney OE. Place name: "Island of the stubborn one."
Pittney

Pitt OE. Place name: "Pit or ditch." Actor Brad Pitt.

Placido Sp. "Serene." Made famous currently by opera star Placido Domingo.
Placedo, Placidus, Placijo, Placyd, Placydo, Plasedo

Plato Gk. "Broad-shouldered." Its occasional use in English-speaking countries may be inspired by admiration for the famous Greek philosopher.
Platon

Platt OF. Place name: "Flat land."
Platte

Pollard ME. "Shorn head." "Poll" was originally a term for head, hence our expression "take a poll." A pollard tree's branches have been cut back to the trunk to promote a bushy growth at the top. Thus the name may either be a place name (for someone who lived near a pollard tree) or a descriptive name (for someone whose head had been closely cropped).
Poll, Pollerd, Pollyrd

Pollock OE. Var. **Pollux**. Artist Jackson Pollock.
Pollack, Polloch

Pollux Gk. "Crown." Along with Castor, one of the Heavenly Twins, the constellation also known as Gemini.

Pomeroy OF. Place name: "Apple orchard." The French word for apple is *pomme*.
Pommeray, Pommeroy

Ponce Sp. "Fifth." Made famous by Spanish explorer Ponce de Leon, but no more common than **Quintus,** its Latin equivalent.

Porfirio Gk. "Purple stone." The English term is "porphyry." Very rare, but borne by one of the 20th century's great playboys, Porfirio Rubirosa, as well as a saint of the 4th century.
Porphirios, Prophyrios

Porter Lat. "Gatekeeper." Occupational name.

Powell OE. Surname related to **Paul**. Author Anthony Powell; Secretary of State Colin Powell.

Powel

Prentice ME. "Apprentice."

Prentis, Prentiss

Prescott OE. Place name: "Priest's cottage." One of the middle names of former President George H.P. Bush, but not widespread.

Prescot, Prestcot, Prestcott

Presley OE. Place name: "Priest's meadow." In the Middle Ages, when these names came into use, the priest was a very important figure in any community. Of course, in the late 20th century the name is associated with another important figure, Elvis Presley.

Presleigh, Presly, Presslee, Pressley, Prestley, Priestley, Priestly

Preston OE. Place name: "Priest's estate." Actor Robert Preston; film director Preston Sturges.

Prewitt OF. "Brave little one."

Prewet, Prewett, Prewit, Pruitt

Price Welsh. "Son of Rhys." **Rhys** is a common Welsh name meaning "ardent."

Brice, Bryce, Pryce

Primo It. "First; firstborn." Number names usually refer to children born with quite a number of older siblings (**Quintus, Octavian**), and tend to indicate exhaustion of the imagination, but Primo may allude to great pride in the firstborn, especially a son. Author Primo Levi.

Preemo, Premo, Prime

Prince Lat. "Prince." As a last name, it may have indicated someone who worked in a prince's household, and occasional first-name use is generally transferred from the last name. There are, of course, exceptions, like the musician formerly known as Prince, who undoubtedly cherished the name for its royal connotations. Comedian Freddie Prinze and actor Freddie Prinze Jr.; theatrical producer Harold Prince.

Printz, Printze, Prinz, Prinze

Proctor Lat. "Official, administrator." Occupational last name.
Prockter, Procter

Prosper Lat. "Fortunate," as in "prosperous." Poet Prosper Mérimée.
Prospero

Pryor Lat. "Monastic leader." A prior is the monk in charge of a monastery, so this might be an occupational name. On the other hand, the tradition of monastic chastity would seem to prevent such a name's being handed down to children.
Prior

Purvis Eng./Fr. "Purveyor." Originally indicated someone who provided food, or provisions.
Purves, Purviss

Quennell OF. Place name: "Small oak."
Quennel
Quentin Lat. "Fifth." Probably used without any consideration of its meaning since so few families extend to five children anymore. Author Quentin Crisp.
Quent, Quenten, Quenton, Quint, Quintin, Quinton, Quintus

Quigley Ir. Gael. Meaning disputed: possibly "Distaff," or "One with messy hair."

Quillan Ir. Gael. "Cub."
Quillen

Quimby ONorse. Place name: "Estate of the woman." A woman's estate would have been quite a rarity in the Old Norse era.
Quinby

Quincy OF. Place name: "Estate of the fifth son." Last name of a prominent Massachusetts family whose name is borne by a town and by the 6th U.S. President, John Quincy Adams. Musician Quincy Jones.
Quin, Quincey, Quinsy

Quinlan Ir. Gael. "Fit, shapely, strong."
Quindlen

Quinn Ir. Gael. Meaning unknown. Very common Irish last name, occasionally transferred to first-name status, especially in the U.S. Actors Anthony Quinn, Aidan Quinn.

Rabi Arab. "Gentle wind."
Rabbi, Rabee
Rad OE. "Adviser."
Radbert OE. "Bright adviser."

Radburn OE. Place name: "Red brook."
Radborn, Radborne, Radbourn, Radbourne, Radburne

Radcliff OE. Place name: "Red cliff." In America, most likely to be associated with the renowned women's college that is now part of Harvard. Actor Daniel Radcliffe.
Radcliffe, Radclyffe, Ratcliff, Ratcliffe

Radford OE. Place name: "Red ford" or "Ford with reeds."
Radferd, Radfurd

Radley OE. Place name: "Red meadow." As in **Radford**, the first element could also refer to reeds.
Radlea, Radlee, Radleigh, Radly

Radnor OE. Place name: "Red shore" or "Reedy shore."

Rafael var. **Raphael** (Heb. "God has healed").

Rafferty Ir. Gael. "Prosperity wielder." Irish last name occasionally used as a first name.
Raferty, Raffarty, Raffertey

Rafi Arab. "Holding high."
Rafee, Raffi, Raffy

Ragnar Nor. "Powerful army" or "Warrior of judgment."
Though this ancient Scandinavian form is very rare in the
U.S., it is related to Germanic names like **Reginald** and
Rainier.
**Ragnor, Rainer, Rainier, Rayner, Raynor, Regner,
Reiner**

Rainart Ger. "Mighty judgment."
**Rainhard, Rainhardt, Reinart, Reinhard, Reinhardt,
Reinhart, Renke**

Rainier Fr. var. **Reginald** (OE. "Counsel power"). Today's
most famous Rainier is the late Grace Kelly's husband,
Prince Rainier of Monaco. Poet Rainer Maria Rilke.
Rainer, Rayner, Raynier

Raleigh OE. Place name: "Meadow of roe deer." Commemorates Sir Walter Raleigh, explorer and court favorite
of Queen Elizabeth I, who is supposed to have spread his
cape over a puddle so she could cross with dry feet. The
city in North Carolina was named for him.
Ralegh, Rawleigh, Rawley, Rawly

Ralph OE. "Wolf-counsel." A name that has been steadily, if
not enormously, popular for the last thousand years (though
today's parents might not recognize it immediately in older
forms like Rathulf or Radolphus). Its greatest vogue in the
U.S. occurred at the turn of the century. Now uncommon.
Poet Ralph Waldo Emerson; consumer activist Ralph
Nader; actors Ralph Macchio, Ralph Fiennes.
Rafe, Raff, Ralf, Raoul, Raul, Rolf, Rolph

Ralston OE. Place name: "Ralph's settlement."

Ramiro Port. "Great judge." Baseball player Manny
Ramirez.
Ramirez

Ramon Sp. Var. **Raymond** (OG. "Counselor-protector").
Given its greatest exposure by the silent-movie star of the
1920s, Ramon Novarro. Baseball player Ramon Martinez.

Ramsay OE. Place name: "Raven island" or "Ram island."
Originally a last name common in Scotland. English

statesman Ramsay McDonald; U.S. Attorney General
Ramsey Clark.

Ramsey

Ramsden OE. Place name: "Ram valley." Like most of
these place names turned last names, this was transferred
to a first name in the 19th century.

Rand OE. "Shield, fighter." Generally a diminutive of **Randolph** and related names.

Randall OE. "Shield-wolf." This is the medieval spoken
form of **Randolph**. Enjoyed some popularity with parents
in the baby boom era. Actor Tony Randall; football player
Randall Cunningham; poet Randall Jarrell.

**Rand, Randal, Randel, Randell, Randey, Randie,
Randl, Randle, Randy**

Randolph OE. "Shield-wolf." From the same root as **Randall**, which has been more popular in the U.S. English
politician Lord Randolph Churchill.

Randal, Randall, Randell, Randolf, Randy

Randy Dim. **Randall, Randolph**. More popular now than
either Randall or Randolph.

Randey, Randi, Randie

Ranger OF. "Forest guardian."

Rainger, Range

Rankin OE. "Little shield" or Celt. "Son of Francis." A last
name found in Scotland and Ireland, rarely transferred as
a first name.

Rankine, Rankinn

Ransford OE. Place name: "Raven ford."

Ransley OE. Place name: "Raven meadow."

Ransleigh, Ransly

Ransom Opinions differ: possibly OE. "Shield's son," possibly a diminutive of **Randolph**. First-name use is mostly
a late-Victorian phenomenon.

Ransome

Raoul Fr. Var. **Ralph** (OE. "Wolf-counsel"). Uncommon
among English-speaking parents. Actor Raul Julia.

Raul, Roul, Rowl

Raphael Heb. "God has healed." The name of one of the
archangels, possibly (because of his name) the one who

stirred the waters at the pool of Bethesda to give it healing powers. Most common in very religious eras (16th and 17th centuries) and the 19th century, which cherished the picturesque. May become more popular (as **Gabriel** has) in the current quest for the unique. Painter Raphael Sanzio; author Raphael Yglesias.

Falito, Rafal, Rafael, Rafaelle, Rafaelo, Rafaello, Rafe, Rafel, Rafello, Raffael, Raffaello, Raphaello, Raphello, Ravel

Rashid Arab. "Righteous, rightly advised." **Rashida** is also used for girls.

Rasheed, Rasheid, Rasheyd

Rasmus Dim. **Erasmus** (Gk. "Loved, desired"). Used occasionally in German-speaking countries.

Ravi Hindi. "Sun." Made familiar to today's parents by the eminent sitar player Ravi Shankar.

Ravee

Rawlins OF. Ultimately a diminutive of **Roland**. A name like this was originally an oral contraction (**Rolandson** to **Rawlinson** to **Rawlins**), then became a last name, and was revived in the late 19th century as a first name.

Rawlinson, Rawson

Ray Dim. **Raymond**. Quite firmly rooted as an independent name, used mostly in the 20th century. Singer Ray Charles; boxer Sugar Ray Leonard; author Ray Bradbury; actors Ray Liotta, Ray Romano.

Rae, Rai, Raye, Reigh

Rayburn OE. Place name: "Roe-deer brook." Painter Henry Raeburn.

Raeborn, Raeborne, Raebourn, Raeburn, Rayborn, Raybourne, Rayburne

Raymond OG. "Counselor-protector." Old Teutonic name that was used in the Middle Ages, then forgotten until a very strong 19th-century revival, especially in America. Though far from fashionable, it is steadily used in a quiet way. Author Raymond Chandler; actors Raymond Massey, Raymond Burr.

Raemond, Raemondo, Raimond, Raimondo, Raimund, Raimundo, Rajmund, Ramon, Ramond, Ramonde,

Ramone, Ray, Rayment, Raymondo, Raymund, Raymunde, Raymundo

Raynor Nor. "Mighty army." An anglicized version of **Ragnar**, and a version of the better-known **Rainier**.

Ragnar, Rainer, Rainier, Rainor, Ranieri, Raynar, Rayner

Read OE. "Red-haired." Descriptive name that long ago became a last name, and thence a first name, especially in the U.S.

Reade, Reed, Reid, Reide

Reading OE. "Son of the red-haired." Also a place name.

Redding, Reeding, Reiding

Redford OE. Place name: "Red ford." Hard to use today without invoking the ultrafamous blond actor, Robert Redford.

Radford, Radfurd, Redfurd

Redley OE. Place name: "Red meadow."

Radley, Redlea, Redleigh, Redly

Redman OE. Obscure: could mean either "Man of counsel" or "Man who rides." Never a common choice for parents.

Redmond Ir. Var. **Raymond.**

Radmond, Radmund, Redmund

Reece Welsh. "Fiery, zealous." The native Welsh form is **Rhys,** and it is very popular in Wales. Actor Roger Rees.

Rees, Reese, Rhys, Rice

Reed OE. "Red-haired." This spelling of the name had a mild flourish of popularity in the baby boom era.

Read, Reade, Reid, Reyd

Reeve ME. Occupational name: "Bailiff." A reeve was an administrator for the king or someone of high position, who collected rents and maintained order on the lord's estates. Actor Christopher Reeve.

Reave, Reeves

Regan Ir. Gael. "Little king." Mostly 20th-century use.

Reagan, Reagen, Regen

Reginald OE. "Counsel power." **Ronald** and **Reynolds** are just two of the names that come from the same source; Reginald's popularity was mainly British and 19th century. Actor Judge Reinhold; baseball star Reggie Jackson; theologian Reinhold Niebuhr.

Naldo, Raghnall, Rainault, Rainhold, Raonull, Raynald, Rayniero, Reg, Reggie, Regin, Reginalt, Reginauld, Reginault, Reginvald, Reginvalt, Regnauld, Regnault, Reinald, Reinaldo, Reinaldos, Reinhold, Reinold, Reinwald, Renaud, Renault, Rene, Reynaldo, Reynaldos, Reynold, Reynolds, Rheinallt, Rinaldo, Ronald

Remington OE. Place name: "Raven-family settlement." Familiar to Americans as a brand of razors. Artist Frederick Remington.

Remy Fr. "From Rheims." Champagne, and the fine brandies made from champagne, are the principal product of Rheims, a town in central France. The name is used—albeit rarely—for both boys and girls. Author Remy Charlip.

Remee, Remi, Remie, Remmey, Remmy

Remus Lat. "Swift." The name of one of the legendary twins (the other was Romulus) who founded Rome. At the turn of the century Joel Chandler Harris's "Uncle Remus" stories (including the famous one about the Tar Baby) were very popular.

Remo

René Fr. "Reborn." The modern form of **Renatus,** which did not survive as a male name. Unlike the female version, René has not really spread beyond French-speaking families, probably because it is well entrenched as a girl's name. Actor René Auberjonois.

Renat, Renato, Renatus

Renfred OE. "Powerful peace."

Renfrew Old Welsh. Place name: "Calm river."

Renny Ir. Gael. "Small and mighty."

Renshaw OE. Place name: "Raven woods."

Renishaw

Renton OE. Place name: "Settlement of the roe deer."

Renzo Dim. **Lorenzo** (Lat. "Laurel"). Interior designer Renzo Mongiardino.

Reuben Heb. "Behold, a son." Old Testament name that

came into general use in the 18th century. Also a sandwich that features corned beef, sauerkraut, and Swiss cheese. Singer Ruben Blades.

Reuban, Reubin, Reuven, Rouvin, Rube, Ruben, Rubin, Rubino, Ruby

Rex Lat. "King." Mostly 20th-century use, possibly influenced by actor Rex Harrison. Probably most common as a name for a dog.

Rexford OE. Place name: "King's ford."

Rey Sp. "King." The Hispanic equivalent of **Rex** or **Leroy**. Not in general use.

Reyes, Reyni

Reynard OF. "Fox" or OG. "Powerful and courageous." Some of the variations (like **Renaud**) come close to variations of the **Reynold/Reginald** names, but are not as common.

Raynard, Reinhard, Reinhardt, Renard, Renaud, Renauld, Rennard

Reynold Var. **Reginald** (OE. "Counsel power"). Probably most familiar in America as a surname, though in the Middle Ages this was the most common form of **Reginald**. Painter Joshua Reynolds.

Reinaldo, Renado, Renaldo, Renato, Renauld, Renault, Reynaldo, Reynolds, Rinaldo

Rhett Var. **Rhys**. Modern parents can hardly use it without thinking of Margaret Mitchell's immortal Rhett Butler, and his great line, "Frankly, my dear, I don't give a damn!"

Rhodes Gk. "Where roses grow." The name of an important Greek island and an important British philanthropist, Cecil Rhodes. He gave his name to both a country (Rhodesia) and a scholarship fund.

Rhoads, Rhodas, Rodas

Rhys Welsh. "Fiery, zealous." This is the native Welsh form of the name that appears more often in English-speaking countries as **Reece**. It is currently very popular in Wales. Actor Roger Rees.

Richard OG. "Dominant ruler." Norman name that went on to be a steady favorite for the last 900 years, with one century (the 19th) of neglect. In the current hunger for the unusual, it is somewhat overlooked, but plenty of parents still choose it. Ricardo is very popular in Spain. English Kings Richard I-III; rock star Little Richard; composer Richard Rodgers; actors Richard Burton, Richard Kiley, Richard Gere, Richard Chamberlain; photographer Richard Avedon; U.S. President Richard Nixon; football player Rich Gannon.

Dick, Dickie, Dicky, Raechard, Ric, Richard, Ricardo, Riccardo, Rich, Richardo, Richart, Richerd, Richie, Rick, Rickard, Rickert, Rickey, Ricki, Rickie, Ricky, Rico, Rikard, Riki, Rikki, Riocard, Ritchard, Ritcherd, Ritchie, Ritchy, Ritchyrd, Ritshard, Ritsherd, Ryszard

Richmond OG. "Powerful protector." Most frequently encountered in the U.S. as a place name, like the capital city of Virginia.

Rick Dim. **Richard, Frederick**. Used independently, though more common as a nickname. Humphrey Bogart's character in *Casablanca* was named Rick. Actors Rick Moranis, Rick Nelson.

Ric, Ricci, Rickey, Rickie, Ricky, Rik, Rikki, Rikky

Rickward OE. "Mighty guardian."

Rickwerd, Rickwood

Rico It. Dim. **Henry** (OE. "Home ruler") via **Enrico**, or dim. **Ricardo**.

Rider OE. "Horseman." Likely to be a transferred last name, for instance a mother's maiden name. Author Rider Haggard; painter Albert Pinkham Ryder.

Ridder, Ryder

Ridge OE. Place name: "Ridge." Referring to a geographical feature in a landscape, as do the following "Ridg-" names.

Rigg

Ridgeway OE. Place name: "Road on the ridge."

Ridgeley OE. Place name: "Ridge meadow."

Ridgeleigh, Ridgeley, Ridglea, Ridglee, Ridgleigh

Ridley OE. Place name: "Red meadow." Film director Ridley Scott.

Riddley, Ridlea, Ridleigh, Ridly

Riley Ir. Gael. "Courageous." Irish last name used as a first name for the last 150 years. Actor John C. Reilly.
Reilly, Ryley

Ring OE. "Ring." Very unusual, though given exposure by author Ring Lardner. Beatles fans will remember that Ringo Starr took his name from the jewelry he favored.
Ringo

Riordan Ir. Gael. "Bard, minstrel."
Rearden, Reardon

Rip Invented name: made famous by actor Rip Torn, who was actually named Elmore. Before his fame, the best-known American Rip was Rip van Winkle, the man who slept for twenty years in Washington Irving's tale.

Ripley OE. Place name: "Shouting man's meadow."
Ripleigh, Riply

Risley OE. Place name: "Meadow with shrubs."
Rislea, Rislee, Risleigh, Risly, Wrisley

Riston OE. Place name: "Settlement near the shrubs." Financier Walter Wriston.
Wriston

Ritter Ger. "Knight." Actor John Ritter.

Roald OG. "Famous and powerful" or "Famous ruler." Rare in English-speaking countries. Polar explorer Roald Amundsen; author Roald Dahl.

Roark Ir. Gael. "Illustrious and mighty." Usually occurs as a last name. This spelling recalls Howard Roark, the protagonist of Ayn Rand's influential novel *The Fountainhead.* Actor Mickey Rourke.
Roarke, Rorke, Rourke, Ruark

Rob Dim. **Robert**. The most common nickname for Robert is probably **Bob,** but Rob may be given more often as an independent name. Actor Rob Lowe.
Robb, Robbie, Robby

Robert OE. "Bright fame." Another staple male name, common for the last millennium and still in the American top fifty. It has steadily drifted out of top-twenty status in the last dozen years. Senator Robert Kennedy; poet Robert Burns; actors Robert DeNiro, Robert Duvall, Rob

Schneider; authors Robert Ludlum, Robert Lawson; General Robert E. Lee; baseball players Roberto Alomar, Roberto Clemente.

Bert, Bertie, Bob, Bobbie, Bobby, Rab, Rabbie, Riobard, Rip, Rob, Roban, Robb, Robben, Robbin, Robbins, Robbinson, Robby, Robers, Roberto, Robertson, Robi, Robin, Robinson, Robson, Robyn, Robynson, Rupert, Ruperto, Ruprecht

Robin Dim. **Robert**. Usually a girl's name in America, though A.A. Milne immortalized his son as Christopher Robin in the "Winnie the Pooh" stories. Actor Robin Williams; TV personality Robin Leach.

Roban, Robben, Robbin, Robbyn, Robyn

Robinson OE. "Son of Robert." More commonly a last name. Singer Smokey Robinson; poet Robinson Jeffers; actor Paul Robeson.

Robbinson, Robeson, Robynson, Robson

Rocco Ger./It. "Rest." The most common form (in America, at least) of the name of a popular saint who cured plague victims. He was especially venerated in Italy, which may be why this version of the name is the most common. **Rocky** is usually a nickname.

Roch, Roche, Rochus, Rock, Rocko, Rocky, Roque

Rochester OE. Place name: "Stone camp or fortress."

Chester, Chet, Rock

Rock Var. **Rocco**. Actor Rock Hudson is the most important precedent for using this name. His original name was Roy Scherer.

Rocky

Rockley OE. Place name: "Rock meadow."

Rocklee, Rockleigh, Rockly

Rockwell OE. Place name: "Rock spring." Illustrators Norman Rockwell, Rockwell Kent.

Rocky Var. **Rocco**. Impossible to use today without invoking Sylvester Stallone's *Rocky* movies.

Rod Dim. **Roderick**. Used sparingly as an independent name. Actors Rod Steiger, Roddy McDowall.

Rodd, Roddie, Roddy

Roderick OG. "Renowned rule." Most commonly used in

Scotland and other parts of Britain; never a great favorite in America.

Broderick, Brodrick, Brodryck, Rhoderick, Rhodric, Rod, Rodd, Rodderick, Roddie, Roddrick, Roddy, Roderic, Roderich, Roderigo, Roderyck, Rodrick, Rodrik, Rodrigo, Rodrigue, Rodrigues, Rodriguez, Rodrique, Rodriquez, Rodryck, Rodryk, Roric, Rorick, Rory, Rurek, Rurik, Ruy

Rodney OE. Place name: "Island near the clearing." Like many last names, this one began intensive use as a first name in the mid-19th century. This mild popularity has endured for some 150 years. Comedian Rodney Dangerfield.

Rodnee, Rodnie

Roe ME. "Roe deer." May originally have been an occupational name indicating an ancestor who hunted or trapped such deer.

Row, Rowe

Rogan Ir. Gael. "Red-head." Irish Gaelic has several names to indicate red hair; but then, the Irish people produce many redheads.

Roger OG. "Renowned spearman." At its most popular in the Middle Ages and the 19th and 20th centuries, but on the wane since the 1950s. Actors Rutger Hauer, Roger Moore; opera singer Ruggiero Raimondi.

Dodge, Hodge, Rodge, Rodger, Rog, Rogelio, Rogerio, Rogers, Rogiero, Rudiger, Ruggero, Ruggiero, Rutger, Ruttger

Roland OG. "Renowned land." **Orlando** is a more common variant in several European languages. **Rowland** was, for a long time, the preferred version in English. The name dates from the Dark Ages, and the most famous Roland was the valorous nephew of Charlemagne, about whom many romantic tales were written.

Lannie, Lanny, Orlando, Roeland, Rolando, Roldan, Roley, Rolland, Rollie, Rollin, Rollins, Rollo, Rolly, Rowe, Rowland

Rolf Var. **Rudolph** (OG. "Famous wolf"). Most common in Scandinavian countries.

Rolfe, Rolle, Rollo, Rolph, Rowland

Roman Lat. "From Rome." The name of several obscure saints and one short-lived pope. The significance of the name no doubt comes from the fact that Rome is the center of the Roman Catholic faith. Film director Roman Polanski; author Romain Gary.

Romain, Romaine, Romanes, Romano, Romanos, Romanus

Romeo It. "Pilgrim to Rome." Cannot be used without reference to the famous romance, and sure to engender a lot of teasing.

Romney Old Welsh. Place name: "Winding river." Painter George Romney.

Romulus Lat. "Man of Rome." Along with Remus, the legendary founder of Rome, though Romulus actually murdered his twin brother in a quarrel over where to situate the city, which he then ruled for 37 years. A rare name. Playwright Romulus Linney.

Romolo

Ronald OE. "Counsel power." Also from the same source as **Reginald** and **Reynold**. Though it was fairly common in the 1940s and 1950s, most parents will associate Ronald with two-term President Ronald Reagan and with clown Ronald McDonald. In spite of these uncool connections, the name is used from time to time.

Ranald, Renaldo, Ron, Ronaldo, Roneld, Ronell, Ronello, Ronnie, Ronny

Ronan Ir. Gael. "Little seal." Mostly Irish use.

Ronson OE. "Son of Ronald."

Rooney Ir. Gael. "Red-haired." Yet another Irish name indicating the traditional Irish coloring. Actor Mickey Rooney.

Roone, Rowan, Rowen, Rowney

Roosevelt Old Dutch. Place name: "Rose field." A name that would be simply an ethnic curiosity if it hadn't been borne by two 20th-century presidents, Theodore and Franklin Delano Roosevelt (who were second cousins).

Roper OE. Occupational name: "Rope maker."

Rory Ir. Gael. "Red." Also occurs as a nickname for **Rod-**

erick. Mostly Scottish use, but the name seems highly eligible for 21st century popularity, since it is unusual without being weird.

Rosario Port. "The rosary." Most common, for obvious reasons, among Catholic families.

Roscoe ONorse Place name: "Woods of the female deer." Tennis star Roscoe Tanner.
Ross, Rosscoe

Roslin Scot. Gael. "Little redhead."
Roslyn, Rosselin, Rosslyn

Ross Scot. Gael. "Headland." A place name in Scotland, and very popular as a first name there, as well. The name (like so many of the *R* names) may also come from the Gaelic word for "red." Presidential candidate Ross Perot.
Rosse, Rossell

Roswell OE. Place name: "Rose spring."

Roth OG. "Red." Could apply to hair or complexion, though England's flaxen-haired Teutonic invaders might have used it more for the former, in sheer surprise. Actor Tim Roth.
Rothe

Rothwell ONorse. Place name: "Red spring."

Rover ME. "Traveler, wanderer." The term "roving" turns up most often in poetry and songs (as in Byron's poem "So, We'll Go No More A-Roving"), and the name is most commonly given to dogs.

Rowan OE. Place name: "Rowan tree." Also possibly another Gaelic name meaning "red." Presumably, since the term applied to so many people, variations in the name were necessary to tell them apart.
Roan, Rohan, Rowe

Rowell OE. Place name: "Roe deer well."

Rowley OE. Place name: "Roughly cleared meadow."
Rowlea, Rowlee, Rowleigh, Rowly

Roxbury OE. Place name: "Rook's town or fortress." "Rook" may have referred to a large population of rooks or crows.
Roxburghe

Roy Gael. "Red" or Fr. "King." Most popular earlier in the

20th century, but hard to use because of the Roy Rogers chain of fast-food restaurants. Cowboy Roy Rogers; actor Roy Scheider.
Rey, Roi, Ruy

Royal OF. "Royal." Scarce as a name.
Royall

Royce Meaning and origin unclear: Some sources offer OF./OE. "Son of the king"; others suggest OG. "Kind fame." The most famous Royce is the man who, along with Mr. Rolls, began turning out England's foremost luxury car.
Roice

Royden OE. Place name: "Rye hill."
Roydan, Roydon

Royston OE. Place name: Not related to **Roy** at all, but a name whose original meaning varied geographically.

Rudd OE. "Ruddy-skinned." Student leader Mark Rudd.

Rudolph OG. "Famous wolf." Parents would have to have very strong feelings about the name to use it, given the enormous fame of Rudolph the red-nosed reindeer. Actor Rudolph Valentino; ballet star Rudolf Nureyev.
Dolph, Raoul, Rodolfo, Rodolph, Rodolphe, Rolf, Rolfe, Rollo, Rolph, Rolphe, Rudey, Rudi, Rudie, Rudolf, Rudolfo, Rudolphus, Rudy

Rudy Dim. "Rud-" names. Well established by singer Rudy Vallee; fashion designer Rudi Gernreich; New York City Mayor Rudy Giuliani.
Rudee, Rudi

Rudyard OE. Place name: "Red paddock." Preempted by English poet and novelist Rudyard Kipling, though fans of the *Just So Stories* or the *Jungle Book* might want to use it.

Ruford OE. Place name: "Red ford" or "Rough ford."
Rufford

Rufus Lat. "Red-haired." Another redhead name, though this one comes from Latin rather than Gaelic. Most common in the 19th century.
Ruffus, Rufous

Rugby OE. "Rook fortress." The name of a famous British school, which in turn gave its name to a famous game.

Rumford OE. Place name: "Wide river-crossing."

Rupert Var. **Robert**. Well established in Britain since the 18th century, but less used here, possibly because to Americans, it has a very English flavor. Actor Rupert Everett; publisher Rupert Murdoch.
  Ruprecht

Rushford OE. Place name: "Ford with rushes."

Ruskin OF. "Little red-haired one." Author John Ruskin.

Russell Fr. "Red-head; red-skinned." Originally a last name, but popular as a first name in the middle of the 20th century. Like most fashions of that era, the name is now somewhat neglected. Philosopher Bertrand Russell; author Russell Baker; actor Russell Crowe.
  Roussell, Russ, Russel

Rusty Fr. "Red-haired." Most commonly a nickname, given when the fact of red hair is well established (which may occur long after a bald baby is given a proper name).

Rutherford OE. "Cattle crossing." Most commonly a family name transferred to first-name use, since passionate admiration for U.S. President Rutherford Hayes seems unlikely to influence parental choice. Use may also be limited by the fact that there is no handy nickname.
  Rutherfurd

Rutland ONorse. Place name: "Land of roots" or "Red land."

Rutley OE. Place name: "Root meadow" or "Red meadow."

Ryan Irish last name. Meaning is unclear, though some sources connect it with "king." Has been very popular in recent years, especially in Scotland and Ireland. Actors Ryan O'Neal, Ryan Philippe; baseball player Ryne Sandberg.
  Rian, Rien, Ryen, Ryon, Ryun

Rycroft OE. Place name: "Rye field."
  Ryecroft

Ryland OE. Place name: "Land where rye is grown."
  Ryeland

S **Saber** Fr. "Sword." The kind of curved sword traditionally used by cavalrymen; also a weapon used in modern-day fencing. Slightly bloodthirsty as a first name.

Sabr, Sabre

Sabin Lat. "Sabine." The Sabines were a tribe living in central Italy around the time Romulus and Remus established the city of Rome. In an effort to provide wives for the citizens of Rome, Romulus arranged the mass kidnapping of the Sabine women, which came to be known (and frequently portrayed in art and literature) as the "Rape of the Sabines." The name is more common in the feminine form, **Sabina**.

Sabeeno, Sabino, Savin, Savino

Sacha Rus. Dim. **Alexander** (Gk. "Defender of mankind"). Cropped up in English-speaking countries in the last 20 years. The "-a" ending in Russian is not necessarily feminine. French singer Sacha Guitry.

Sascha, Sasha, Sashenka

Sadler OE. Occupational name: "Harness maker." Like most last names turned first names, this one was first transferred in the 19th century.

Saddler

Safford OE. Place name: "Willow river crossing."

Said Arab. "Happy." Currently popular in Arabic countries and also used in Northern and eastern Africa. Actor Saeed Jaffrey.

Saeed, Saiyid, Sayeed, Sayid, Syed

Salim Arab. "Tranquility."

Saleem, Salem, Selim

Salton OE. Place name: "Manor settlement" or "Willow settlement."

Salvatore It. "Savior." Used mostly by families of Latinate descent. Artist Salvador Dali.
 Sal, Salvador, Salvator, Salvidor, Sauveur, Xavier, Xaviero, Zavier, Zaviero

Sam Dim. **Samuel** or **Samson.** Occasionally used on its own, more commonly a nickname. Playwright Sam Shepard; actor Sam Waterston; singer Sammy Davis, Jr.
 Samm, Sammey, Sammie, Samy

Samson Heb. "Sun." In the Old Testament, Samson was the warrior whose strength ebbed away when his hair was cut by Delilah. The name was used in the Middle Ages, and the Puritans kept it current with their fondness for Old Testament names, but it has not been fashionable for several hundred years.
 Sam, Sampson, Sansom, Sanson, Sansone, Shem

Samuel Heb. "Told by God." A judge and prophet in early Israel; two Old Testament books are named for him. The name was used, predictably, by the Puritans and has never really faded since then, though it peaked in the 19th century. In contrast to lukewarm U.S. use, this is a top-ten name in England. Opera singer Samuel Ramey; lexicographer Samuel Johnson; playwright Samuel Beckett; author Samuel Clemens (Mark Twain); actor Samuel L. Jackson.
 Sam, Sammie, Sammy, Samuele, Samuello, Samwell, Shem

Sanborn OE. Place name: "Sandy stream."
 Sanborne, Sanbourn, Sanburn, Sanburne, Sandborn, Sandbourne

Sancho Lat. "Sacred." Don Quixote's sidekick was called Sancho Panza, which is a little joke, since "Panza" is Spanish slang for "belly."
 Sanche, Sanctio, Sancos, Sanzio, Sauncho

Sanders ME. "Son of Alexander." (Gk. "Defender of mankind.")
 Sanderson, Sandor, Saunders, Saunderson, Sandros

Sandor Hung. Var. **Alexander** (Gk. "Defender of mankind"). Novelist Sandor Marai.
 Sandros, Xandros

Sanditon OE. "Sandy settlement."

Sandy Dim. **Alexander** (Gk. "Defender of mankind"). Sometimes also given as a nickname based on a person's coloring, like **Rusty**. Apparently red or reddish hair is unusual enough to warrant this kind of name, but corresponding names for blonds or brunets don't seem to exist.
Sandey, Sandie, Sandino

Sanford OE. Place name: "Sandy ford." Acting teacher Sanford Meisner.
Sandford, Sandfurd

Santiago Sp. "Saint James." Catholics are traditionally less reluctant to use religious names than Protestants, routinely naming children **Salvatore, Socorro,** and even **Jesus,** as well as choosing the names of individual saints.
Sandiago, Sandiego, Santeago, Santiaco, Santigo

Santo It./Sp. "Holy." Also a nickname for full saints' names.
Santos

Sargent OF. Occupational name: "Officer." Painter John Singer Sargent; politician Sargent Shriver.
Sarge, Sergeant, Sergent, Serjeant

Saturnin Sp. "Saturn." A "saturnine" temperament is moody or sullen, and people born under the sign of Saturn (Capricorns) are generally considered painstaking, reliable, and reserved.
Saturnino

Saul Heb. "Asked for." The name of the first king of Israel, and also the name of the apostle Paul before his conversion to Christianity. Overlooked in the 16th-century revival of Old Testament names, at its peak in the late 19th century. Author Saul Bellow.
Saulo, Shaul, Sol, Sollie

Saville Fr. "Willow town." Savile Row, in London, is the worldwide source for fine men's tailoring.
Savil, Savile, Savill, Savylle

Sawyer ME. Occupational name: "Wood-worker." Most familiar as the name of Mark Twain's boy hero, *Tom Sawyer.*

Saxon OE. "Knife, sword." Used for one of the Germanic

tribes that fought with short-bladed weapons. The name may also refer to origin in the German area of Saxony, which probably took its name from those effective daggers.
Saxe, Saxen

Sayer Welsh. "Woodworker." Football star Gale Sayers.
Sayers, Sayre, Sayres

Scanlon Ir. Gael. "Little trapper."
Scanlan, Scanlen

Schuyler Dutch. "Shield, protection" or "Scholar." Harks back to the Dutch settlers who brought the name to America in the 17th century.
Schuylar, Skuyler, Skylar, Skyler, Skylor

Scott OE. "Scotsman." Use is emphatically 20th century, and while the name is not fashionable it certainly is familiar to parents and nursery school teachers in our era. Actors Scott Glenn, Scott Caan; authors Scott Peck, F. Scott Fitzgerald, Scott Turow; musician Scott Joplin; basketball player Scottie Pippen.
Scot, Scottie, Scotto, Scotty

Seabert OE. "Shining sea."
Seabright, Sebert, Seibert

Seabrook OE. Place name: "Stream near the sea."
Seabrooke

Seamus Ir. Var. **James** (Heb. "He who supplants"). "Shamus" is old-fashioned American slang for a detective, possibly because the urban police force has traditionally been heavily Irish. Poet Seamus Heaney.
Seumas, Seumus, Shamus

Sean Ir. Var. **John** (Heb. "God is gracious"). Spread outside of Ireland only in the 20th century. Quite heavily used now, perhaps influenced by the popularity of actors Sean Connery and Sean Penn. A top-ten name in Ireland. Basketball player Shawn Kemp; actors Sean Hayes, Sean Astin, Sean Bean; musician and entrepreneur Sean ("Puffy" or "P. Diddy") Combs.
Shane, Shaughn, Shaun, Shawn

Searle OE. "Armor." Cartoonist Ronald Searle.

Seaton OE. Place name: "Town near the sea."
Seeton, Seton

Sebastian Lat. "From Sebastia" (an ancient city). Saint Sebastian, an early Christian martyr, was killed in a hail of arrows, and was a favorite subject for Old Master painters. (He is now patron of soldiers.) The name has never been common, though the British have used it somewhat since the 1940s, possibly influenced by a character in Evelyn Waugh's popular *Brideshead Revisited.* In France **Sebastien** is very popular. Track star Sebastian Coe.
Bastian, Bastien, Seb, Sebastiano, Sebastien, Sebestyen, Sebo

Sedgley OE. Place name: "Sword meadow." Could indicate a kind of coarse, sharp reedlike grass growing in a meadow, or that the meadow belonged to (or was frequented by) a swordsman. In all cases, refers to a long-ago meadow.
Sedgeley, Sedgely

Sedgwick OE. Place name: "Sword place." As with Sedgley, the sword could refer to grass or an actual weapon.
Sedgewick, Sedgewyck, Sedgwyck

Seeley OE. "Blessed." From the same Germanic root as Selig.
Sealey, Seely, Seelye

Sefton OE. Place name: "Town in the rushes."

Seger OE. "Sea fighter." Musician Pete Seeger.
Seager, Segar, Seeger

Segundo Sp. "Second." Not common: parents usually have enough imagination to come up with at least two proper names.
Secondo

Selby OE. Place name: "Manor village."
Selbey, Shelbey, Shelbie, Shelby

Seldon OE. Place name: "Willow valley."
Selden, Sellden, Shelden

Selig OG. "Blessed."
Seligman, Seligmann, Zelig

Selwyn OE. "Manor-friend." Alternatively, an offshoot of **Silvanus.** Mostly 19th-century use.
Selwin, Selwinn, Selwynn, Selwynne

Senior OF. "Lord." Hard to use in these days when it has come to mean any individual older than 65.

Sennett Fr. "Elderly." Related to **Senior**. Comedian Mack Sennett.

Sennet

Septimus Lat. "Seventh." Most common in the 19th century, when very large families were the norm.

Seraphim Heb. "Ardent." The seraphim are the highest-ranking angels in Heaven (above angels, archangels, cherubim, etc.). They have six wings and are noted for their zealous love. There have been two Saints Seraphim, one a 17th-century Italian, one an 18th-century Russian mystic.

Sarafino, Saraph, Serafin, Serafino, Seraph, Seraphimus

Sereno Lat. "Tranquil." Though the feminine form, **Serena,** is somewhat popular, the masculine version is very rare.

Cereno

Sergio Lat. "Servant, attendant." Strongly associated with Russia, perhaps because of composers Rachmaninoff and Prokofiev, yet it comes from a Latin name and was used by an early pope. This Spanish form is the most common one in the U.S. Impresario Serge Diaghilev; film director Sergio Leone.

Seargeoh, Sergei, Sergey, Sergi, Sergio, Sergios, Sergiu, Sergiusz, Serguei, Sirgio, Sirgios

Seth Heb. "Set, appointed." In the Old Testament, Adam and Eve's third son (after Cain and Abel). Passed over in the Puritan revival of biblical names, but included to some extent in the late-20th-century revival of the same. Actor Seth Green.

Severin Lat. "Severe."

Severino, Severinus, Seweryn

Severn OE. "Boundary." The Severn is an important river running through southern England.

Seward OE. "Sea guardian" or "Victory guardian." Largely 19th century.

Sewerd, Siward

Sewell OE. "Sea strong."
Sewald, Sewall

Sexton ME. Occupational name: "Church custodian." The sexton (or sacristan) is charged with the upkeep of a church building.

Sextus Lat. "Sixth." Less common than **Septimus** or **Octavius,** though five popes have used it. The first one, oddly enough, was actually Christendom's seventh pope.
Sesto, Sixto, Sixtus

Seymour OF. "From Saint Maur." Indicates an ancestor who came from a village called Saint Maur, most probably in Normandy. Quite a popular name in the 19th century, but virtually invisible today.
Seamore, Seamor, Seamour, Seymore

Shadrach Heb. Meaning unknown. Old Testament name: one of three Hebrew men (along with Meshach and Abednego) thrown into a fiery furnace by King Nebuchadnezzar and rescued by an angel. Used steadily in the 16th–19th centuries, but now rare.
Shad, Shadrack

Shakil Arab. "Good-looking, well-developed." The root of Shaquille O'Neal's name, and more accurate than his parents could ever have predicted.
Shakeel, Shakill, Shakille, Shaqueel, Shaquil, Shaquille

Shalom Heb. "Peace." Related to Solomon.
Sholom, Solomon

Shamus Var. Seamus (Ir. Var. **James:** Heb. "The supplanter").

Shanahan Ir. Gael. "Wise, clever." Football coach Mike Shanahan.

Shandy Possibly OE. "Boisterous, high-spirited."
Shandey

Shane Var. Sean (Ir. Var. **John:** Heb. "The Lord is gracious"). Popularity in the 1950s and 1960s probably depended on the film *Shane.* Now losing ground. Screenwriter Shane Black.
Shaine, Shayn, Shayne

Shanley Ir. Gael. "Small and ancient." Playwright John Patrick Shanley.
Shannley

Shannon Ir. Gael. "Old, ancient." The name of an important river, county, and airport in Ireland, used as a first name in this century. Most popular among families with Irish roots, and more common for girls. Football player Shannon Sharpe.
Shanan, Shanen, Shannan, Shannen, Shanon

Shaquille Modern re-spelling of **Shakil** (Arab. "Well-developed, good-looking"). Known the world over as the name of basketball megastar Shaquille O'Neal.
Shaq, Shaqeell, Shaqueel, Shaquil

Sharif Arab. "Honest." Actor Omar Sharif.
Shareef

Shaw OE. Place name: "Copse, grove of trees."

Shawn Var. Sean. This version is not as common as the Irish spelling, **Sean**. Basketball player Shawn Kemp.
Shawnel, Shawnell

Sheehan Ir. Gael. "Small and tranquil."

Sheffield OE. Place name: "Crooked meadow."

Shelby OE. Place name: "Village on the ledge." Author Shelby Foote.
Shelbey, Shelbie

Sheldon OE. Place name: "Steep valley," or possibly "Flat-topped hill." Most common in the middle of the 20th century. Author Sidney Sheldon.
Shelden, Sheldin

Shelley OE. Place name: "Ledge meadow." Last name made famous by the poet Percy Bysshe Shelley. Much more commonly used for girls at the moment.
Shelly

Shelton OE. Place name: "Ledge village."

Shem Heb. "Fame." The name of Noah's eldest son in the Old Testament. (Ham and Japheth were the other two.) None of the sons' names are as popular as that of their father, and though the entire human race descends, according to the Bible, from these three men and their wives, the wives are never named at all.

Shepherd OE. Occupational name: "Shepherd." Mostly 19th-century use, very uncommon now. *Pooh* illustrator Ernest Shepard.

Shep, Shepard, Shephard, Shepp, Sheppard, Shepperd

Shepley OE. Place name: "Sheep meadow."

Sheplea, Shepleigh, Shepply, Shipley

Sherborn OE. Place name: "Bright stream."

Sherborne, Sherbourn, Sherburn, Sherburne

Sheridan Ir. Gael. Unclear meaning, possibly "Wild man." Used mostly in Britain. Critic Sheridan Morley; playwright Richard Brinsley Sheridan; Civil War General Philip Sheridan.

Sheredan, Sheridon, Sherridan

Sherlock OE. "Bright hair." Irresistibly reminiscent of Arthur Conan Doyle's fictional detective, Sherlock Holmes.

Sherlocke, Shurlock

Sherman OE. Occupational name: "Shear man." Around the time when last names were coming into being, England's great export was wool. The wool business has given the modern world a number of occupational names, like Sherman, **Shepherd, Fuller,** and **Weaver**. Civil War general William Tecumseh Sherman.

Scherman, Schermann, Shearman, Shermann

Sherwin ME. "Bright friend."

Sherwind, Sherwinn, Sherwyn, Sherwynne

Sherwood OE. Place name: "Shining forest." Sherwood Forest, a real forest in central England, was the home of the legendary bandit/hero Robin Hood. Playwright Robert Sherwood; Author Sherwood Anderson.

Sherwoode, Shurwood

Shipton OE. Place name: "Sheep village" or "Ship village."

Shlomo Var. Solomon (Heb. "Peaceable").

Shelomi, Shelomo, Shlomi

Sidney OE. "From Saint Denis." Famous English last name turned first name in the 18th century, very fashionable in the late 19th century, now little used for boys. Author Sid-

ney Sheldon; film director Sydney Pollack; actor Sidney
Poitier.
Sid, Sydney

Siegfried OG. "Victory peace." The hero of the last two of
Wagner's "Ring" cycle of operas, son of Siegmund, husband of Brunhilde.

Sigmund OG. "Victorious protector." Another character
from the "Ring" cycle, son of the god Wotan. He fathers
Siegfried on his own sister, Sieglinde. The other famous
Sigmund is the father of psychoanalysis, Sigmund Freud.
A name with many weighty connotations.
**Seigmond, Segismond, Siegmund, Sigismond,
Sigismondo, Sigismund, Sigismundo, Sigismundus,
Sigmond, Szygmond**

Sigwald OG. "Victorious leader."
Siegwald

Silas A contraction of **Silvanus**. New Testament name used
in the Puritan era and occurring since then. Has an old-
fashioned air that may appeal to parents of the 21st century.
**Silvan, Silvano, Silvaon, Silvanus, Silvio, Sylas,
Sylvan**

Silvanus Lat. "Wood dweller." Also a New Testament
name, but never as widely adopted as its spinoff, **Silas**.
Silvain, Silvano, Silvio, Sylvanus, Sylvio

Silvester Lat. "Wooded." Original form of the name we
know as **Sylvester**.
Silvestre, Silvestro, Sylvester

Simon Heb. "Listening intently." Prominent New Testament name, one of the twelve apostles. A common name
from the Middle Ages through the 18th century, then revived early in the 20th century. To Americans, it has a
rather English air. Simeon, the Old Testament version, has
never been as common. Orchestra conductor Simon Rat-
tle; Latin American freedom fighter Simón Bolívar.
**Shimon, Si, Sim, Simen, Simeon, Simmonds,
Simmons, Simms, Simone, Simonson, Simpson,
Symms, Symon, Syms, Szymon**

Sinclair OF. Place name: "From Saint Clair." Still much more familiar as a last name. Authors Sinclair Lewis, Upton Sinclair.
Sinclare, Synclair

Siraj Arab. "Light, beam."

Skelly Ir. Gael. "Bard."
Scully

Skerry ONorse. Place name: "Stony isle."

Skip Scan. "Ship boss." The term that has come down to us is "skipper," for the captain of a ship or boat. Skip occurs more commonly as a nickname.
Skipp, Skipper

Slade OE. Place name: "Valley." Art collector Felix Slade.
Slaide, Slayde

Slater OE. Occupational name: "Hewer of slates." Actor Christian Slater.

Slavin Ir. Gael. "Mountain man."
Slawin, Slavin, Sleven

Sloan Ir. Gael. "Man of arms." An Irish last name that has become well entrenched in Britain and the U.S. Sometimes makes the leap to first-name status, perhaps as a maternal maiden name. Novelist Sloan Wilson.
Sloane

Smedley OE. Place name: "Flat meadow."
Smedleigh, Smedly

Smith OE. Occupational name: "Blacksmith." This extremely common last name occurs as a first name, but parents would be unlikely to use it unless it was a family name. Economist Adam Smith; Mormon leader Joseph Smith; Smithsonian founder James Smithson.
Smithson, Smitty, Smyth, Smythe, Smythson

Snowden OE. Place name: "Snowy peak." The name of a mountain in Wales, and the title (Earl of Snowdon) of the late Princess Margaret's ex-husband.
Snowdon

Socrates Gk. Meaning unknown. The name of the great Greek philosopher, used mostly by Greek families.
Sokrates

Solomon Heb. "Peaceable." In the Old Testament, the wise king of Israel. Used in the Middle Ages and the 18th century, but currently a far from common choice.
Salmon, Salomo, Salomon, Salomone, Shalmon, Sol, Solaman, Sollie, Soloman

Somerset OE. Place name: "Summer settlement." A county in England, and a last name given prominence as a first name by author and playwright Somerset Maugham.
Sommerset, Summerset

Somerton OE. Place name: "Summer town."
Somervile, Somerville

Sorrell OF. "Red-brown." A term now used to describe the color of a horse, perhaps applied long ago to the color of an ancestor's hair.
Sorel, Sorrel

Southwell OE. Place name: "South well."

Spalding OE. Place name: "Divided field." More commonly a last name, rarely transferred to first-name use. Performance artist Spalding Gray.
Spaulding

Spear OE. Occupational name: "Spear-man." Names are sometimes a window into the concerns of a former era, and a number of names from the war-torn Anglo-Saxon age have to do with weapons.
Speare, Spears, Speer, Speers, Spiers

Spencer ME. Occupational name: "Provisioner." Used for the person in a large household who dispensed food and drink. Usually a last name, but occurs as a first name, more commonly in Britain. Actors Spencer Tracy, John Spencer; poet Edmund Spenser.
Spence, Spenser

Spiridon Gk. "Basket." The name of a 4th-century Cypriot sheep farmer who became a bishop and a popular Greek saint. The name is little used outside Greek communities. U.S. Vice President Spiro Agnew.
Speero, Spero, Spiridion, Spiro, Spiros, Spyridon, Spyros

Squire ME. Occupational name: "Knight's companion." In

more modern terms, perhaps, an aide-de-camp. First-name use mostly 19th century.

Squier, Squiers, Squires, Squyre, Squyres

Stacy Dim. **Eustace** (Gk. "Fertile"). More common as a female name. Actor Stacy Keach.

Stacey, Stacie

Stafford OE. Place name: "Landing place ford." As with many of these place/last names, used mostly in the 19th century.

Stafforde, Staford

Stanbury OE. Place name: "Stone fortification."

Stanberry, Stanbery, Stanburghe, Stansberry, Stansburghe, Stansbury

Stancliff OE. Place name: "Stony cliff."

Stancliffe, Stanclyffe, Stanscliff, Stanscliffe

Standish OE. Place name: "Stony parkland." The Pilgrims' military leader was Miles Standish, whose courtship Longfellow immortalized in a poem.

Stanfield OE. Place name: "Stony field."

Stansfield

Stanford OE. Place name: "Stony ford." Familiar as the name of the great California railroad magnate Leland Stanford, who founded the university that bears his name. Composer Charles Stanford.

Stamford, Standford

Stanislaus Slavic. Possibly "glorious camp or stand." The patron saint of Poland, Saint Stanislaus, was an 11th-century bishop and martyr.

Stana, Stanek, Stanicek, Stanislas, Stanislav, Stanislaw, Stannes, Stanousek, Stasio

Stanley OE. Place name: "Stony field." It is not clear why some place names, like **Sidney** and Stanley, became popular enough so that they made the transition to common first names, while others, like **Stanford** or **Sinclair,** remain primarily last names. As with Sidney, Stanley's transformation to a first name was the result of great popularity at the turn of the century. Filmmaker Stanley Kubrick; actor Stanley Tucci.

Stan, Stanlea, Stanlee, Stanly

Stanmore OE. Place name: "Stony lake." On the evidence of this group of "Stan-" names, stones seem to have occupied a great deal of Anglo-Saxon man's attention, perhaps because they had to be cleared from the earth before it could be farmed effectively.
Stanmere

Stanton OE. Place name: "Stony village."
Stanten, Staunton

Stanway OE. Place name: "Stony roadway."
Stanaway, Stannaway, Stannway

Stanwick OE. "Dweller at the rocky village."
Stanwicke, Stanwyck

Stanwood OE. Place name: "Stony woods."

Starr ME. "Star." Beatle Ringo Starr; football player Bart Starr.

Stavros Gk. "Crowned." Related to **Stephen,** and currently popular in Greece. Greek plutocrat Stavros Niarchos.

Steadman OE. Occupational name: "Farmstead occupant."
Steadmann, Stedman

Steel OE. "Like steel." In the rough times when the name was coined, this would have been quite a compliment. TV character Remington Steele.
Steele

Stein Ger. "Stone." Skiing champion Stein Erickson.
Steen, Sten, Steno, Stensen, Stenssen

Stephen Gk. "Crowned." As the name of Christianity's first martyr (Saint Stephen, who was stoned to death), common until the late 18th century. A slow decline was reversed in the middle of the 20th century, and **Steven** is still going very strong after a long period of great popularity. Though the "ph-" spelling is traditional, the "v-" is much more common. Actors Stephen Collins, Steve Martin, Steve McQueen, Steve Buscemi; songwriter Stephen Foster; physicist Stephen Hawking; author Stephen King; filmmaker Steven Spielberg; musician Stevie Wonder; computer entrepreneur Steven Jobs; film and stage director Stephen Daldry.
Esteban, Estefan, Estevan, Etienne, Staffan, Steban, Steben, Stefan, Stefano, Steffen, Steffon, Stephan,

Stephanus, Stephens, Stephenson, Stephon, Stevan, Steve, Steven, Stevenson, Stevie, Stevy

Sterling OE. "Genuine, first-rate." As in sterling silver. Not common, but has potential for 21st century popularity. Race-car driver Stirling Moss; sports commentator Sterling Sharpe.
Stirling

Sterne ME. "Stern, unbending"; Ger. "Star." Authors Laurence Sterne, Thomas Stearns Eliot; violinist Isaac Stern.
Stearn, Stearne, Stearns, Stern

Stewart OE. Occupational name: "Steward." An early variant of **Stuart,** which finally became the more popular form of the name. It is more common as a first name than many occupational names (**Baker, Shepherd, Carpenter**), but has never really become a standard first name either. Actors Jimmy Stewart, Patrick Stewart, Steward Townsend.
Steward, Stuart

Stillman OE. "Silent man." Filmmaker Whit Stillman.

Stockley OE. Place name: "Tree-stump field." Like the stones in the "Stan-" names, tree stumps would be a hindrance to efficient farming, and thus worthy of note and commemorated in last names.

Stockton OE. Place name: "Tree-stump settlement."

Stockwell OE. Place name: "Tree-stump well."

Stoddard OE. "Horse guard" or "Horse herder." Occupational name.
Stoddart

Storm OE. "Tempest; storm." The almost too appropriate name of meteorologist Storm Field.

Strahan Ir. Gael. "Minstrel, sage." Football player Michael Strahan.
Strachan

Stratford OE. Place name: "Street river-crossing."
Strafford

Strong OE. "Powerful." Originally a name that would characterize its bearer. In the last name, the meaning is lost.

Struthers Ir. Gael. Place name: "Near the brook."
Struther

Stuart OE. Occupational name: "Steward." The steward would administer a large feudal household. This was the name of kings of Scotland and England, often considered the most romantic ruling family. (Long curls, a taste for luxury, a reputation for womanizing, and a couple of beheadings all added to the romance.) Most popular in the middle of the 20th century. Portrait painter Gilbert Stuart.
Steward, Stewart

Styles OE. Place name: "Stile." A stile is a set of stairs placed over a wall so it can be crossed easily on foot—an important feature in a rural landscape.
Stiles

Suffield OE. Place name: "Southern field."

Sulaiman Arab. "Peaceable." The Arabic version of **Solomon**. The Turkish sultan Suleiman the Magnificent brought civilization in his country to new heights, but contemporaneous Western rulers would never have characterized him as living up to his name.
Suleiman, Suleyman

Sullivan Ir. Gael. "Black-eyed." Composer Arthur Sullivan; TV host Ed Sullivan; architect Louis Sullivan.
Sullavan, Sullevan, Sully

Sully OE. Place name: "South meadow." Painter Thomas Sully.
Sulleigh, Sulley

Sutcliff OE. Place name: "Southern cliff."
Sutcliffe

Sutherland Scan. "Southern land." Sutherland is the name of a county in northern Scotland, which was nevertheless to the south of the Nordic people who called it that.
Southerland

Sutton OE. Place name: "Southern settlement."

Sven Scan. "Youth." Currently popular in Sweden, but not much used in English-speaking countries.
Svein, Sveinn, Svend, Swain, Swen, Swensen, Swenson

Sweeney Ir. Gael. "Small hero."
Sweeny

Swinburne OE. Place name: "Swine stream." Swine, or pigs, were also an important feature of life in the days when last names were being formed. Poet Algernon Swinburne.
Swinborn, Swinbourne, Swinburn, Swinbyrn, Swynborne

Swinford OE. Place name: "Swine ford."
Swynford

Swinton OE. Place name: "Swine settlement."

Sylvester Lat. "Wooded." In spite of a distinguished past, the name is now associated with a cartoon cat and an extremely muscular actor, Sylvester Stallone.
Silvester, Sly

Tab Several origins are proposed, including OG. "Shining, brilliant" and ME. "Drummer." But the name would be merely a curiosity without the career of fifties teen idol Tab Hunter, whose given name was Arthur.
Tabb, Taber, Tabor

Tabor Hung. "Encampment" or Heb. "Misfortune, bad luck."
Taber, Taibor, Tavor, Taybor, Tayber

Tabib Turkish. "Doctor."
Tabeeb

Tad Dim. **Thaddeus** (meaning unknown). Also Old Welsh. "Father." Also used as a nickname in the U.S., where "tad" is slang for "small," probably from "tadpole."
Tadd, Thad

Tadeo Sp. Var. **Thaddeus** (meaning unknown).
Taddeo, Tadzio

Taggart Ir. Gael. "Son of the priest."
Taggert

Tahir Arab. "Pure, unsullied."
   Taheer
Tait ONorse. "Cheerful, gay."
   Tate, Tayte
Tal Heb. "Rain, dew."
   Tahl, Talor
Talbot Meaning unknown. An aristocratic last name in England, used as a first name since the 19th century. Tennis star Billy Talbert.
   Talbert, Talbott, Tallbot, Tallbott
Tanner OE. Occupational name: "Leather tanner." Hides need to be tanned, or treated with a substance containing tannin, before they become leather. Fairly well used, though its popularity has been waning since the late 1990s. Artist Henry Ossawa Tanner.
   Tan, Tanier, Tannen, Tanney, Tannie, Tannis, Tannon
Tanton OE. Place name: "Still river settlement."
Tarleton OE. "Thor's settlement." Margaret Mitchell fans will remember the Tarleton twins, admirers of Scarlett O'Hara, in the early pages of *Gone With the Wind*.
Tarrant Old Welsh. "Thunder."
   Tarrent
Tate ME. "Happy, cheerful." Related to Norwegian **Tait**.
   Tait, Taitt, Tayte
Tavish Ir. Gael. "Twin."
   Tavis, Tevis
Taylor ME. Occupational name: "Tailor." Like many occupational names, this was first used as a given name in the 19th century. It has recently become much more popular. In the mid-1990s it was a top-ten girls' name, which may have disqualified it as a choice for boys. Film director Taylor Hackford; football player Lawrence Taylor; singers James and Livingston Taylor.
   Tailer, Tailor, Tayler
Teague Ir. Gael. "Bard, poet." This name and its variants are experiencing a little flicker of popularity among parents who want to be adventurous in their choice of names.
   Teagan, Tegan, Teger, Teigan, Teige, Teigen, Teigue
Ted Dim. **Theodore** (Gk. "Gift of God") or **Edward** (OE.

"Wealthy defender"). Rarely used as an independent name. Parents tend to give the longer rather than the shorter version of a name, even if they have decided ahead of time to use the diminutive form. Newscaster Ted Koppel; actor Ted Danson.

Tedd, Teddey, Teddie, Teddy

Tedmund OE. "Protector of the land."

Tedmond

Telford OF. "Iron-piercer."

Telfer, Telfor, Telfour, Tellfer, Tellfour

Tempest Fr. "Storm." Occurs as an aristocratic English last name, and occasionally as a first name, though few parents could wish for a baby's personality to fit the name.

Tempestt

Templeton OE. Place name: "Temple settlement." Also the name of the rat in *Charlotte's Web,* a point that the young are sure to seize on.

Temp, Temple, Templeten

Tennant OE. "Tenant, renter." Last name used as first name.

Tenant, Tennent

Tennessee Cherokee place name, used for the state. Made famous by playwright Tennessee Williams (whose given name was Thomas) and likely to be used by parents in homage, or perhaps in nostalgia for a childhood home.

Tennyson ME. "Son of Dennis." Used by 19th-century parents in homage to British Poet Laureate Alfred, Lord Tennyson.

Tenny

Terence Lat. Clan name of unknown meaning, though some sources propose "Smooth" or "Polished." Early Christian name that was never widely adopted until the late 19th century, and even then did not become a standard choice. The most common spelling today is **Terrance**. Actor Terence Stamp; playwright Terrence McNally; priest Terence Cardinal Cooke.

Tarrants, Tarrance, Tarrenz, Terencio, Terrance, Terrence, Terrey, Terri, Terris, Terrious, Terrius, Terron, Terronce, Terry

Terrell OG. "Following Thor." Thor, the god of thunder, was a crucial figure in Norse mythology. The son of Odin, the chief god, Thor was the benevolent intercessor for mankind. His name is an element in many names that have come down to us, the most notable being "Thursday." Football players Terrell Davis, Terrell Owens.
Tarrall, Terrall, Terrel, Terrill, Terryal, Terryl, Terryll, Tirrell, Tyrrell

Terry Dim. **Terence**. Lat. Clan name. Used for both boys and girls, almost as frequently as Terence itself. Football player Terry Bradshaw; filmmaker Terry Gilliam.
Terrey, Terri, Terrie

Tex Modern name of the Lone Star state, used occasionally as a first name. It has a rakish aura, no doubt from association with cowboys and the Wild West.

Thaddeus Aramaic. Meaning unclear, though "courageous" and "praise" have been suggested. He was one of the more obscure of the twelve apostles, but even this distinction has not popularized the name. Jude is another form of the name.
Tad, Tadd, Taddeo, Taddeusz, Tadeo, Tadio, Tadzio, Thad, Thaddaios, Thaddaos, Thaddaeus, Thaddaus, Thadeus, Thady

Thane OE. "Landholder." In Old England a thane fit, socially, between the serfs and the nobility. He held his own land, but owed service to his lord. Rare even as a last name.
Thaine, Thayne

Thatcher OE. Occupational name: "Roof thatcher." Very soon this name will be free of any associations with British Prime Minister, Margaret Thatcher.
Thacher, Thatch, Thaxter

Thaw OE. "Melt." Found more often as a last name.

Theobald OG. "Courageous people." Unusual, though some of its foreign variants like **Thibault** are more common in their countries of origin.
Dietbald, Dietbold, Ted, Teddy, Teobaldo, Thebault, Theo, Thibaud, Thibault, Thibaut, Tibold, Tiebold, Tiebout, Tybald, Tybalt, Tybault

Theodore Gk. "Gift of God." Early Christian name and saint's name, but only mildly popular until President Theodore Roosevelt brought it to prominence. (The teddy bear, of course, is named for him.) The name is now neither popular nor unpopular. Authors Theodore Dreiser, Theodore Sturgeon; painter Théodore Rousseau.

Fedor, Feodor, Fyodor, Teador, Ted, Teddie, Teddy, Tedor, Teodoor, Teodor, Teodoro, Theo, Theodor, Theodorus, Theodosios, Theodosius, Todor, Tudor

Theodoric OG. "People's ruler." This is the original form of **Dietrich** and the more common **Derek** or **Dirk**. In this version it is extremely rare.

Derek, Derrick, Dieter, Dietrich, Dirck, Dirk, Rick, Ted, Teodorico, Thedric, Thedrick

Theophilus Gk. "Loved by God." A New Testament name that is very rare, though Thornton Wilder entitled one of his most popular novels *Theophilus North.* French author Théophile Gautier.

Teofil, Teofilo, Théophile

Thierry Fr. Var. **Theodoric**. Not, as one might suppose, the French version of **Terry**. Fashion designer Thierry Mugler.

Thomas Aramaic. "Twin." One of the apostles was known as Doubting Thomas because he refused to recognize the risen Christ unless he could see and feel the marks of the crucifixion. In spite of this skeptical example, the name has been hugely popular since the 12th century martyrdom of Thomas à Becket. Other Saints Thomas include Thomas Aquinas and Thomas More, but the name has been so widely used that it has no religious aura to it. The recent vogue for unusual names has somewhat eclipsed this old standard but it is still one of the basic names for boys born in America, and a top-ten name in England. President Thomas Jefferson; inventor Thomas Edison; actors Tom Cruise, Tom Hanks; dancer Tommy Tune; fashion designer Tom Ford.

Tam, Tamas, Tamhas, Thom, Thoma, Thomason, Thomson, Thompson, Tom, Tomas, Tomaso, Tomasso, Tomasz, Tome, Tomek, Tomey, Tomie, Tomislaw, Tomkin, Tomlin, Tommaso, Tommey, Tommie, Tommy

Thor ONorse. "Thunder." The Norse god of thunder, Thor, holds an important place in the Norse pantheon, but in the Anglo-Saxon world the name appears more often in derivative forms, as in **Terrell**. Explorer Thor Heyerdahl.

Thorin, Thorvald, Tor, Tore, Torre, Tyrus

Thorald ONorse. "Follower of Thor."

Terrell, Terrill, Thorold, Torald, Tyrell

Thorbert ONorse. "Thor's brightness."

Torbert

Thorburn ONorse. "Thor's bear."

Thorbern, Thorbjorn

Thorley OE. Place name: "Thor's meadow" or "Thorn meadow."

Thorlea, Thorlee, Thorleigh, Thorly, Torley

Thormond OE. "Defended by Thor." Senator Strom Thurmond.

Thurman, Thurmond, Thurmund

Thorndike OE. Place name: "Thorny bank."

Thorndyck, Thorndyke

Thorne OE. Place name: "Thorn thicket."

Thorn

Thornley OE. Place name: "Thorny meadow."

Thornlea, Thornleigh, Thornly

Thornton OE. Place name: "Thorny village or town." Used as a first name since the 19th century. Writer Thornton Wilder.

Thorpe OE. Place name: "Hamlet, village." Athlete Jim Thorpe.

Thorp

Thurlow OE. Place name: "Thor's hill."

Thurloe

Thurston Scan. "Thor's stone." Parents who have watched a lot of old sitcoms might shy away from a name that recalled Thurston Howell, the effete millionaire castaway on "Gilligan's Island." Social critic Thorstein Veblen.

Thorstan, Thorstein, Thorsten, Thurstain, Thurstan, Thursten, Torsten, Torston

Tibor Slavic. "Sacred place."

Tiernan Ir. Gael. "Lord."

Tiarnan, Tiarney, Tierney

Tilden OE. Place name: "Fertile valley." Statesman Samuel Tilden; tennis champion William Tilden.

Tillden, Tildon

Tilford OE. Place name: "Fertile ford."

Till Ger. "People's ruler." Another form of **Theodoric,** vaguely familiar to American ears from the German legends about Till Eulenspiegel, inspiration for an opera by Richard Strauss.

Thilo, Tillman, Tilmann

Tilton OE. Place name: "Fertile estate." All of these "Til-" names were last names, used occasionally as first names starting in the 19th century.

Timothy Gk. "Honoring God." New Testament name, correspondent with Saint Paul. Scanty use until the 18th century, then increased gradually to the middle of the 20th. After a baby boom peak, it has faded to steady but unspectacular use. Radical thinker Timothy Leary; actors Timothy Hutton, Tim Allen, Tim Roth; hockey player Teemu Selanne; basketball player Tim Duncan.

Tim, Timmo, Timmy, Timmothy, Timo, Timofei, Timofeo, Timofey, Timon, Timoteo, Timothé, Timotheo, Timothey, Timotheus, Tymmothy, Tymon, Tymoteusz, Tymothy

Tino Sp. Dim. **Agostino** and other "-tin" names. Baseball player Tino Martinez.

Teeno, Teino, Tyno

Titus Lat. Unknown meaning. New Testament character. Use is mostly 18th and 19th centuries. Has nothing to do, in spite of its sound, with titans or giants.

Tito, Titos

Tobias Heb. "The Lord is good." Old Testament name that faded after the Puritans used it, and was revived in the 19th century. The diminutive, **Toby,** is slightly more common now, though still very unusual. Author Tobias Wolff.

Thobey, Thobie, Thoby, Tobe, Tobee, Tobey, Tobi, Tobia, Tobiah, Tobie, Tobin, Tobit, Toby, Tobyn

Toby Dim. **Tobias.** Actor Tobey Maguire.

Thobey, Thobie, Thoby, Tobe, Tobee, Tobey, Tobi, Tobie

Todd ME. "Fox." Used mostly in this century, and fashionable for a spell in the 1970s. Still quite steadily used; much more popular than Tobias, for instance. Hockey player Todd Bertuzzi.

Tod

Tom Dim. **Thomas** (Aramaic. "Twin"). Most common in the 19th century as an independent name. Actors Tom Cruise, Tom Hanks.

Thom, Tomm, Tommy

Tomlin OE. "Little Tom."

Tomalin, Tomlinson

Tommy Dim. **Thomas**. Given with some regularity as a first name. Baseball player Tommy John; actor Tommy Lee Jones; fashion designer Tommy Hilfiger; musician Tommy Lee.

Tony Dim. Anthony (Lat. "Beyond price"). Used independently only since the middle of the 20th century. Actors Tony Curtis, Tony Danza; singer Tony Bennett.

Toney, Tonie

Tor Nor. "Thunder." Var. **Thor**. Also, Hebrew for "Turtledove."

Thor

Torquil ONorse. "Thor's kettle." Used in Scandinavian countries and a tiny bit in Britain.

Thirkell, Thorkel, Torkel, Torkel, Torkill

Torr OE. Place name: "Tower."

Tor

Torrance Ir. Gael. Place name: "Little hills."

Tore, Torin, Torr, Torrence, Torrens, Torrey, Torrin, Torry

Townley OE. Place name: "Town meadow."

Townlea, Townlee, Townleigh, Townlie, Townly

Townsend OE. Place name: "End of town."

Townshend

Tracy OF. Place name. Almost always a girl's name now. Author Tracy Kidder; basketball player Tracy McGrady.

Trace, Tracey, Treacy

Trahern Welsh. "Strength of iron." Poet Thomas Traherne.
Trahearn, Trahearne, Traherne

Travis OF. Occupational name: "Toll taker." Most common in the U.S. Fictional Detective Travis Magee.
Traver, Travers, Traviss, Travys

Tremain Celt. Place name: "Stone house." Popular among African-American families.
Tramain, Tramaine, Tramayne, Tremaine, Tremayne

Trent Lat. "Gushing waters." Name of an important river in England, thus a place name. U.S. Senator Trent Lott; football player Trent Dilfer.
Trenten, Trentin, Trenton

Trevor Welsh. "Large homestead." Use expanded outside of Wales in the mid-Victorian era, but the name was most popular in the middle of the 20th century. Actor Trevor Howard.
Trefor, Trevar, Trever

Trey ME. "Three." Related to the French *trois* for "three." Actor Trey Hunt.
Trai, Traye, Tre

Tristan Welsh. The name's Welsh meaning is unclear, but since *triste* is French for "sad," that explanation is often given. Tristan, in the medieval legends, is the knight who is in love with Isolde, wife of his uncle. The tale has been told in many forms, including an epic poem by Tennyson and an opera by Wagner. Currently very popular in Spain.
Tris, Tristam, Tristram

Trowbridge OE. Place name: "Bridge by the tree."

Troy Ir. Gael. "Foot-soldier." The name of the famous Greek city where the Trojan wars were fought, and a fairly common place name in America (as in Troy, NY). Actor Troy Donahue may have been behind the name's surge of popularity in the 1960s and 1970s. Jane Fonda named one of her children Troy. Football player Troy Aikman.
Troi, Troye

Truman OE. "Loyal one." Unusual as a last name or a first name, in spite of the greatly admired author Truman Capote or U.S. President Harry S. Truman.
Trueman, Trumaine, Trumann

Trumble OE. "Powerful."
   Trumball, Trumbell, Trumbo, Trumbull

Tucker OE. Occupational name: "Fabric pleater." Another occupational name relating to one of medieval Britain's principal industries, the woolen trade.
   Tuck, Tuckerman

Tudor Welsh. Var. **Theodore** (Gk. "Gift of God"). Famous as the name of the English dynasty of kings.

Turner ME. Occupational name: "Wood-worker." "Turning" referred to use of a lathe, which provided the decorative elements on much furniture in the 16th and 17th centuries. Painter J.M.W. Turner.

Twain ME. "Divided in two." The most famous bearer of this name, the American writer Mark Twain, took it from the calls of riverboatmen. His original name was Samuel Clemens.
   Twaine, Twayn

Twyford OE. Place name: "Double river crossing."

Tyler OE. Occupational name: "Maker of tiles." The name of one of the country's less memorable presidents (John Tyler, 1841–1845). Still, the name rocketed up popularity charts in the 1990s, with no clear prompting from popular culture. After a spell in the top ten it is beginning to drift out of fashion.
   Tilar, Ty, Tylar, Tylor

Tynan Ir. Gael. "Dark, dusky."
   Tienan, Tynell, Tynen, Tynin, Tynnen, Tynnin, Tynon

Tyrone Ir. Gael. "Land of Owen." Given prominence almost entirely by the actors Tyrone Power, Sr., and Jr., around the middle of the 20th century. Football player Tyrone Wheatley.
   Tirone, Tirohn, Tirown, Tyron

Tyson OF. Meaning unclear, though "spark, firebrand" has been suggested. Parents may use it in admiration of the boxing star (and firebrand) Mike Tyson.
   Thyssen, Tiesen, Tycen, Tyssen

Ubadah Arab. "Serves God."

Udell OE. Place name: "Valley of yew trees." Politician Morris Udall.

Dell, Eudel, Udel, Udall, Yudale, Yudell

Udo Dim. **Ulric**.

Udolf OE. "Wolf-wealth."

Udolfo, Udolph

Ugo It. Var. **Hugh** (OG. "Mind, intellect").

Ulf OG. "Wolf." More common in the Scandinavian countries.

Ulmer OE. "Fame of the wolf."

Ullmar, Ulmar

Ulric OG. "Power of the wolf" or "Power of the home." Used in Britain before the Norman invasion, but barely known in the last 900-odd years. Actor Skeet Ulrich.

Rick, Udo, Ullric, Ulrich, Ulrick, Ulrik

Ulysses Lat. Var. **Odysseus**, which may mean "wrathful." American use was spurred by the presidency of Civil War hero Ulysses S. Grant. Now rare.

Ulises, Ulisse

Umberto It. Var. **Humbert** (OG. "Renowned Hun"). A royal name in Italy, though very scarce in English-speaking countries. Author Umberto Eco.

Unwin OE. "Nonfriend."

Unwinn, Unwyn

Upton OE. Place name: "Upper settlement." Mostly last-name use. Author Upton Sinclair.

Upwood OE. Place name: "Upper forest."

Urban Lat. "From the city." We have a modern word, "urbane," from the same root. Apparently in ancient times city-dwellers had better manners than their rural contemporaries. Though the name was used by eight popes, it is scarce today in English-speaking countries.

Urbain, Urbaine, Urbane, Urbano, Urbanus

Uriah Heb. "The Lord is my light." Prominent Old Testament name at its most popular in the 19th century, though literary parents will be reminded of the smarmy, hand-wringing Uriah Heep in Dickens's *David Copperfield.* Dickens may have killed off the name, in fact; it is very scarce today.

    Uri, Uria, Urias, Urija, Urijah, Uriyah, Yuri, Yuria

Uriel Heb. "Flame of God." The Muslim version of the name is Israfil; he is the Muslim angel of music and appears in the Koran along with Gabriel and Michael. In Christian terms he is one of seven named archangels.

Usamah Arab. "Like a lion."

Uziel Heb. "Strength, power."

    Uzziah, Uzziel

Vachel OF. "Small cow." Something of a curiosity, brought to public notice by the poet Vachel Lindsay.

    Vachell

Vail OE. Place name: "Valley." Famous now as a ski resort in Colorado. Generally a transferred last name.

    Bail, Bale, Vaile, Vaill, Vale

Val Dim. Valentine. Actor Val Kilmer.

Valdemar OG. "Renowned leader."

    Waldemar

Valentine Lat. "Strong." This name and **Valerian** come from the same root. Valentine is used for both boys and girls, although the early Christian martyr for whom the holiday is named was male.

    Val, Valentijn, Valentin, Valentinian, Valentino, Valentinus, Valentyn

Valerian Lat. "Strong, healthy." Far less common than the feminine version, **Valerie**. Designer Valerian Rybar; conductor Valery Gergiev.
Valerien, Valerio, Valerius, Valery, Valeryan

Van Dutch. "Of." A particle of many Dutch names, as in **Vandyke**. Also possibly a nickname for **Evan**. Originally may have been used as a nickname for children with transferred Dutch last names, but it became generally popular in the middle of the 20th century. Neglected now. Pianist Van Cliburn; actor Van Johnson.
Vann, Von, Vonn

Vance OE. Place name: "Marshland." Author Vance Packard; diplomat Cyrus Vance.

Vandyke Dutch. Place name: "Of the dyke." The New York area was originally settled by Dutch colonists, and a few Dutch names survive, though not many are used as first names. A "Vandyke" is also the name of a small beard or goatee, from the beards portrayed in portraits by the 17th-century Flemish painter Anthony Van Dyck. Actor Dick Van Dyke.

Vanya Rus. Dim. **John** (Heb. "The Lord is gracious") via **Ivan**. Rare outside of Russia.

Vardon OF. Place name: "Green knoll." The second half of the name comes from the French word that gives us "dune."
Varden, Verdon, Verdun

Varick OG. "Leader who defends."
Varrick, Warick, Warrick

Vasilis Gk. "Royal, kingly." More familiar in its anglicized form, **Basil**. Painter Wassily Kandinsky.
Vasileios, Vasilij, Vasily, Vaso, Vasos, Vassilij, Vassily, Vasya, Wassily

Vaughn Welsh. "Small." Appeared as a first name at the turn of the 20th century, at its peak popularity in the baby boom era. Never especially common, though. Actors Robert Vaughn, Vince Vaughn; composer Ralph Vaughan Williams.
Vaughan

Vere Fr. Place name of unknown meaning. It was an upper-class last name in England, and took on near-caricature connotations of nobility, especially after Tennyson published "Lady Clara Vere de Vere," a poem praising the simple values of simple folk. (It contains the famous line "Kind hearts are more than coronets.") Vere has not been used much in the self-consciously democratic U.S.

Vernon OF. Place name: "Alder grove." A Norman name that took root as an English last name and, by the 19th century, a first name. Statesman Vernon Jordan.

Lavern, Vern, Vernal, Verne, Vernen, Vernin, Verney

Verrill OF. "Loyal" or OG. "Masculine."

Verill, Verrall, Verrell, Verroll, Veryl

Victor Lat. "Conqueror." Extremely common in Christian Rome, as was its female form, **Victoria**. Revived during the reign of Queen Victoria, but not very popular (except among her numerous descendants and godchildren). It was used most during the baby boom era, but not very widely. Cinematographer Vittorio Storaro; film director Vittorio de Sica; actor Victor Mature; author Victor Hugo.

Vic, Vick, Victorien, Victorin, Vidor, Viktor, Vitorio, Vittorio, Vittorios

Vilmos Hung. "Determined fighter." Cinematographer Vilmos Szigmond.

Vincent Lat. "Conquering." From the same root as **Victor**, but used much more steadily since early Christian days. It has not suffered neglect, but neither has it ever been truly popular. Saint Vincent de Paul, a 17th-century priest, founded an order of missionary brothers, and the Saint Vincent de Paul Society, an international charitable organization, was founded in his honor in the 19th century. Painter Vincent Van Gogh; film director Vincente Minnelli; actors Vincent Gardenia, Vince Vaughn, Vin Diesel, Vincent D'Onofrio, Vinnie Jones; football coach Vince Lombardi; basketball player Vince Carter.

Vicente, Vicenzio, Vincenzo, Vin, Vince, Vincens, Vincentius, Vincents, Vincenty, Vincenz, Vincenzio, Vincenzo, Vincien, Vinicent, Vinnie, Vinny, Vinzenz, Wincenty

Vine OE. Occupational name: "Vineyard worker."

Vinson OE. "Son of Vincent."

Virgil Lat. Clan name: possibly meaning "staff bearer." (The staff would have been part of official insignia in ancient Rome.) The name is usually homage to the Roman author of *The Aeneid.* Composer Virgil Thomson.
Verge, Vergil, Vergilio, Virgilio

Vito Lat. "Alive." Generally used by Italian families. St. Vitus was an early martyr whose legend held that he could cure epilepsy and another disorder known as "St. Vitus' dance."
Vital, Vitale, Vitalis, Vitaly, Vitas, Vitus, Witold

Vivian Lat. "Full of life." Used occasionally for boys in Britain, but an American infant named Vivian would be assumed to be a girl.
Viviani, Vivien, Vivyan, Vyvian, Vyvyan

Vladimir Slavic. "Renowned prince." Popular in Russia. Pianist Vladimir Horowitz; opera singer Vladimir Hvorostovsky.
Vladamir, Vladimeer, Wladimir, Wladimyr

Vladislav Old Slavic. "Splendid rule."

Volker Ger. "People's defender." From the German word that gives us "folk."

Volney OG. "Spirit of the folk."

 Wade OE. Place name: "River ford." Transferred last name with a certain popularity in old southern families, after Confederate General Wade Hampton.
Waddell, Wadell, Wayde

Wadley OE. Place name: "Ford meadow."
Wadleigh, Wadly

Wadsworth OE. Place name: "Village near the ford."

Transferred last name of a family that has long been prominent on the American cultural scene. Poet Henry Wadsworth Longfellow.

Waddsworth

Wagner Ger. Occupational name: "Wagon-builder." New York City Mayor Robert Wagner; composer Richard Wagner.

Waggoner, Wagoner

Wainwright OE. Occupational name: "Wagon-builder." Quite a mouthful as a first name, and most likely to be used when it's a family name, such as a mother's maiden name.

Wainright, Wainewright, Wayneright, Waynewright, Waynright

Waite ME. Occupational name: "Guard, watchman." In other words, one who waited for something to happen. Christmas carolers used to be known as "waits" because the custom of singing carols originated with bands of watchmen who would sing a tune to mark the passing hours of the night. Actor/musician Tom Waits.

Waights, Waits, Wayte

Wakefield OE. Place name: "Damp field."

Wakeley OE. Place name: "Damp meadow."

Wakelea, Wakeleigh, Wakely

Wakeman OE. Occupational name: "Watchman." Or one who was awake when others slept. All too appropriate for most babies.

Wake

Walcott OE. Place name: "Cottage by the wall." Could originally have referred to the great Roman wall that still stands in the north of England.

Wallcot, Wallcott, Wolcott

Waldemar OG. "Renowned ruler." Many of these Old German names (**William** is another) are actually made up of two particles that are both nouns: in this case they are "fame" and "power."

Valdemar

Walden OE. Place name: "Wooded valley." Could also be another variant of one of the Old German names that include the "Wald-" ("power") element, like **Walter**. Many literature-loving parents may think of Thoreau's book and the pond *Walden.*

Waldenn, Waldi, Waldon

Waldo Dim. **Waldemar,** etc. The "-o" ending is a particularly Germanic diminutive. Possibly also a German place name: "Forest meadow." Though more common than some of the longer forms like Waldemar, it's still unusual. Poet Ralph Waldo Emerson.

Waldron OG. "Powerful raven."

Walford OE. Place name: "Brook ford." Composer Walford Davies.

Walfred OG. "Ruler of peace."

Walfried

Walker OE. Occupational name: "Cloth-walker." The era that saw the rise of last names was also the great English era of the wool trade, giving us such cloth-manufacturing names as **Fuller, Dyer,** and **Weaver**. In that medieval era, workers trod on the wool to cleanse it of impurities. Author Walker Percy; photographer Walker Evans.

Wallace OE. "Welshman." Originally a Scottish name, used to identify foreigners from the south. Like many last names, it was most popular as a first name in the 19th century. Poet Wallace Stevens; actor Wallace Beery.

Wallach, Wallas, Wallie, Wallis, Wally, Walsh, Welch, Welsh

Waller OE. Occupational name: "Wall maker" or OG. "Powerful one."

Wally Dim. **Walter, Wallace,** etc. Actors Wally Shawn, Wally Cox.

Walter OG. "People of power" or "Army of power." Norman name that took root strongly in Britain and has been used quite steadily for the last 900 years (with the occasional century of neglect). Not particularly fashionable now. Cartoonist Walt Disney; poet Walt Whitman; journalist Walter Cronkite; actors Walter Brennan, Walter Matthau.

Gaultier, Gauthier, Gautier, Gualterio, Gualtiero, Valter, Valther, Walder, Wally, Walt, Walther, Wat, Watkins

Walton OE. Place name: "Walled town." Composer William Walton; entrepreneur Sam Walton.

Walworth OE. Place name: "Walled farm."

Walwyn OE. "Welsh friend."
Walwin, Walwinn, Walwynn, Walwynne, Welwyn

Warburton OE. Place name: "Long-standing fortress town."

Ward OE. Occupational name: "Watchman." Like many of these occupational or place names turned last names, Ward was revived as a first name in the 19th century. It is still somewhat more common as a first name than most other occupational names (**Smith, Baker, Turner,** etc.). Author Ward Just.
Warde, Warden, Worden

Wardell OE. Place name: "Watchman's hill."

Wardley OE. Place name: "Watchman's meadow."
Wardlea, Wardleigh

Ware OE. "Watchful, aware."

Warfield ME. Place name: "Field by the weir." A weir is a kind of enclosure built into a stream to trap fish.

Warford ME. "Ford near the weir."

Warley ME. "Meadow near the weir."

Warner OG. "Fighting defender." Philosopher Wernher Erhardt; U.S. Senator John Warner.
Werner, Wernher

Warren OE. "Watchman" or ME. "Park warden." A warren was originally an area devoted to breeding game, especially rabbits. By extension, the word is now used to describe human dwellings that resemble the haphazard and overcrowded rabbits' tunnels. As a name, Warren was used in the late 19th century and given a boost by the career of President Warren G. Harding. Actor Warren Beatty; U.S. Supreme Court Chief Justice Warren Burger; football player Warren Sapp.
Ware, Waring, Warrin, Warriner

Warton OE. Place name: "Town near the weir."
Wharton

Warwick OE. Place name: "Buildings near the weir." Football player Warrick Dunne.
Warick, Warrick

Washburn OE. Place name: "Flooding stream."
Washborn, Washbourne, Washburne

Washington OE. Place name: Possibly "Clever man's settlement." Author Washington Irving, born in 1783, was in all likelihood named for the first U.S. president, but the name has not been used as much as one might think, possibly because of its length. Educator Booker T. Washington.

Watson OE. "Son of Walter." Last name used as a first name primarily in the 19th century. Most famous as the name of the sidekick to whom Sherlock Holmes perpetually condescended: "Elementary, my dear Watson." IBM founder Thomas Watson.

Waverley OE. Place name: "Meadow of quivering aspens."
Waverlee, Waverley

Wayland OE. Place name: "Land by the path." Singer Waylon Jennings.
Way, Waylan, Waylen, Waylin, Waylon, Weylin

Wayne OE. Occupational name: "Wagon builder or driver," as in **Wainwright**. Its period of greatest popularity coincided with the popularity of the actor Marion Morrison, better known as John Wayne. Performer Wayne Newton; hockey player Wayne Gretzky.
Wain, Wayn

Webb OE. Occupational name: "Weaver." Mostly 19th-century use. Actors Clifton Webb, Jack Webb.
Web, Weber, Webster

Webley OE. Place name: "Weaver's meadow."
Webbley, Webbly, Webly

Welborne OE. Place name: "Spring-fed stream." Not, alas, indicative of patrician origins.
Welborn, Welbourne, Welburn, Wellborn, Wellbourn, Wellburn

Welby OG. Place name: "Well-farm." A television series about an avuncular doctor named Marcus Welby was very popular in the early 1970s.
Welbey, Welbie, Wellbey, Wellby

Weldon OE. Place name: "Well-hill."
Welden, Welldon

Welford OE. Place name: "Well-ford."
Wellford

Wellington OE. Place name of unclear meaning. Has aristocratic connotations, no doubt from the famous Duke of Wellington, who defeated Napoleon and gave his name to tall, waterproof boots and filet of beef wrapped in pastry.

Wells OE. Place name: "Wells." The name of a famous cathedral town in western England. First-name use was mostly 19th century. Baseball player David Wells.

Welton OE. Place name: "Well-town."

Wenceslaus Old Slavic. "Glorious garland." King Wenceslas, the patron saint of the Czech Republic, was a 10th-century monarch of Bohemia and a martyr for the faith. The famous Christmas carol (written in the 19th century) refers to an entirely imaginary episode, but the name would be unknown to us without it.
Wenceslas, Wenzel, Wiencyslaw

Wendell OG. "Wanderer." Quite rare. Politician Wendell Willkie.
Wendall, Wendel

Wentworth OE. Place name: "Pale man's settlement."

Werner OG. "Defense army." Closely related to **Warner**. Use is mostly confined to the U.S.
Verner, Warner, Wernhar, Wernher

Wesley OE. Place name: "Western meadow." Used in honor of John and Charles Wesley, who founded the Methodist church in the 18th century. Actors Wesley Snipes, Wes Bentley.
Wesly, Wessley, Westleigh, Westley

Westbrook OE. Place name: "Western stream." This group of place names illustrates one way last names came into use: They described the location of someone's dwelling. Fencer Peter Westbrook.
Brook, Brooke, Wesbrook, West, Westbrooke

Westby OE. Place name: "Western farmstead."
Westbey, Westbie

Westcott OE. Place name: "Western cottage."
Wescot, Wescott, Westcot

Weston OE. Place name: "Western settlement." Photographer Edward Weston.
Westen, Westin

Wetherby OE. Place name: "Wether-sheep farm." A wether is a male sheep that has been castrated; a bell-wether is a wether who wears a bell and leads a flock. Again, the importance of the wool trade in England when last names were formed gives these "Wether-" names unusual prominence.
Weatherbey, Weatherbie, Weatherby, Wetherbey, Wetherbie

Wetherell OE. Place name: "Wether-sheep corner."
Weatherell, Weatherill, Wetherill, Wethrill

Wetherly OE. Place name: "Wether-sheep meadow."
Weatherley, Weatherly, Wetherleigh, Wetherley

Wharton OE. Place name: "Shore or bank settlement." Author William Wharton.
Warton

Wheatley OE. Place name: "Wheat field." Football player Tyrone Wheatley.
Wheatlea, Wheatleigh, Wheatly

Wheaton OE. Place name: "Wheat settlement."

Wheeler OE. Occupational name: "Wheel maker."

Whistler OE. Occupational name: "Whistler or piper." Artist James Whistler.

Whitby OE. Place name: "White farm." All of these "Whit-" names are more commonly last names, though some were used more regularly as first names in the 19th century.
Whitbey, Whitbie

Whitcomb OE. Place name: "White valley." Poet James Whitcomb Riley.
Whitcombe, Whitcumb

Whitelaw OE. Place name: "White hill." Diplomat Whitelaw Reid.
Whitlaw

Whitfield OE. Place name: "White field."

Whitford OE. Place name: "White ford."

Whitley OE. Place name: "White meadow." Author Whitley Streiber.

Whitlock OE. "White lock of hair."

Whitman OE. "White man." The description would refer to hair or complexion. Poet Walt Whitman.

Whitmore OE. Place name: "White moor."
Whitmoor, Whittemore, Witmore, Wittemore

Whitney OE. Place name: "White island." Last name that was annexed as a girl's name in the 1980s. It became much more popular for girls than it ever was for boys. Railroad millionaire William Collins Whitney; inventor Eli Whitney.

Whittaker OE. Place name: "White field." The last part of the name may refer to an acre of land. Actor and director Forrest Whittaker.
Whitacker, Whitaker

Wickham OE. Place name: "Village paddock."

Wilbert OG. "Brilliant and resolute." Not the same as **Wilbur,** despite the similar sound. Used sporadically in the 19th and 20th centuries.
Wilburt

Wilbur OG. Last name of obscure meaning. Probably confused with **Wilbert** over the years. E.B.White fans will associate it with the protagonist of *Charlotte's Web,* Wilbur the Pig. Aviator Wilbur Wright.
Wilber, Willbur

Wiley OE. Place name: "Water meadow." Indicates a meadow that would be flooded from time to time.
Willey, Wylie

Wilford OE. Place name: "Willow-ford." Actor Wilford Brimley.

Wilfred OE. "Purposeful peace." Like **Waldemar,** another name whose two elements are both nouns (in this case "will" and "peace"), to the confusion of the translator. Neglected after the Norman invasion, but revived in the 19th century to some popularity, which never spread as far as the U.S. Author Wilfred Sheed.
Wilfredo, Wilfrid, Wilfried, Wilfryd, Will, Willfred, Willfredo, Willfrid, Willfried, Willfryd

Wilkinson OE. "Son of little Will."
Wilkins, Willkins, Willkinson

Willard OG. "Bold will." Most common in the U.S., though far from a household word. TV weatherman Willard Scott.
Willerd

William OG. "Will-helmet." Another two-noun name, more often translated as "resolute protection" or the like. Given a great boost in Norman England by William the Conqueror and succeeding English kings. Between the 17th and 20th centuries, one of the top handful of boy's names. Its popularity faded somewhat in the middle of the 20th century but by the end, it was one of the top two dozen boys' names in America. Its popularity may have been partially prompted by the example of Prince William of Wales. Playwright William Shakespeare; actors William Hurt, Willem Dafoe, Billy Crudup, Bill Pullman; film director Wim Wenders; poet William Blake; author William Faulkner; U.S. Presidents William H. Harrison, William H. Taft, William McKinley, Bill Clinton.
Bill, Bille, Billie, Billy, Guglielmo, Guillaume, Guillermo, Liam, Vilhelm, Villem, Wilek, Wiley, Wilhelm, Wilhelmus, Wilkes, Wilkie, Wilkinson, Will, Willem, Willhelmus, Willi, Williamson, Willie, Willis, Willkie, Wills, Willson, Willy, Wilmar, Wilmot, Wilmott, Wilson, Wim

Willoughby OE. Place name: "Willow farm."
Willoughbey, Willoughbie, Willughby

Wilmer OG. "Determined fame."
Wilmar, Willmar, Willmer, Wylmer

Wilson OE. "Son of Will." Last name turned first name, possibly in compliment to President Woodrow Wilson. Composer Robert Wilson; Beach Boy Brian Wilson.
Willson

Wilton OE. Place name: "Well settlement."

Windsor OE. Place name: "Riverbank with a winch." Famous from the town and castle of that name in England, and above all from the fact that it is the British royal family's last name. Also the name of a standard way to tie a

necktie, invented by the Duke of Windsor, who was a great dandy.
Winsor, Wyndsor

Winfield OE. "Friend's field." Baseball player Dave Winfield; Civil War general Winfield Scott.
Winnfield, Wynfield, Wynnfield

Wingate OE. Place name: "Winding gate." May refer to a gate like a turnstile.

Winslow OE. Place name: "Friend's hill." Painter Winslow Homer.

Winston OE. Place name: "Friend's town" or "Wine's town." For modern parents, recalls both English statesman Winston Churchill and a popular brand of cigarettes.
Winsten, Winstonn, Wynstan, Wynston

Winthrop OE. Place name: "Friend's village." In the U.S., it hearkens back to the Puritan governor of Massachusetts, John Winthrop, and his numerous Bostonian descendants.

Winton OE. Place name: "Friend's settlement." Closely related to **Winston**. Musician Wynton Marsalis.
Wynton

Wolcott OE. Place name: "Wolf's cottage." Wolf, in this case, would be a first name. Oliver Wolcott of Connecticut signed the Declaration of Independence.

Wolfe OG. "Wolf." Irish patriot Wolfe Tone.
Wolf, Wolff, Wolfhart, Woolf, Wulf, Wulfe

Wolfgang OG. "Wolf gait." A very Germanic name that would not be considered by English-speaking parents without the fame of composer Wolfgang Amadeus Mozart.

Woodrow OE. "Row by the woods." "Row" could refer to a row of houses or trees or bushes (as in a hedgerow). The name has been given prominence beyond the usual place name by admirers of U.S. President Woodrow Wilson.
Woody

Woodward OE. Place name: "Woods warden." Actor Edward Woodward.
Woodard

Woody Dim. **Woodrow**, etc. A particularly American name adopted by actor, director, and writer Allen Konigsberg, now better known as Woody Allen. Folk singer Woody Guthrie.

Worth OE. Place name: "Fenced farm." Used since the 19th century.

Worthey, Worthing, Worthington, Worthy

Wright OE. Occupational name: "Carpenter." Again, mostly 19th-century use. The astounding feats of aviators Orville and Wilbur Wright apparently did not inspire parents to use their name in homage. Painter Joseph Wright of Derby; architect Frank Lloyd Wright.

Wyatt OF. "Small fighter." Last name occasionally used as a first name, notably by Wild West Sheriff Wyatt Earp.

Wiatt, Wye, Wyeth

Wycliff OE. Place name: "White cliff." Musician Wycliffe Jean.

Wycliffe

Wylie OE. "Clever, charming, full of wiles." Literary agent Andrew Wylie.

Wiley, Wye

Wyndham OE. Place name: Either "Wyman's hamlet" or "Hamlet near the winding way." Used as a first name in the 19th century and into the 20th, but very unusual today. Author Wyndham Lewis.

Windham, Wynndham

Wynn Welsh. "Fair, white" or OE. "Friend." Used more frequently for girls in the past few years, but still uncommon. Gambling entrepreneur Steve Wynn.

Win, Winn, Wynne

Xan Dim. **Alexander** (Gk. "Defender of mankind").

Xanthus Gk. "Golden-haired."
Xanthos

Xavier Basque. "New house." Most often found as a middle name following **Francis,** in honor of Saint Francis Xavier, a 16th-century Jesuit missionary who took Christianity to the East Indies and Japan. Bandleader Xavier Cugat; baseball player Javier Lopez.
Javier, Saviero, Savion, Savyon, Xaviell, Xayvion, Xever, Zavier

Xenophon Gk. "Foreign voice." Xenophon was a Greek historian of the 4th century B.C.
Xeno

Xenos Gk. "Hospitality."
Zeno, Zenos

Xerxes Per. "Monarch." Xerxes was the title of several Persian rulers. One (in the 5th century B.C.) made war on the Greeks and also appears in the biblical Apocrypha as Ahasuerus, husband of Esther.

Ximenes Sp. Var. **Simon** (Heb. "Listening intently").
Jimenes, Jimenez, Ximenez

Yaakov Heb. Var. **Jacob** ("He who supplants"). Comedian Yakov Smirnov.
Iago, Yaacob, Yachov, Yacov, Yago, Yakob, Yakov

Yale OE. Place name: "Fertile moor." Familiar as the name of one of the Ivy League universities, founded by Elihu Yale.
Yael

Yancy Origin unclear. Several sources suggest this was an Indian word for "Englishman," and propose that this was the origin of the word "Yankee." But the *Facts on File Dictionary of First Names* claims the name is used to honor a Southern proslavery politician of the 19th century. Rare, in any case. Football player Yancey Thigpen.
Yance, Yancey, Yantsey

Yannis Gk. Var. **John** (Heb. "The Lord is gracious").
Ioannis, Yanni, Yannakis

Yaphet Heb. "Comely." Actor Yaphet Koto.
Japhet, Japheth, Yapheth

Yardley OE. Place name: "Fenced meadow."
Yardlee, Yardlea, Yardleigh, Yardly, Yarley, Yeardley

Yasahiro Jap. "Serene."

Yasir Arab. "Well to do." Palestinian leader Yasser Arafat.
Yaseer, Yasr, Yasser

Yates ME. Place name: "The gates." Poet W.B. Yeats.
Yeats

Yazid Arab./Swahili. "Becoming greater."
Yazeed

Yehudi Heb. "Praise." Related to the feminine **Judith,** as well as to **Jude.** Violinist Yehudi Menuhin.
Judah, Yechudi, Yechudit, Yehuda, Yehudah, Yehudit

Yeoman ME. "Attendant, servant."
Youman

Yĭtzhak Heb. Var. **Isaac** ("laughter"). Violinist Itzhak Perlman.
Itzak, Izaak, Yitzchak

Yochanan Heb. "The Lord is gracious." A form of **John**.
Johanan, Yohannan

York OE. Place name: "Boar settlement" or "yew settlement." Used as a title (Duke of York) in the English royal family for several hundred years. A bit difficult to use as a first name.
Yorick, Yorrick, Yorke

Yule OE. "Winter solstice." The time of year around Dec. 21, the pagan winter feast. Now, of course, it means Christmas. Rarely used, even for Christmas babies.
Euell, Ewell

Yuri Rus. Var. **George** (Lat. "Farmer").
Yurii, Yury

Yusuf Var. **Joseph** (Heb. "The Lord increases"). Currently very popular in Arabic-speaking countries. The "-uf" ending is more typically Arab, the "-ef" ending more often Hebrew.
Yosef, Yoseff, Yusef, Yusuff

Yves Fr. Var. **Ivo** (OG. "Yew wood"). Since yew wood was used for bows, the name may have been an occupational one meaning "archer." This form is almost exclusively found in France. Singer and actor Yves Montand; fashion designer Yves Saint Laurent.
Evo, Ives, Ivo, Yvo, Yvon

Zachariah Heb. "The Lord has remembered." Biblical name occurring in both Old and New Testaments. As might be expected, it was revived by the Puritans and found fairly constantly through the 19th century. The numerous phonetic variations hint at its current popularity.

Zacaria, Zacarias, Zacary, Zaccaria, Zaccariah, Zaccheus, Zach, Zachaios, Zacharia, Zacharias, Zacharie, Zachary, Zacheriah, Zachery, Zacheus, Zack, Zackariah, Zackerias, Zackery, Zak, Zakarias, Zakarie, Zakariyyah, Zakery, Zecheriah, Zekariah, Zekeriah, Zeke

Zachary Heb. "The Lord has remembered." The most popular form of **Zachariah,** one of the top two dozen names for boys in the country. President Zachary Taylor.

Zaccary, Zaccery, Zacharie, Zachery, Zackarey, Zackary, Zackery

Zadok Heb. "Fair, righteous."

Zadoc, Zaydok

Zahir Arab. "Brilliant." Currently popular in English-speaking countries.

Zale Gk. "Sea-strength."

Zayle

Zalman Heb. "Peaceable." The more common form in English is **Solomon.** Author Salman Rushdie.

Salman, Zalomon

Zane Derivation and meaning unclear. May be a variation of **John** (Heb. "The Lord is gracious"), or a version of a Scandinavian last name. Made famous by author Zane Grey, who wrote many novels about the Wild West, among them *Riders of the Purple Sage.*

Zain, Zayne

Zared Heb. "Trap."

Zebediah Heb. "Gift of Jehovah." In the New Testament, the father of apostles John and James. The name is all but obsolete today.

Zeb, Zebedee, Zebediah

Zebulon Heb. "To give honor to." Old Testament name of one of Jacob's sons. Extremely rare.

Zebulen, Zebulun, Zevulon, Zevulun

Zedekiah Heb. "The Lord is just." Name of an Old Testament king of Judah. Mostly 19th-century use.

Zed, Zedechiah, Zedekias

Zeke Heb. "Strength of God." Dim. **Ezekiel**. Ezekiel was an important Old Testament prophet.

Zelig Yiddish. "Blessed, holy." In German, "selig" means holy. Movie buffs will remember a Woody Allen movie in which a character named Zelig turns up at many different historic events.
   Selig, Zeligman, Zelik

Zenas Gk: "Hospitable."
   Zenios, Zenon

Zephaniah Heb: "Precious to the Lord." A minor Old Testament prophet. Sparing 19th-century use.
   Zeph, Zephan

Zero Arab. "Void." A rather daunting name for a baby, though actor Zero Mostel seems to have survived it.

Zeus Gk. "Living." The name of the chief of the Olympian gods, who was also father of many gods and goddesses including Athena, Ares, Apollo, and Artemis.

Zindel Yiddish. Var. **Alexander** (Gk. "Defender of mankind").
   Zindil

Ziv Heb. "Full of life, glorious, splendid."
   Ziven, Zivon

Zoltan Hung. "Life." Composer Zoltan Kodaly.

Zuhayr Arab. "Small blossoms."
   Zuhair

Zuriel Heb. "The Lord my rock."